Delivery in the Periviable Period

Editors

BRIAN M. MERCER
KEITH J. BARRINGTON

CLINICS IN PERINATOLOGY

www.perinatology.theclinics.com

Consulting Editor
LUCKY JAIN

June 2017 • Volume 44 • Number 2

ELSEVIER

1600 John F. Kennedy Boulevard • Suite 1800 • Philadelphia, Pennsylvania, 19103-2899

http://www.theclinics.com

CLINICS IN PERINATOLOGY Volume 44, Number 2
June 2017 ISSN 0095-5108, ISBN-13: 978-0-323-53025-5

Editor: Kerry Holland
Developmental Editor: Casey Potter

Clinics in Perinatology (ISSN 0095-5108) is published quarterly by Elsevier Inc., 360 Park Avenue South, New York, NY 10010-1710. Months of issue are March, June, September, and December. Business and Editorial Offices: 1600 John F. Kennedy Blvd., Ste. 1800, Philadelphia, PA 19103-2899. Customer Service Office: 3251 Riverport Lane, Maryland Heights, MO 63043. Periodicals postage paid at New York, NY and additional mailing offices. Subscription prices are $299.00 per year (US individuals), $532.00 per year (US institutions), $350.00 per year (Canadian individuals), $651.00 per year (Canadian institutions), $433.00 per year (international individuals), $651.00 per year (international institutions), $100.00 per year (US students), and $195.00 per year (Canadian and international students). International air speed delivery is included in all Clinics subscription prices. All prices are subject to change without notice. **POSTMASTER:** Send address changes to *Clinics in Perinatology*, Elsevier Health Sciences Division, Subscription Customer Service, 3251 Riverport Lane, Maryland Heights, MO 63043. **Customer Service: Telephone: 1-800-654-2452** (U.S. and Canada); **1-314-447-8871** (outside U.S. and Canada). **Fax: 1-314-447-8029. E-mail: journalscustomerservice-usa@elsevier.com** (for print support); **journalsonlinesupport-usa@elsevier.com** (for online support).

Reprints. For copies of 100 or more, of articles in this publication, please contact the Commercial Reprints Department, Elsevier Inc., 360 Park Avenue South, New York, NY 10010-1710. Tel. 212-633-3874; Fax: 212-633-3820; E-mail: reprints@elsevier.com.

Clinics in Perinatology is also published in Spanish by McGraw-Hill Interamericana Editores S.A., P.O. Box 5-237, 06500 Mexico D.F., Mexico.

Clinics in Perinatology is covered in *MEDLINE/PubMed (Index Medicus) Current Contents, Excepta Medica, BIOSIS and ISI/BIOMED.*

Contributors

CONSULTING EDITOR

LUCKY JAIN, MD, MBA
Richard W. Blumberg Professor and Interim Chairman, Emory University School of
Medicine, Department of Pediatrics, Executive Medical Director and Interim Chief
Academic Officer, Children's Healthcare of Atlanta, Atlanta, Georgia

EDITORS

BRIAN M. MERCER, BA, MD, FRCSC, FACOG
Professor and Chairman, Department of Reproductive Biology, Case Western Reserve
University, Chairman, Department of Obstetrics and Gynecology, The MetroHealth
System, Cleveland, Ohio

KEITH J. BARRINGTON, MB, ChB
Professor, Department of Pediatrics, Chief of Neonatology, Sainte-Justine Hospital,
University of Montreal, Montreal, Quebec, Canada

AUTHORS

CANDE V. ANANTH, PhD, MPH
Virgil G. Damon Professor of Obstetrics and Gynecology, College of Physicians and
Surgeons, Columbia University, Professor, Department of Epidemiology, *Joseph L.
Mailman* School of Public Health, Columbia University, New York, New York

EDWARD F. BELL, MD
Professor, Department of Pediatrics, University of Iowa, Iowa City, Iowa

RENEE D. BOSS, MD, MHS
Associate Professor, Division of Neonatology, Johns Hopkins School of Medicine, Berman
Institute of Bioethics, Baltimore, Maryland

SUNEET P. CHAUHAN, MD
Professor, Department of Obstetrics, Gynecology, and Reproductive Sciences,
McGovern Medical School, University of Texas, Houston, Texas

PO-YIN CHEUNG, MBBS, PhD
Centre for the Studies of Asphyxia and Resuscitation, Royal Alexandra Hospital,
Department of Pediatrics, University of Alberta, Edmonton, Alberta, Canada

EDWARD K. CHIEN, MD, MBA
Associate Professor, Department of Reproductive Biology, Case Western Reserve
University, Division of Maternal Fetal Medicine, Department of Obstetrics and
Gynecology, The MetroHealth System, Cleveland, Ohio

AFIF EL-KHUFFASH, FRCPI, MD, DCh
Consultant Neonatologist, The Rotunda Hospital, Honorary Clinical Associate Professor, Department of Paediatrics, School of Medicine, Royal College of Surgeons in Ireland, Dublin, Ireland

KELLEY BENHAM FRENCH, MJ, BA, BS
Professor of Practice in Journalism, The Media School, Indiana University, Bloomington, Indiana

TING TING FU, MD
Neonatal and Pulmonary Biology Fellow, Perinatal Institute, Cincinnati Children's Hospital Medical Center, Cincinnati, Ohio

NATHALIE GAUCHER, MD, PhD
Department of Pediatrics and Clinical Ethics, Sainte-Justine Research Center, Sainte-Justine Hospital, University of Montreal, Montreal, Quebec, Canada

KELLY S. GIBSON, MD
Assistant Professor, Department of Reproductive Biology, Case Western Reserve University, Division of Maternal Fetal Medicine, Department of Obstetrics and Gynecology, The MetroHealth System, Cleveland, Ohio

MARLYSE F. HAWARD, MD
Department of Pediatrics, Albert Einstein College of Medicine, The Children's Hospital at Montefiore, New York, New York

ANNIE JANVIER, MD, PhD
Department of Pediatrics and Clinical Ethics, CHU Sainte-Justine Research Center, Palliative Care Unit, Sainte-Justine Hospital, University of Montreal, Montreal, Quebec, Canada

STEPHANIE K. KUKORA, MD
Clinical Lecturer, Division of Neonatal-Perinatal Medicine, Department of Pediatrics and Communicable Diseases, University of Michigan, Ann Arbor, Michigan

JEAN-CLAUDE LAVOIE, PhD
Associate Professor, Division of Neonatology, Department of Pediatrics, Associate Professor, Department of Nutrition, Faculty of Medicine, Research Center, Centre Hospitalier Universitaire Sainte-Justine, University of Montreal, Montreal, Quebec, Canada

THUY MAI LUU, MD, MSc
Clinical Assistant Professor of Pediatrics, Division of General Pediatrics, Faculty of Medicine, Research Center, Centre Hospitalier Universitaire Sainte-Justine, University of Montreal, Montreal, Quebec, Canada

PATRICK J. McNAMARA, MD, MSc
Associate Scientist, Physiology and Experimental Medicine, Staff Neonatologist, The Hospital for Sick Children, Professor of Paediatrics and Physiology, University of Toronto, Toronto, Ontario, Canada

KERA McNELIS, MD
Neonatal and Pulmonary Biology Fellow, Perinatal Institute, Cincinnati Children's Hospital Medical Center, Cincinnati, Ohio

BRIAN M. MERCER, BA, MD, FRCSC, FACOG
Professor and Chairman, Department of Reproductive Biology, Case Western Reserve University, Chairman, Department of Obstetrics and Gynecology, The MetroHealth System, Cleveland, Ohio

IBRAHIM MOHAMED, MD, MSc
Clinical Associate Professor of Pediatrics, Division of Neonatology, Faculty of Medicine, Research Center, Centre Hospitalier Universitaire Sainte-Justine, University of Montreal, Montreal, Quebec, Canada

ASMA NOSHERWAN, MBBS
Centre for the Studies of Asphyxia and Resuscitation, Royal Alexandra Hospital, Department of Pediatrics, University of Alberta, Edmonton, Alberta, Canada

ANNE MONIQUE NUYT, MD
Professor of Pediatrics, Division of Neonatology, Faculty of Medicine, Research Center, Centre Hospitalier Universitaire Sainte-Justine, University of Montreal, Montreal, Quebec, Canada

KATRYN PAQUETTE, MD
Fellow, Division of Neonatology, Department of Pediatrics, Faculty of Medicine, Research Center, Centre Hospitalier Universitaire Sainte-Justine, University of Montreal, Montreal, Quebec, Canada

RAVI MANGAL PATEL, MD, MSc
Assistant Professor, Division of Neonatal-Perinatal Medicine, Department of Pediatrics, Children's Healthcare of Atlanta, Emory University School of Medicine, Atlanta, Georgia

ANTOINE PAYOT, MD, PhD
Department of Pediatrics and Clinical Ethics Unit, Palliative Care Unit, Sainte-Justine Research Center, Sainte-Justine Hospital, University of Montreal, Montreal, Quebec, Canada

BRENDA POINDEXTER, MD, MS
Professor of Pediatrics, Director of Clinical and Translational Research, Perinatal Institute, Cincinnati Children's Hospital Medical Center, Cincinnati, Ohio

MUHAMMAD ONEEB REHMAN MIAN, PhD
Post-Doctoral Fellow, Department of Biomedical Sciences, Fetomaternal and Neonatal Pathologies Axis, Research Center, Centre Hospitalier Universitaire Sainte-Justine, University of Montreal, Montreal, Quebec, Canada

KATE ROBSON, MEd
Canadian Premature Babies Foundation, Toronto, Ontario, Canada

MATTHEW A. RYSAVY, MD, PhD
Resident Physician, Department of Pediatrics, University of Wisconsin Hospital and Clinics, Madison, Wisconsin

GEORG M. SCHMÖLZER, MD, PhD
Centre for the Studies of Asphyxia and Resuscitation, Royal Alexandra Hospital, Department of Pediatrics, University of Alberta, Edmonton, Alberta, Canada

KRISTIN SOHN, MD
Fellow in Neonatal-Perinatal Medicine, Department of Pediatrics, University of California Davis, Sacramento, California

THEOPHIL A. STOKES, MD
Assistant Professor of Pediatrics, Associate Fellowship Director, Neonatal-Perinatal Medicine, Department of Pediatrics, Uniformed Services University of the Health Sciences, Walter Reed National Military Medical Center, Bethesda, Maryland

JON E. TYSON, MD, MPH
Michelle Bain Distinguished Professor and Director, Center for Clinical Research and Evidence-Based Medicine, McGovern Medical School, The University of Texas Health Science Center at Houston, Houston, Texas

MARK A. UNDERWOOD, MD, MAS
Chief, Division of Neonatology, Professor, Department of Pediatrics, University of California Davis, Sacramento, California

Contents

> Parents and doctors look at a baby from fundamentally different perspectives. Every prognosis expands or contracts a universe for a doctor or a parent. When the clinician and the parent come together to make a life-and-death decision, language matters.

> Periviable birth carries a high risk of fetal and newborn death, and the potential for life-long complications in survivors. The family at risk for periviable birth should receive objective, accurate, and up to date information regarding fetal, newborn, and maternal risks and outcomes with delivery or with continued pregnancy. This article describes the various descriptive terms for delivery near the limit of viability, considers the evolving limit of viability over time, and highlights the importance of adjusted counseling with brief pregnancy prolongation and/or changing clinical circumstances within the periviable period.

> Periviable births are those occurring from 20 0/7 through 25 6/7 weeks of gestation. Among and within developed nations, significant variation exists in the approach to obstetric and neonatal care for periviable birth. Understanding gestational age–specific survival, including factors that may influence survival estimates and how these estimates have changed over time, may guide approaches to the care of periviable births and inform conversations with families and caregivers. This review provides a historical perspective on survival following periviable birth, summarizes recent and new data on gestational age–specific survival rates, and addresses factors that have a significant impact on survival.

> Preterm birth severely disrupts the normal developmental maturation of organ systems, resulting in lasting adverse effects. High blood pressure,

sulfate, progesterone, and tocolytics may also improve outcome. Studies specifically evaluating these interventions are needed.

Extremely low birth weight (ELBW) infants are particularly vulnerable at birth, and stabilization in the delivery room (DR) remains challenging. After birth, ELBW infants are at high risk for the development of thermal dysregulation, respiratory insufficiency, and hemodynamic instability due to their immature physiology and anatomy. Although successful stabilization facilitates the transition and reduces acute morbidity, suboptimal care in the DR could cause long-term sequelae. This review addresses the challenges in stabilization in the DR and current neonatal resuscitation guidelines and recommendations.

The management of the hemodynamic status of critically ill preterm infants, particularly around the periviable period, remains a significant challenge in the neonatal intensive care unit for a multitude of reasons. The causes of hemodynamic compromise in this population are heterogeneous and usually superimposed on the complex physiologic processes that occur during transition from fetal to neonatal life. This review outlines the unique nature of low blood flow states in this population and present an overview of the current methods for identification and assessment of hemodynamic compromise.

With advancements in the care of preterm infants, the goals in nutritional care have expanded from survival and mimicking fetal growth to optimizing neurodevelopmental outcomes. Inadequate nutritional support may be a risk factor for major complications of prematurity; conversely, higher disease burden is a risk for growth restriction. Early complete parenteral nutrition support, including intravenous lipid emulsion, should be adopted, and the next challenge that should be addressed is parenteral nutrition customized to fit the specific needs and metabolism of the extremely preterm infant. Standardized feeding protocols should be adopted.

Colonization of the extremely preterm infant's gastrointestinal tract and skin begins in utero and is influenced by a variety of factors, the most important including gestational age and environmental exposures. The composition of the intestinal and skin microbiota influences the developing innate and adaptive immune responses with short-term and long-term consequences including altered risks for developing necrotizing

PROGRAM OBJECTIVE
The goal of *Clinics in Perinatology* is to keep practicing perinatologists, neonatologists, obstetricians, practicing physicians and residents up to date with current clinical practice in perinatology by providing timely articles reviewing the state of the art in patient care.

TARGET AUDIENCE
Perinatologists, neonatologists, obstetricians, practicing physicians, residents and healthcare professionals who provide patient care utilizing findings from *Clinics in Perinatology*.

LEARNING OBJECTIVES
Upon completion of this activity, participants will be able to:
1. Review nutrition, medical, and surgical interventions for preterm infants.
2. Discuss strategies for caring for preterm infants and their families in the NICU.
3. Recognize long-term health impacts of preterm birth.

ACCREDITATION
The Elsevier Office of Continuing Medical Education (EOCME) is accredited by the Accreditation Council for Continuing Medical Education (ACCME) to provide continuing medical education for physicians.

The EOCME designates this enduring material for a maximum of 15 *AMA PRA Category 1 Credit*(s)™. Physicians should claim only the credit commensurate with the extent of their participation in the activity.

All other healthcare professionals requesting continuing education credit for this enduring material will be issued a certificate of participation.

DISCLOSURE OF CONFLICTS OF INTEREST
The EOCME assesses conflict of interest with its instructors, faculty, planners, and other individuals who are in a position to control the content of CME activities. All relevant conflicts of interest that are identified are thoroughly vetted by EOCME for fair balance, scientific objectivity, and patient care recommendations. EOCME is committed to providing its learners with CME activities that promote improvements or quality in healthcare and not a specific proprietary business or a commercial interest.

The planning committee, staff, authors and editors listed below have identified no financial relationships or relationships to products or devices they or their spouse/life partner have with commercial interest related to the content of this CME activity:
Cande V. Ananth, PhD, MPH; Keith J. Barrington, MB, CHB; Edward F. Bell, MD; Renee D. Boss, MD, MHS; Suneet P. Chauhan, MD; Po-Yin Cheung, MBBS, PhD; Edward K. Chien, MD, MBA; Afif El-Khuffash, FRCPI, MD, DCh; Anjali Fortna; Kelley Benham French, MJ, BA, BS; Ting Ting Fu, MD; Nathalie Gaucher, MD, PhD; Kelly S. Gibson, MD; Marlyse F. Haward, MD; Kerry Holland; Lucky Jain, MD, MBA; Annie Janvier, MD, PhD; Stephanie K. Kukora, MD; Jean-Claude Lavoie, PhD; Thuy Mai Luu, MD, MSc; Patrick J. McNamara, MD, MSc; Kera McNelis, MD; Brian M. Mercer, BA, MD, FRCSC, FACOG; Ibrahim Mohamed, MD, MSc; Subhalakshmi Vaidyanathan; Asma Nosherwan, MBBS; Anne Monique Nuyt, MD; Katryn Paquette, MD; Ravi Mangal Patel, MD, MSc; Antoine Payot, MD, PhD; Brenda Poindexter, MD, MS; Casey Potter; Muhammad Oneeb Rehman Mian, PhD; Kate Robson, MEd; Matthew A. Rysavy, MD, PhD; George M. Schmölzer, MD, PhD; Kristin Sohn, MD; Theophil A. Stokes, MD; Jon E. Tyson, MD, MPH; Mark A. Underwood, MD, MAS; Kate Widmeier; Amy Williams.

UNAPPROVED/OFF-LABEL USE DISCLOSURE
The EOCME requires CME faculty to disclose to the participants:
1. When products or procedures being discussed are off-label, unlabelled, experimental, and/or investigational (not US Food and Drug Administration [FDA] approved); and
2. Any limitations on the information presented, such as data that are preliminary or that represent ongoing research, interim analyses, and/or unsupported opinions. Faculty may discuss information about pharmaceutical agents that is outside of FDA-approved labelling. This information is intended solely for CME and is not intended to promote off-label use of these medications. If you have any questions, contact the medical affairs department of the manufacturer for the most recent prescribing information.

TO ENROLL
To enroll in the *Clinics in Perinatology* Continuing Medical Education program, call customer service at 1-800-654-2452 or sign up online at http://www.theclinics.com/home/cme. The CME program is available to subscribers for an additional annual fee of $235 USD.

METHOD OF PARTICIPATION

In order to claim credit, participants must complete the following:

1. Complete enrolment as indicated above.
2. Read the activity.
3. Complete the CME Test and Evaluation. Participants must achieve a score of 70% on the test. All CME Tests and Evaluations must be completed online.

CME INQUIRIES/SPECIAL NEEDS

For all CME inquiries or special needs, please contact elsevierCME@elsevier.com.

CLINICS IN PERINATOLOGY

FORTHCOMING ISSUES

September 2017
Quality Improvement
Heather C. Kaplan and Mushish Gupta, *Editors*

December 2017
Minimally Invasive Neonatal Surgery
Mark Wulkan and Hanmin Lee, *Editors*

March 2018
Endocrinology
Andrew Muir and Susan Rose, *Editors*

RECENT ISSUES

March 2017
Human Milk for Preterm Infants
Francis B. Mimouni and
Berthold Koletzko, *Editors*

December 2016
Non-Invasive Ventilation
Bradley Yoder and Haresh Kirpalani, *Editors*

September 2016
Birth Asphyxia
Beena B. Kamath-Rayne and
Alan H. Jobe, *Editors*

ISSUE OF RELATED INTEREST

Obstetrics and Gynecology Clinics of North America, June 2015 (Vol. 42, Issue 2)
Best Practices in High-Risk Pregnancy
Lynn L. Simpson, *Editor*
Available at: http://www.obgyn.theclinics.com/

Foreword

Confronting the Limits of Viability

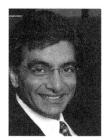

Lucky Jain, MD, MBA
Consulting Editor

There are stories that we all like to tell, many of which are permanently etched in our memories. One such story is from nearly thirty years ago, while as a freshly minted neonatologist, I was confronted with a clinical and ethical dilemma that I vividly remember in excruciating detail even to this day. A mother had presented in advanced labor with a fetus of 24-weeks' gestation. Delivery was imminent, allowing for only a hurried discussion of choices. Both parents were physicians and were diametrically split on what they wanted us to do. Put in an uncomfortable position of brokering an agreement, I opted for resuscitation, hoping that the progress of the infant would guide us as to how far we should go with the care. Things are never as simple as we would like them to be however; one thing led to the other, and the infant had every known complication of extreme prematurity. The young parents were devastated. Mom ended up dropping out of her residency training, and the father moved to the west coast to pursue a fellowship. At her second visit to the developmental clinic, our little NICU graduate had clear signs of spastic diplegia, was blind from retinopathy of prematurity, and had missed most cognitive milestones. I struggled with many aspects of this case, and for many years have relived the traumatic experience every time I was confronted with a similar infant at the limit of viability.

Over the years, our confidence in caring for these tiny babies has grown as well as our ability to predict outcomes. **Fig. 1** shows recent data from the National Institute of Child Health and Human Development (NICHD) Neonatal Research Network with remarkable gains over the past decade, particularly in survival of 23-week infants (article by Ravi Mangal Patel and colleagues, "Survival of Infants Born at Periviable Gestational Ages," in this issue). Similar improvements have been reported from several other countries.[1] However, there is wide variability in outcomes raising the issue of inconsistent care practices and overall approach to care.[2] Centers with the highest survival numbers also report the highest rates of antenatal steroids, resuscitation, surfactant use, and so forth, reflecting a more consistent and comprehensive approach to the care being offered.[2] Neurodevelopment outcomes have also improved. A recent study[3] showed

Clin Perinatol 44 (2017) xv–xvii
http://dx.doi.org/10.1016/j.clp.2017.03.002
0095-5108/17/© 2017 Published by Elsevier Inc.
perinatology.theclinics.com

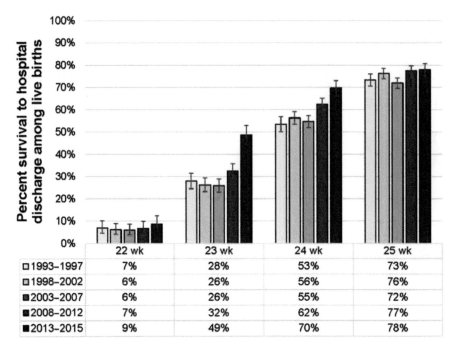

	22 wk	23 wk	24 wk	25 wk
□ 1993–1997	7%	28%	53%	73%
□ 1998–2002	6%	26%	56%	76%
■ 2003–2007	6%	26%	55%	72%
■ 2008–2012	7%	32%	62%	77%
■ 2013–2015	9%	49%	70%	78%

Gestational age

Fig. 1. Survival from 1993 through 2015 following live birth in the NICHD Neonatal Research Network. (*Data from* Stoll BJ, Hansen NI, Bell EF, et al. Trends in care practices, morbidity, and mortality of extremely preterm neonates, 1993-2012. JAMA 2015;314(10):1039–51, for 1993-2012; and Courtesy with permission of the NICHD Neonatal Research Network, Bethesda, MD, USA for 2013-2015.)

that among 22- to 24-week preterm infants, the percentage of infants who survived without neurodevelopmental impairment increased from 16% to 20% (adjusted relative risk, 1.59 [confidence interval, 1.28 to 1.99]).

So where does this discussion lead us? A decade ago, obstetricians and neonatologists were convinced that 24 weeks reflected a biologic barrier in fetal development below which survival without significant impairment was going to be improbable.[4] The same is now being said for infants at 23 weeks of gestation. Care continues to evolve, and we learn from the care we provide for these tiny babies. These and many other issues are the focus of our attention in this issue of the *Clinics in Perinatology*. Drs Mercer and Barrington are to be congratulated for bringing together a superb set of state-of-the-art articles on this topic. As always, I am grateful to the editors, authors, and the publishing team at Elsevier (Kerry Holland and Casey Potter) for creating a masterful issue of the *Clinics in Perinatology* on this important topic.

Lucky Jain, MD, MBA
Department of Pediatrics
Emory University School of Medicine
Children's Healthcare of Atlanta
2015 Uppergate Drive
Atlanta, GA 30322, USA

E-mail address:
ljain@emory.edu

REFERENCES

1. Ancel PY, Goffinet F, Group E-W, et al. Survival and morbidity of preterm children born at 22 to 34 weeks' gestation in France in 2011: results of the EPIPAGE-2 cohort study. JAMA Pediatr 2015;169(3):230–8.
2. Carlo W, McDonald SA, Fanaroff AA, et al, Eunice Kennedy Shriver National Institute of Child Health and Human Development Neonatal Research Network. Association of antenatal corticosteroids with mortality and neurodevelopmental outcomes among infants born at 22-25 weeks' gestation. JAMA 2011;306:2348–58.
3. Younge N, Goldstein RF, Bann CM, et al. Survival and neurodevelopmental outcomes among periviable infants. N Eng J Med 2017;376:617–28.
4. Raju TN, Mercer BM, Burchfield DJ, et al. Periviable birth: executive summary of a joint workshop by the Eunice Kennedy Shriver National Institute of Child Health and Human Development, Society for Maternal-Fetal Medicine, American Academy of Pediatrics, and American College of Obstetricians and Gynecologists. Obstet Gynecol 2014;123(5):1083–96.

Preface

Delivery in the Periviable Period

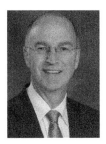
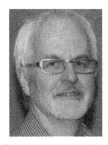

Brian M. Mercer, BA, MD, FRCSC, FACOG   Keith J. Barrington, MB, ChB
Editors

Care of the woman at risk for delivery near the limit of viability is one of the most challenging issues faced by obstetricians and neonatologists. For the asymptomatic woman at risk for early preterm birth based on chronic risk factors or prior obstetrical outcomes, there is often opportunity for extensive counseling, joint decision making, and interventions to prevent or delay early delivery. Unfortunately, such interventions are too often not successful.

When early preterm birth is imminent or urgently required as a result of acute clinical circumstances, obstetric efforts are often focused on optimizing fetal condition and preparing for inevitable delivery. Depending on clinical urgency, the neonatologist may or may not have the opportunity to fully counsel the patient and her family regarding important aspects of newborn outcomes, available interventions, and options regarding care of the critically ill infant, or to obtain their input regarding management after birth of the infant. For both obstetrician and neonatologist, successful delay of delivery provides the opportunity for more detailed discussion with the patient and family, but also introduces the need to adapt counseling to potentially rapidly evolving maternal and fetal condition as well as rapidly changing potential for infant mortality and serious complications with relatively brief pregnancy prolongation and anticipated fetal responses to prenatal interventions such as antenatal corticosteroid and magnesium sulfate administration. When delivery occurs, initial newborn status and response to resuscitative interventions further impact the potential for survival and major morbidities and necessitate repeated reevaluation and counseling of the family.

The woman and family at risk for delivery of the infant near the limit of viability need to assimilate complex and unexpected information, often in a short period of time, so that they can actively participate in their care, adjust their understanding as circumstances change, and participate in interventions that may impact their current health and pregnancy outcome as well as future pregnancies.

All of this occurs within the context of newly available interventions to enhance pregnancy and newborn outcomes, and a progressive decline in the "limit of viability": the

Clin Perinatol 44 (2017) xix–xx
http://dx.doi.org/10.1016/j.clp.2017.03.001   **perinatology.theclinics.com**
0095-5108/17/© 2017 Published by Elsevier Inc.

state of fetal maturity at which there is potential for survival outside the uterus. Because of this, obstetric and newborn providers must be ready to adapt their understanding, counseling, and interventions in the face of a changing state of knowledge.

We thank the authors of this issue of *Clinics in Perinatology*, who have helped to bring together a collaborative and inclusive effort between medical disciplines. In addition to seeking insights from obstetricians and neonatologists with expertise in care and counseling, we have invited input from ethicists and families affected by delivery near the limit of viability. We trust that their insights in addition to the information provided herein will help to inform your clinical practice, educational efforts, and counseling and stimulate further discussion to enhance the care of our patients and their families.

Brian M. Mercer, BA, MD, FRCSC, FACOG
Department of Reproductive Biology
Case Western Reserve University
Department of Obstetrics and Gynecology
The MetroHealth System
Suite G267, 2500 MetroHealth Drive
Cleveland, OH 44109, USA

Keith J. Barrington, MB, ChB
Department of Pediatrics
University of Montreal
Sainte-Justine Hospital
3175 Chemin Côte-Sainte-Catherine
Montreal, QC H3T 1C5, Canada

E-mail address:
keith.barrington@umontreal.ca (K.J. Barrington)

Care of Extremely Small Premature Infants in the Neonatal Intensive Care Unit

A Parent's Perspective

 CrossMark

Kelley Benham French, MJ, BA, BS

KEYWORDS

- Extremely small premature infant • Neonatal intensive care unit
- Life-and-death decisions

KEY POINTS

- Parents and doctors look at a baby from fundamentally different perspectives.
- Every prognosis expands or contracts a universe for a doctor or a parent.
- When the clinician and the parent come together to make a life-and-death decision, language matters.

My daughter was born twiggy and translucent as a baby bird; her eyes fused shut, mouth agape. Through her chest, we could see her flickering heart.

She arrived at 23 weeks and 6 days: the threshold between viability and futility, between everything and nothing. For me, after 5 years of infertility, she came at the trembling membrane between motherhood and despair. The doctors made it clear that no matter what they did, she would probably end up broken or dead.

Juniper French spent 196 days in the neonatal intensive care unit (NICU) at All Children's Hospital (now Johns Hopkins All Children's Hospital) in St. Petersburg, Florida. In that time, my husband and I were reborn, too, morphing into entirely new people with new perspectives and new roles to play. Part of what shaped us were the dozens of conversations we had with the doctors and nurses who led, prodded, encouraged, guided, and steered us along.

Each of those conversations shifted the tectonic plates beneath our lives. Some had the power to salvage our family or destroy it. We saw the doctors and nurses studying our faces, trying to determine what we could handle. How much science? How much hope?

Disclosure: K.B. French is the author of the book, *Juniper: The Girl Who Was Born Too Soon*, published by Little, Brown.

The Media School, Indiana University, 601 E Kirkwood Avenue, Bloomington, IN 47405, USA
E-mail address: kbfrench@indiana.edu

Clin Perinatol 44 (2017) 275–282
http://dx.doi.org/10.1016/j.clp.2017.01.008

We studied their faces, too, noting the lines of their worry and the weight of their responsibility, as we tried to figure out what they were hiding. Our primary nurse, Tracy, had a habit of wearing a mask when she didn't want us to know how scared she was.

One cardiologist, explaining a clot in our daughter's heart, drew a square, divided it into 4, and said, "This is a heart." I realized he probably had to talk to parents every day who truly did not know what a heart looks like or what it does.

Doctors have impossible conversations every day, I realized. But the skills that make someone a good doctor are not the same as those that make a good teacher, counselor, interpreter, or therapist. We needed all of those things. Training in communication skills can be inadequate in neonatal fellowship programs.[1] Even in the unit, the conversations tend to be heavy on medical information but skirt the harder stuff: long-term outcomes, right and wrong, quality of life.[2] It's hard to imagine, given the complexity of the task and the stakes of the job, that any training could ever be enough.

Many times, before our daughter's birth and after, her life hung on how a conversation unfolded. How unsettling, then, to discover later that the tone, content, and style of those talks varied so wildly depending on which member of the medical team showed up.

I'd like to describe some of the conversations that rerouted our lives. Each is worth revisiting, for they all held such staggering and beautiful power.

THE DECISION

The first took place a day before our daughter was born. I had been in and out of the hospital since the 20th week of pregnancy, when I'd begun to bleed. I was wired to monitors and haunted by the lullabies that played over the intercom in the labor and delivery unit. Every time a healthy, squawking newborn entered the world, those lullabies reminded me mine would likely be born only to die.

I was cramping and bleeding, inverted in the bed. Magnesium sulfate pumped through my veins, making me feel like I was scalding from the inside out. A neonatologist visited my husband and me to explain the odds. I had never seen a neonatologist, even on TV. He was professional and compassionate, and I could see that the conversation was not easy for him.

He dutifully plodded through the relevant acronyms: IVH, PVH, NEC, ROP, CLD, RDS. A head-to-toe litany of disability. He appeared to be following a standard, if unofficial script, covering all bases. Our daughter could be damaged to any degree in any corner of her body or mind. He worked his way from the brain to the heart and lungs and gut, from cerebral palsy to nearsightedness.

Looking back, it reminds me of the absurd humor of a Cialis commercial. How immediate is the threat of the 8-hour erection, and is now the best time to consider it?

While my daughter is about to be pulled into the bright cold air and made to breathe, is asthma something I should be thinking about, or should we focus on the odds she'll spend her life on a ventilator? The information was a fire hose of calamity.

He delivered the numbers: 53% chance of death no matter what; 80% chance of death or moderate to severe disability. He talked a lot about morbidity.

He said more, but when he left, what remained in my head was that figure: *Eighty percent.*

I saw an 80% chance that she would die or live in misery. That she would look at me with stoned eyes that asked: Why did you do this to me? I saw an 80% chance that my marriage would collapse, that medical debt would destroy us, that any hope for future children would dissolve.

I saw a pistol with 5 chambers, 4 bullets. Russian roulette for my daughter's life. Would I gamble on 20%?

Hold on, a statistician or scientist might say. *That's misinterpreting the numbers.* But parents are not statisticians. They are panicked and sleep deprived and displaced. Some of us sputtered through high school math. Some don't speak the language. In the first hazy nauseating days in the NICU, we are not rational beings.

After my baby was out of the hospital, I found an interpreter in Dr John Lantos, the brilliant pediatric bioethicist. He told me some things I wish I'd known sooner.

The statistics the doctor had quoted were correct. That haunting number, 80%, came from the National Institute of Child Health and Human Development's neonatal outcome estimator,[3] which accounts for variables such as gestational age, gender, and antenatal steroids. They are also of limited use.

The number I needed to know, Lantos explained, was not the percent chance she would die *or* be disabled. Because if we chose not to intervene, the odds she would die were 100%. The number we needed to know was *if she lived*, what were the odds she would be okay?

That number was closer to 50%.[4] That is a bet I would have taken with far greater confidence.

Parents and doctors look at a baby from fundamentally different perspectives. The doctor sees a patient who will experience x number of morbidities before discharge. The parent sees an extension of their body and their family, a child who will occupy their home and the far reaches of their heart, who will expand their understanding of what it means to be alive. Every prognosis expands or contracts a universe.

When the clinician and the parent come together to make a life-and-death decision, language matters. Doctors have their own language, freighted with insider meaning and designed for other doctors.

Morbidity. That oft-repeated word clung to me like a reaper.

What did it mean? Deafness? Wheelchair? Toaster head?

It comes from "morbid": *gruesome, ghastly, suggesting the horror of death or decay*. At its root is the Latin *mori*: *to die*.

Morbidity is not a word parents need to hear. It simply means something different to a parent than it means to a doctor.

Another standard phrase seemed bland enough: "Do you want everything done?"

But that phrase, too, is code. The doctor's years of expertise had imbued the phrase with specifics: Ventilator. Surfactant. TPN.

Even as he described those measures, our frazzled layman's brains struggled to fill in the gaps. Would they batter our baby with CPR, fracturing her ribs? Would they prolong her suffering? When was it all too much?

If we agreed to "do everything," would the doctors assume we also meant "at any cost?"

The doctor said the choice was ours. I wanted to shake him and make him tell us what to do, and my husband wanted to punch him in the mouth. Surely the neonatologist, with his decades of training and experience, knew more than we did. Surely he was in a stronger state of mind.

He couldn't make the call for us, of course, because he would not have to raise or bury the child. And he couldn't put meaning into the statistics. So my husband and I sat up all night, trying to muster the courage to let our daughter die.

THE STORYTELLER

The next morning, we requested a second consultation. The NICU should have automatically sent someone to follow up with us, whether we asked for it or not. Bizarre as it may sound, it can be hard to summon a doctor. The power differential is daunting.

Nurses and residents act as a shield. Face-to-face communication skills are rusty in the Smartphone age. Time with an actual physician is so fleeting that the pressure on the patient to remember every question and extract every ounce of wisdom is overwhelming. We were professional adults with a dying baby, and we hated to bother the doctor again.

We were disappointed when, instead of the doctor we had seen the night before, a nurse practitioner arrived. She turned out to be a gift. Her tone, experience, and perspective helped us see a more complete picture. She knew the numbers too, but she didn't focus on them. Instead, she told stories.

She told stories of babies she'd known who had survived against great odds and of babies whose parents had unintentionally tortured them with futile procedures. She told us that we didn't have to decide right away—that we could intervene, and if things went south, we could withdraw support.

"It's a process," she said.

It took a lot of people to save our daughter's life, but she was the first.

I've staked my career on the belief that words have power. I never felt it more acutely than I did that day. Stories, in particular, have power. Stories give meaning to the random events that we endure. Stories breathe life into statistics.

The stories that Diane Loisel told us allowed us to imagine ourselves as the protagonists, to envision a future for our daughter and for ourselves. We saw a way to be the kind of parents we had always hoped to be, even if only for an hour, or a day.

Diane didn't lecture; she asked questions. Those questions allowed us to articulate how the choices fit our values. This approach is known as narrative ethics and is described by Geisler[5] this way:

> Narrative ethics centers the ethical dilemma squarely in the patient's life, and recognizes the patient as the author of his or her own life story…. To do what is right and good for someone requires a reliable understanding of what is best for that person within the context of his or her lived life.

Geisler quotes the poet Stephen Schmidt: "When you come into my room, you need to know my heart."

THE PAPERWORK

Once the decision had been made to resuscitate, we started signing consent forms. Consent forms are worth addressing, because they are part of the way parents and doctors communicate. They purportedly protect the patient and the hospital, and they ensure a somewhat consistent message when human interaction is so fraught and subjective.

Signing those forms was my first official act as a mother. The responsibility made my cheeks hot. But I didn't read a single page. The only thing I remember about any of those forms was how it felt to write next to my name that I was someone's mom.

I casually surveyed my friends who have had children in NICUs. None of them ever read a form, either.

A few years ago, I watched with interest as the medical community got into in a furious debate about consent forms used in important pediatric research. Critics of the landmark SUPPORT trial of oxygen therapies said the research put kids at risk and the consent forms didn't do their jobs.

I listened to hours of debate on my laptop as unquestionably smart people agonized over verbiage, evoked Tuskegee, and asked, "How many babies must die?" It seemed absurd.

In all the bluster, an essential truth was lost. All babies born so young are experiments. The rest is just paperwork.

I didn't need a 7-page document to tell me my daughter was dying. And the boilerplate language didn't mean that the actual care delivered was routine or consistent.

In the real world, critically sick babies are treated by a constantly rotating team. Some doctors are plain smarter or more experienced than others. We can tell. Some doctors know the baby better than others. Some treat aggressively and some don't. One doctor is pro-life. One has disabled kids. One was unexpectedly widowed. All of these factors influence how they talk to parents, how they assess quality of life, and how they interpret risk.

Our baby didn't hover inside an oxygen saturation target dictated by protocols. She cascaded wildly. Gunk in a tube or even a loud noise or a song she didn't like would send her crashing. Everyone who entered her room had a different threshold for when to intervene. Sometimes a doctor would turn the oxygen up, and as soon as he or she was gone, the nurse would turn it back down.

Yet we talk about the "standard of care" as though it were something pure and tangible and logical.

We listened to doctors debate whether to give our daughter a drug that was never tested in babies so small, or whether to try an intervention no one had tried before, or take a wild guess on the dose for a 2-pound baby.

Our baby had to go first. Somebody's baby always has to go first.

I don't even remember all the things I consented to. Was I informed? More than most. Was I informed enough? Of course not.

I had not slept in days. I was scared out of my mind. I had the mental capacity of a drunk being chased by bears. No form can protect a parent in a situation like that.

In the time we lived in the NICU, we learned to accept risk. There may be risk to participating in a certain study, but there is also risk to not participating. There may be risk to clinical intervention. But the risk of not intervening, in our case, was 100%.

Second-guessing and finger wagging over consent forms should not hamstring important research. Already overwhelmed parents shouldn't be offered false choices. Consent forms for nonnegotiable interventions such as PICC lines should be dealt with as wordlessly as possible, so parents can save their bandwidth for decisions that matter. Parents and practitioners must accept that at the frontier of human possibility, no form can make medicine a safe or predictable endeavor.

No matter what the forms say, the human interaction will always matter more. If a doctor or nurse I trusted asked me for a signature, I gave it. Those people, some of whom I had known mere minutes or hours, could have talked me into signing away anything, even my child's life. It does not comfort me to know that academics and researchers argue about what the paperwork says, because the paperwork is for lawyers, not for parents.

I want them to do the research that saves lives and do a better job explaining themselves to my face.

THE RESEARCHER

The first time a doctor pulled up a chair to talk to us, our baby was 2 months old. Until then, our conversations were hallway or bedside stand-up affairs, 10 minutes or less. We were startled and impressed when Dr Rajan Wadhawan, on his first day on service, scheduled an appointment to review our child's progress. It made us feel like he cared enough and respected us enough to engage.

At the meeting, he methodically reviewed the obstacles she faced, in order of urgency. Clot in her heart, chylothorax, ventilator dependence, retinopathy, on and on.

I cut to what I needed to know: "Could she still be a normal kid?" I asked. "Could she still go to kindergarten?"

He couldn't say. But instead of shrugging me off, he took time to walk us through the indicators. He cited the most relevant research—including the SUPPORT study—and by now, we were ready to learn. We were past the initial trauma. We had acclimated to the vocabulary of the unit, even the metric system.

Dr Raj, as everyone called him, told us something I wished I'd known sooner. He said studies show parents do have power over their children's long-term outcomes. Kids from 2-parent families and kids who receive services in early childhood have a huge advantage.[6] The brain adapts, and we can help.

That was the first time a doctor had really told us, in a way that we could absorb, how much we mattered. In the beginning, we had only our paralysis and guilt. We couldn't hold or feed our daughter. We went home each night without her. But here was hard evidence—backed by numbers—that we had a role to play. Given that some parents fade away and disappear when their babies are born ill, surely that information would have been just as important in the early days as the stats on ROP.

I didn't want false hope, but there is plenty of real hope in the research. Let us in on it.

THE MOTHER

So that brings me to the last conversation that changed us, and saved us, and in many ways defined our experience in the NICU. Our baby was dying. She was on an oscillating ventilator at 100%. Her blood pressure was low, her saturations were low, and she was slipping away in front of our eyes.

Our doctor, Fauzia Shakeel, had to decide whether to send her to surgery. The surgeon didn't want to operate because she said the operation would kill our daughter. The neonatologist explained as best she could and asked us what we wanted.

Again, we were desperate for guidance. But there was no guidance in the research or in the doctor's clinical experience. We didn't know it at the time, but this particular doctor had a saying: "Look at the baby."

She reminds herself and her colleagues that the answers are not always in the monitors. That the technology is not a substitute for human instinct.

So Dr Shakeel looked at our daughter, who had just opened her eyes for the first time. Something she saw there told her to send Juniper to surgery.

Then, the doctor pulled up a chair and sat down with us and talked to us for almost an hour. She didn't ask us to make any more decisions; she just told stories. She told about her own kids having spent time in the hospital and knowing what it's like to stare at a monitor. She spoke as a mother. She told us about babies she'd known before. She allowed us to imagine a future with our daughter, and she helped us paint a picture for ourselves, where we were good parents to our little girl for whatever amount of time she had left.

This was not about transferring information or calculating odds. It was a threshold crossed. It was the moment I made a friend for life, no matter how the surgery turned out. It was the moment I looked past a white coat and saw a human being, full of complexity and knowledge and expertise, sure, but also faith.

"Where there's life," she told us, "there's hope."

I saw that it would take a great deal more than drugs and monitors to save my child. It would take people like her. Every time Juniper was yanked back from the edge of death, it was a human being paying attention, and not a monitor, that made the difference. It was a gut call. Sometimes those calls were mine. Usually they were not.

People smarter than me will debate what the forms should say, and what the script should be when a baby comes crashing into the world at the threshold of viability and the doctor has to walk into the room and confront the shattered parents on the worst day of their lives.

If I were writing the script, though, here is what it might say:

Your baby is not finished developing. That means every part of their body is weak, from their lungs to their brain. Your baby is so early that trying to save her will take everything we've got. We need to talk you through what is going to happen, because you're going to have to help us decide how to proceed. We can resuscitate her when she's born and see how she does, or you might decide just to hold her until she dies. There's no right or wrong choice. You have to think about what works for your family, and we will support you either way.

Statistics always lag a little behind what is actually happening in the NICU, but the best statistics we have tell us that about half of babies just like yours will die no matter what. Usually babies who are going to die do so in the first few days. But about half of them live. And of the ones who live, about half turn out just fine. They go to college. They join the gymnastics team. They grow up healthy.

The other half of the kids who live will have some challenges. They might go home on a feeding tube or oxygen support, which they could outgrow later. We see them come back to the hospital when they are 3 and they get the flu and need help recovering. Many will catch up with their peers by the time they start school. Some will have issues their whole lives. Cerebral palsy, developmental delays and autism are all possibilities.

A lot depends on what happens in the first couple of weeks. We'll be watching for bleeding in the brain – that can tell us a lot. We'll be very concerned about infection, especially in the intestines. And we'll be watching to see if the lungs can grow and function on their own.

If you do decide you want us to treat your baby, we will keep you informed at every step. There will be opportunities in the first week or so to withdraw support if things are not going well. A lot of parents find that very hard to consider once they have met their child. If your baby suffers massive bleeding in the brain, we will talk to you then about quality of life. This is a process, and we will work through these questions together.

You and your baby are in the best place you can be. We know a lot about how to help these babies, and we can let you talk to other parents who have been through this, and we can let you meet some other kids who started out just like your child.

I want you to know that you have a lot of power here. There are a lot of unknowns, but we do know that your baby can hear your voice and that your presence means a lot. Your breast milk, your touch and your voice are powerful medicine. One of the strongest indicators of how a very early baby will turn out is whether they have an involved parent.

If you decide to go forward, it will feel terrifying, and it will also feel beautiful and sacred. You'll be a different person in a few weeks than you are right now, and that's okay.

You don't have to resuscitate. A lot of parents don't, and you're still great parents if you choose not to. I can talk more about what the next few months in the NICU might look like, or I can talk about what it might be like if you choose to just hold your baby when she's born and let her go.

Do you want to keep talking, or should I come back in a couple of hours? Who else would you like to talk to? Can I leave you some reading material? If you read something on the internet, let's talk about it, because not all the things you read apply to your baby. I'd like you to have the best information available.

I'd talk more about long-term outcomes than short term morbidity. I'd narrow the focus of the initial conversation and widen the circle of support.

The conversation doesn't have to end with any script, though, and it must be more than a warning, more than a lecture. It helps when clinicians tell stories and ask questions and drop the jargon and the euphemisms. It helps when parents can talk and stumble over their words and contradict themselves and not feel rushed. It helps to know it all doesn't have to be decided in a single hour, that the doctor will be back in the morning.

The science and the research and the paperwork and the numbers all matter. But the person parents need most in that moment is someone who understands the research so well that she has the confidence to step out from behind the statistics and the paperwork, pull up a chair, and look a parent square in the eye.

REFERENCES

1. Boss R, Hutton N, Donoghue PK, et al. Neonatologist training to guide family decision making for critically ill infants. Arch Pediatr Adolesc Med 2009;163:783–8.
2. Bastek TK, Richardson DK, Zupancic JA, et al. Prenatal consultation practices at the border of viability: a regional survey. Pediatrics 2005;116:407–13.
3. Tyson JE, Parikh NA, Langer J, et al, National Institute of Child Health and Human Development Neonatal Research Network. Intensive care for extreme prematurity—moving beyond gestational age. N Engl J Med 2008;358:1672–81.
4. Wood NS, Marlow N, Costeloe K, et al. Neurologic and developmental disability after extremely preterm birth. EPICure Study Group. N Engl J Med 2000;343: 378–84.
5. Geisler SL. The value of narrative ethics to medicine. J Physician Assist Educ 2006;17:54–7.
6. Ment L, Vohr B, Allan W, et al. Change in cognitive function over time in very low-birth-weight infants. JAMA 2003;289(6):705–11.

Periviable Birth and the Shifting Limit of Viability

 CrossMark

Brian M. Mercer, BA, MD, FRCSC

KEYWORDS

- Periviable birth • Limit of viability • Patient counseling

KEY POINTS

- When periviable birth is anticipated, the obstetrician and pediatricians should provide coordinated and consistent counseling that incorporates up to date and accurate information based on estimated gestational age and other specific relevant factors.
- When brief pregnancy prolongation occurs in a patient who remains at risk for periviable birth, the obstetrician and pediatrician should adjust their counselling regarding potential outcomes according to individual clinical circumstances.
- Obstetricians and pediatricians should recognize that the limit of viability continues to decline. Currently available data suggest potential survival of infants born and resuscitated at 22 weeks' of gestation.

Preterm birth near the limit of viability is a grave circumstance that carries a high risk of fetal and newborn death, and the potential for severe life-long complications among those who do survive. Brief delay in delivery early in pregnancy can have a dramatic effect on outcomes; those delivering before the limit of viability suffering certain death regardless of postnatal interventions, and those delivering soon after the limit of viability having rapidly increasing potential for survival with brief pregnancy prolongation. All infants born soon after the limit of viability require intensive resuscitation and prolonged neonatal intensive care unit (NICU) care. Regardless of the odds against them, many families choose aggressive intervention for fetal benefit, many mothers willingly attempt pregnancy prolongation despite risks due to the underlying medical and/or obstetric condition leading to preterm birth, and many mothers willingly accept the risks of surgical interventions (eg, potential classical cesarean) for fetal benefit. Because of the potential for evolving and increasing maternal risks with attempted pregnancy prolongation in this timeframe, and because newborn risks and potential outcomes change rapidly with advancing gestational age, it is important that the family be provided objective, accurate, and up-to-date information regarding fetal, newborn,

Disclosure Statement: None.
Department of Obstetrics & Gynecology, The MetroHealth System, Suite G267, 2500 MetroHealth Drive, Cleveland, OH 44109, USA
E-mail address: bmercer@metrohealth.org

Clin Perinatol 44 (2017) 283–286
http://dx.doi.org/10.1016/j.clp.2017.02.002
0095-5108/17/© 2017 Elsevier Inc. All rights reserved.
perinatology.theclinics.com

and maternal risks and outcomes and that this counseling adapt to changing clinical circumstances.

There is considerable overlap in descriptive terms for very early preterm birth (**Table 1**)[1-7] but none of these fully reflects all relevant issues to these newborns. In 2014, the Society for Maternal-Fetal Medicine, *Eunice Kennedy Shriver* National Institute of Child Health and Human Development, American Academy of Pediatrics, and American College of Obstetricians and Gynecologists published proceedings of a jointly sponsored workshop. They recognized that there is no ideal definition for very early delivery but developed a consensus definition of periviable birth as delivery occurring from 20 0/7 weeks to 25 6/7 weeks of gestation, reflecting the gestational age range in which survival ranges from 0% to more than 50%.[7] This group recognized that the division between 1 week and the next is an arbitrary cut-off that fails to reflect continuous growth and maturation; that gestational age and fetal weight estimates are not always accurate; that other factors, including fetal sex, plurality, and antenatal treatments (eg, antenatal corticosteroids, magnesium sulfate for neuroprotection, antibiotic treatment), can affect outcomes; and that individual newborn responses to resuscitation cannot be predicted before birth. The workshop participants agreed that development of accurate and precise predictive models for newborn outcomes are needed. However, currently available predictive models are not highly accurate. As such, gestational age remains a mainstay for patient counseling before delivery and was the basis for guidance offered regarding interventions for threatened and imminent delivery in the periviable period.

Table 1 Various descriptive terms for delivery and birth near the limit of viability	
	Criteria
Birth weight specific descriptions of early preterm birth	
Very low birth weight	<1500 g
Extremely low birth weight	<1000 g
Micropreemie or Micropremie	Variably defined <1 $^3/_4$ lb or <3 lb, or <1000 g, or <26 or <29 wk of gestation
Gestational age specific descriptions of early preterm birth	
Midtrimester or second trimester	13th to 27th wk of pregnancy, 4th through 6th mo of pregnancy
Remote from term	No consistent definition
Early preterm	No consistent definition
Extremely low gestational age	No consistent definition
Extreme preterm	<28 wk of gestation
Very preterm	28 through 31 6/7 wk of gestation
Newborn outcome specific descriptions of early preterm birth	
Previable	Not sufficiently developed to survive outside the uterus
Marginal viability	23 0/7 through 26 6/7 wk of gestation
Threshold of viability	At or before 25 wk of gestation or <750 g, 23–25 wk of gestation
Periviable	20 0/7 through 25 6/7 wk of gestation

Data from Refs.[1-7]

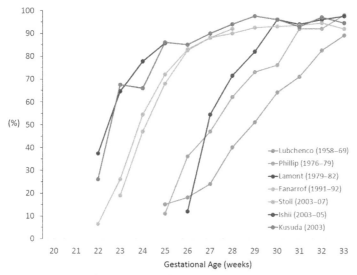

Fig. 1. Changing pattern of survival according to gestational age at birth over time. (*Data from* Refs.[8–15])

Critical to family counseling is an understanding that newborn outcomes change not only with advancing gestational age and the newborn's condition at birth but that these outcomes have also changed over years and continue to do so. Although gestational age and birth weight are constants, newborn outcomes at a given gestational age and birth weight are not. Before the early 1980s, death with delivery at or before 25 weeks of gestation was virtually assured[8,9] (**Fig. 1**). However, since that time, with the development of NICUs, ventilator and feeding technologies, and advances in treatments such as antenatal corticosteroid and surfactant therapies, there has been a progressive increase in newborn survival at any given gestational age near the limit of viability.[10–13] Studies published within the last decade have consistently reported survival rates of 5% to 7% after birth at 22 weeks of gestation.[12,13] Of note, however, several recent reports have reported dramatically higher survival rates of approximately 25% to 35% with delivery at 22 weeks[14,15]; rates similar to those seen at 23 weeks in the 1990s and 2000s. Potential reasons for this variation may include differences in reporting, such as single vs multicenter, definition of mortality (neonatal, at discharge, infant), inclusion criteria (all live births, resuscitated newborns, NICU admissions), as well as local practices and protocols for withholding or withdrawing aggressive newborn care.

Both obstetricians and pediatricians have a history of underestimating newborn survival and intact survival, with this error being greater near the limit of viability.[16] Recognizing this and the changing pattern of survival over time, it is particularly important that physicians be aware of current outcomes, accept the potential that the limit of viability will continue to decline, and collaborate in providing consistent, accurate and up to date information to patients at risk for periviable birth.

REFERENCES

1. ICD-10 International statistical classification of diseases and related health problems: Tenth revision. Geneva (Switzerland): World Health Organization; 2008.

Available at: http://apps.who.int/classifications/icd10/browse/2016/en. Accessed March 5, 2017.

2. Available at: www.micropreemies.com/. Accessed February 5, 2017.

3. Merriam Webster Medical Dictionary. Available at: www.merriam-webster.com/medical. Accessed February 5, 2017.

4. Available at: www.who.int/mediacentre/factsheets/fs363/en/. Accessed February 5, 2017.

5. Rennie JM. Perinatal management at the lower margin of viability. Arch Dis Child 1996;4:214–8.

6. Perinatal care at the threshold of viability. American Academy of Pediatrics, Committee on Fetus and Newborn, American College of Obstetricians and Gynecologists, Committee on Obstetric Practice. Pediatrics 1995;96:974–6.

7. Raju TN, Mercer BM, Burchfield DJ, et al. Periviable birth: executive summary of a joint workshop by the Eunice Kennedy Shriver National Institute of Child Health and Human Development, Society for Maternal-Fetal Medicine, American Academy of Pediatrics, and American College of Obstetricians and Gynecologists. Obstet Gynecol 2014;123:1083–96.

8. Lubchenco LO, Searls DT, Brazie JV. Neonatal mortality rate: relationship to birth weight and gestational age. J Pediatr 1972;81:814–22.

9. Philip AG, Little GA, Polivy DR, et al. Neonatal mortality risk for the eighties: the importance of birth weight/gestational age groups. Pediatrics 1981;68:122–30.

10. Lamont RF, Dunlop DPM, Crowley P, et al. Spontaneous preterm labour and delivery at under 34 weeks' gestation. BMJ 1983;286:454–7.

11. Fanaroff AA, Wright LL, Stevenson DK, et al. Very-low-birth-weight outcomes of the National Institute of Child Health and Human Development Neonatal Research Network, May 1991 through December 1992. Am J Obstet Gynecol 1995;173:1423–31.

12. Stoll BJ, Hansen NI, Bell EF, et al. Neonatal outcomes of extremely preterm infants from the NICHD Neonatal Research Network. Pediatrics 2010;126:443–56.

13. Rysavy MA, Li L, Bell EF, et al. Eunice Kennedy Shriver National Institute of Child Health and Human Development Neonatal Research Network. Between-hospital variation in treatment and outcomes in extremely preterm infants. N Engl J Med 2015;372:1801–11.

14. Kusuda S, Fujimura M, Sakuma I, et al, Neonatal Research Network, Japan. Morbidity and mortality of infants with very low birth weight in Japan: center variation. Pediatrics 2006;118:e1130–8.

15. Ishii N, Kono Y, Yonemoto N, et al, Neonatal Research Network, Japan. Outcomes of infants born at 22 and 23 Weeks' gestation. Pediatrics 2013;132:62–71.

16. Morse SB, Haywood JL, Goldenberg RL, et al. Estimation of neonatal outcome and perinatal therapy use. Pediatrics 2000;105:1046–50.

Survival of Infants Born at Periviable Gestational Ages

Ravi Mangal Patel, MD, MSc[a],*, Matthew A. Rysavy, MD, PhD[b],
Edward F. Bell, MD[c], Jon E. Tyson, MD, MPH[d]

KEYWORDS

- Mortality • Perinatal epidemiology • Preterm infant • Resuscitation • Stillbirth

KEY POINTS

- Estimates of gestational age–specific survival vary significantly across hospitals, regions, and countries and are influenced by a number of factors that can make unbiased comparisons challenging.
- Survival among live periviable births at 22 to 25 weeks of gestation has incrementally improved since the 1950s, with continued gains over the past decade.
- Provision of active treatment, particularly at 22 and 23 weeks of gestation, varies widely among centers and countries, and this variation has a substantial impact on reported survival rates.
- Improved reporting of survival rates for periviable births may yield a better understanding of birth outcomes for periviable births occurring at 20 to 25 weeks of gestation.

INTRODUCTION

Periviable births comprise a particularly high-risk group of patients cared for by obstetricians, neonatologists, and other caregivers. Periviable birth is currently defined as delivery occurring from 20 0/7 through 25 6/7 weeks of gestation.[1,2] This review provides a historical perspective into survival of periviable births, summarizes recent and new data on gestational age–specific survival rates, and reviews factors that can have a significant impact on survival. As this review is focused on survival, we do not

Conflicts of Interest: The authors have no conflicts of interest to report.
[a] Division of Neonatal-Perinatal Medicine, Department of Pediatrics, Children's Healthcare of Atlanta, Emory University School of Medicine, 2015 Uppergate Drive Northeast, 3rd Floor, Atlanta, GA 30322, USA; [b] Department of Pediatrics, University of Wisconsin Hospital and Clinics, 600 Highland Avenue, Madison, WI 53792, USA; [c] Department of Pediatrics, University of Iowa, 200 Hawkins Drive, 8811 JPP, Iowa City, IA 52242, USA; [d] Center for Clinical Research and Evidence-Based Medicine, McGovern Medical School, The University of Texas Health Science Center at Houston, 6431 Fannin Street, MSB2.106, Houston, TX 77030, USA
* Corresponding author.
E-mail address: rmpatel@emory.edu

Clin Perinatol 44 (2017) 287–303
http://dx.doi.org/10.1016/j.clp.2017.01.009
0095-5108/17/© 2017 Elsevier Inc. All rights reserved.

discuss additional outcomes among surviving periviable infants, such as disability, but acknowledge the importance of considering such outcomes alongside estimates of mortality to inform understanding about prognosis.

HISTORICAL PERSPECTIVES

The survival of extremely low birth weight (ELBW; birth weight ≤1000 g) infants, including periviable infants, has improved consistently over the past 7 decades. In the 1940s, death was the expected outcome for all ELBW infants born in developed nations around the world.[3] Beginning in the 1950s and 1960s, the probability of survival for ELBW infants among several centers in the United States and the United Kingdom increased to 10% to 30% as understanding of neonatal physiology improved and the provision of neonatal intensive care became more common and more advanced.[3,4] In the 1970s, multiple reports from the United States and international centers demonstrated improved survival rates for ELBW and extremely preterm infants.[3] A single-center study from Illinois of 100 ELBW infants born between 1974 and 1976 and admitted to the neonatal intensive care unit (NICU) reported survival rates of 10% for infants weighing 501 to 750 g and 48% for infants weighing 751 to 1000 g.[5] A multicenter study of live births from 1976 to 1978 in New York City reported a survival rate of approximately 50% for singleton live births weighing 501 to 1250 g born at level-3 centers.[6] In a population-based study from England and Wales, survival of liveborn infants weighing less than 1000 g increased from 16% in 1964 to 23% in 1975.[7]

In the late 1980s and mid-1990s, prospective cohort studies from the National Institute of Child Health and Human Development (NICHD) Neonatal Research Network (NRN)[8] and EPICure[9] were among the first to systematically evaluate periviable birth outcomes on a relatively large scale in the surfactant era of neonatology. The NICHD NRN reported outcomes of 1804 very low birth weight (VLBW; birth weight 501–1500 g) live births at 8 academic centers in the United States from 1989 to 1990.[8] The estimated survival for liveborn infants in this cohort was 18% at less than 23 weeks of gestation, 15% at 23 weeks, 54% at 24 weeks, and 59% at 25 weeks. The EPICure study collected outcomes for periviable live births across all maternity units in the United Kingdom and Ireland in 1995 (n = 4004) and reported survival rates of 40% for births between 20 and 25 weeks of gestation.[9] Similar to the NICHD NRN study, the EPICure study reported survival approaching 20% for infants born before 24 weeks of gestation and survival greater than 60% for infants at 25 weeks of gestation.

In the early part of the twenty-first century, data from the NICHD NRN for periviable live-births from 2003 to 2007 suggested that improvements in survival had plateaued, with no increases in survival rates over the period.[10] However, more recent reports from the NICHD NRN (**Fig. 1**) and other centers in the United States,[11–13] as well as from several other developed nations around the world,[14–19] demonstrate incremental improvements in survival following periviable birth, continuing trends established more than half a century ago. These studies are discussed in detail in this article.

ESTIMATES OF GESTATIONAL AGE–SPECIFIC SURVIVAL

During the past 5 years, large cohort studies from developed nations in North America,[11–13,20,21] South America,[22] Europe,[14,15,23–25] Asia,[18,19,26] and Australia[27] have reported estimates of gestational age–specific survival following periviable birth. Direct comparisons of estimated survival rates among these studies are limited, however, by potential biases introduced from differences in the data sources, ascertainment of death, selection of denominators, and definitions of live birth.[28] Recommendations

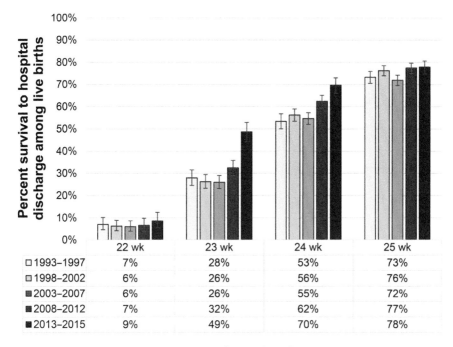

	22 wk	23 wk	24 wk	25 wk
☐ 1993–1997	7%	28%	53%	73%
☐ 1998–2002	6%	26%	56%	76%
▪ 2003–2007	6%	26%	55%	72%
▪ 2008–2012	7%	32%	62%	77%
▪ 2013–2015	9%	49%	70%	78%

Gestational age

Fig. 1. Survival from 1993 through 2015 following live birth in the NICHD Neonatal Research Network. Includes all participating centers. Liveborn infants were included regardless of whether active treatment was initiated. Whisker bars indicate 95% CIs calculated with the Clopper-Pearson method. (*Data from* Stoll BJ, Hansen NI, Bell EF, et al. Trends in care practices, morbidity, and mortality of extremely preterm neonates, 1993-2012. JAMA 2015;314(10):1039–51, for 1993-2012; and *Courtesy with permission of* the NICHD Neonatal Research Network, Bethesda, MD, USA for 2013-2015.)

to improve reporting of birth outcomes have recently been published with the goal of providing more clinically meaningful and comparable estimates of survival.[29] These recommendations emphasize the importance of reporting standardized information on the source population and outcomes measured, including the timing of assessment, and measures of statistical uncertainty, such as 95% confidence intervals (CIs), when reporting on periviable birth outcomes. With the aforementioned caveats that studies have varied in their methodology and reporting, estimates of gestational age–specific survival for select population-based and multicenter studies that report outcomes among periviable live births or infants admitted to the NICU (**Table 1**) are shown in **Fig. 2**.

These studies show a wide variation in survival rates following live birth at periviable gestational ages, ranging from 0% to 37% at 22 weeks, 1% to 64% at 23 weeks, 31% to 78% at 24 weeks, and 59% to 86% at 25 weeks of gestation. The variation in survival rates following periviable birth among cohorts in developed nations (see **Fig. 2**) is much greater in magnitude than the increases in survival over time within the NICHD NRN (see **Fig. 1**). Variation in approaches to perinatal care and other factors that may explain the large amount of variation in periviable survival are discussed later in this article. In general, we have categorized this variation as resulting from between-study differences in national and institutional recommendations and guidelines for

Table 1
Recent studies reporting gestational age–specific survival following periviable birth

Study (Publication Year)	EPICure (2012)[14]	EXPRESS (2009)[83]	EPIPAGE-2 (2015)[15]	Victoria (2016)[27]	NICHD NRN[a]	Japan NRN (2013)[18]	SNN (2016)[24]	Pediatrix (2016)[20]	CNN (2013)[21]
Study type	Population-based cohort studies				Center-based cohort studies				
Source population	National	National	National (except 1 region, 2% of births)	Regional	18 network centers	48 tertiary centers	15 NICUs (95% of births in nation)	362 NICUs	National network of NICUs
Country	UK	Sweden	France	Australia	US	Japan	Switzerland	US	Canada
Year(s)	2006	2004-2007	2011	2010-2011	2013-2015	2003-2005	2009-2012	1997-2013	2010-2011
Sample size[b] (at 22-25 wk)	2034 (1454)	707 (501)	5169 (641)	541 (279)	2430	1057 (1057)	3068 (450)	64,896 (17,085)	6106 (1208)
GA inclusion	22-26 wk	<27 wk[c]	22-34 wk	22-27 wk	22-25 wk	22-25 wk	23-31 wk	22-29 wk	23-30 wk
Minimal BW inclusion	400 g	None	None	None	401g	None	None	None	None
Inception (denominator reported by study)	Live birth or stillbirth	Live birth or stillbirth	Live birth, stillbirth or TOP	Live birth	Live birth	Live birth	Live birth	NICU admission	NICU admission
Denominator for Fig. 2	Live births	Live births						Infants admitted to center	
Outborn, % of denominator	14.7% - Included	16.5% - Included	21.0% - Included	15.5% - Included	Not reported	9.3% - Included	4.9% - Included	18.5% - Excluded	18.1% - Included
Exclusions	TOP	TOP, birth outside country	No verbal consent	TOP, birth defects	Outborn	Admitted after 28 d, birth defects	TOP, birth defects	Outborn, transfer, birth defects	Multiple[d]
Survival assessment[e]	Survival to d/c	Survival to 1 y	Survival to d/c	Survival to d/c	Survival to d/c	Survival to d/c	Survival to d/c	Survival to d/c	Survival to d/c

Abbreviations: BW, birth weight; CNN, Canadian Neonatal Network; d/c, hospital discharge; EPIPAGE-2, Etude Epidémiologique sur les Petits Ages Gestationnels 2; EX-PRESS, Extremely Preterm Infants in Sweden Study; GA, gestational age; NICHD, National Institute of Child Health and Human Development; NICU, neonatal intensive care unit; NRN, Neonatal Research Network; SNN, Swiss Neonatal Network; TOP, termination of pregnancy.

[a] Data on mortality among inborn live births from 2013 to 2015 courtesy of the NICHD NRN.

[b] Sample size of live births for year(s) listed; number of periviable births in **Fig. 2** noted in parentheses.

[c] Stillbirths at 22 0/7 to 26 6/7 included; no lower gestational age bounds for live births.

[d] Infants declared moribund, infants receiving palliative care, infants with lethal birth defects, infants with missing birth date or missing/ambiguous gender.

[e] For consistency, survival to hospital discharge reported in **Fig. 2** if it could be determined from reported outcomes, although some studies also reported longer-term survival to 1 year or beyond.

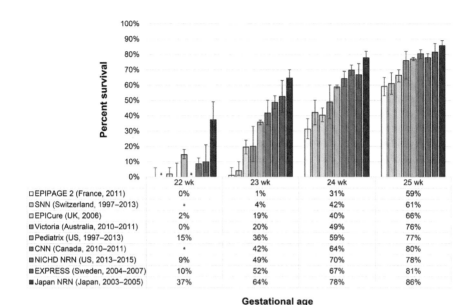

	22 wk	23 wk	24 wk	25 wk
□ EPIPAGE 2 (France, 2011)	0%	1%	31%	59%
▨ SNN (Switzerland, 1997–2013)	ᵃ	4%	42%	61%
□ EPICure (UK, 2006)	2%	19%	40%	66%
▨ Victoria (Australia, 2010–2011)	0%	20%	49%	76%
▨ Pediatrix (US, 1997–2013)	15%	36%	59%	77%
▪ CNN (Canada, 2010–2011)	ᵃ	42%	64%	80%
▪ NICHD NRN (US, 2013–2015)	9%	49%	70%	78%
▪ EXPRESS (Sweden, 2004–2007)	10%	52%	67%	81%
▪ Japan NRN (Japan, 2003–2005)	37%	64%	78%	86%

Gestational age

Fig. 2. Gestational age–specific survival following live birth by study type. Data are shown for population-based cohorts (*gray hues*), center-based cohorts reporting survival for live births (*blue hues*) and center-based cohorts reporting survival for infants admitted to the NICU (*orange hues*). Characteristics of the data sources are reported in **Table 1**. Whisker bars indicate 95% CIs calculated with the Clopper-Pearson method. ᵃ Estimates not reported by the study.

perinatal care, cohort characteristics, maternal-infant characteristics, and antenatal and postnatal treatment, including decisions about the initiation and withdrawal of care.

RECOMMENDATIONS AND GUIDELINES FOR PERINATAL CARE

Some of the variation in survival observed in **Fig. 2** may be attributable to variation in the approach to perinatal care based on guideline statements from professional organizations and scientific societies. In a systematic review of 31 national or international guidelines for perinatal care of periviable births in highly developed countries, there was substantial variation in recommendations. Sixty-eight percent of guideline statements supported comfort care at 22 weeks of gestation and 65% supported active treatment and resuscitation at 25 weeks of gestation.[30] At 23 and 24 weeks of gestation, there was more variability among recommendations, including for comfort care, routine active treatment, individualized care, and active treatment based on parental wishes. Many of these guidelines statements include reporting of country-specific survival rates, although as we discuss later in this article, substantial within-country variation in survival rates have also been reported.

In the United States, a recent consensus statement by the American College of Obstetricians and Gynecologists and the Society for Maternal-Fetal Medicine provides general guidance regarding obstetric and neonatal active treatment for fetuses and infants at periviable gestational ages.[2] At 20 to 21 weeks of gestation, provision of antenatal corticosteroids, cesarean delivery for fetal indication, and neonatal assessment for resuscitation are not recommended. At 22 weeks of gestation, the authors recommend that clinicians "consider" neonatal assessment for resuscitation but do not recommend antenatal corticosteroids or cesarean delivery. At 23 weeks of gestation, the investigators recommend that clinicians consider all general measures of neonatal and obstetric active treatment but do not give a firm recommendation for any of them. At 24 weeks of gestation, cesarean delivery should be considered, and all other measures of neonatal and obstetric active treatment are recommended. At 25 weeks of gestation, cesarean delivery and other active neonatal and obstetric measures are recommended. Given the recent publication of this guideline statement in the United States, it is too soon to assess the effect of these recommendations on clinical practice.

ADDITIONAL FACTORS INFLUENCING SURVIVAL RATES FOR PERIVIABLE INFANTS
Cohort Selection

Differences in the conduct of cohort studies are important to understand when interpreting and comparing gestational age–specific survival rates. This is particularly relevant when studies use different numerators (eg, death in the delivery room, death before 28 days, death before hospital discharge, death before 1 year) and denominators (eg, fetus alive at maternal admission and >20 weeks of gestation, all live births, inborn live births, live births receiving active treatment, infants admitted to the NICU) to estimate mortality rates (**Fig. 3**). The appropriate numerator and denominator depend on the relevant period at risk.[29] For a woman pregnant with a fetus alive at 20 weeks of gestation, studies reporting outcomes with a denominator of infants admitted to the NICU do not reflect all of the potential birth outcomes of her fetus (see **Fig. 3**). Likewise, a high stillbirth rate may be obscured by reporting outcomes only among live births, and a high delivery room death rate could be obscured by reporting only outcomes for infants admitted to the NICU (**Fig. 4**). In contrast, if the population of interest is infants receiving active treatment after live birth, the stillbirth rate has ordinarily been assumed to be irrelevant. However, exclusion of stillbirths can lead to imperfect risk adjustment when comparing populations that differ in prenatal and antepartum care and the proportion of fetuses at high risk for death after birth.

Study selection criteria, particularly with regard to selection of infants based on admission to a hospital or birth within a geographic population, decisions regarding the inclusion of outborn infants in hospital-based studies, and the exclusion of infants born below a lower bounds of birth weight or with the diagnosis of a birth defect, can impact the estimated mortality rates.

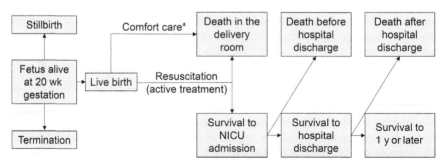

Fig. 3. Potential birth outcomes for a fetus alive at 20 weeks of gestation. [a] Although uncommon, survival to NICU admission may occur following initial provision of comfort care.

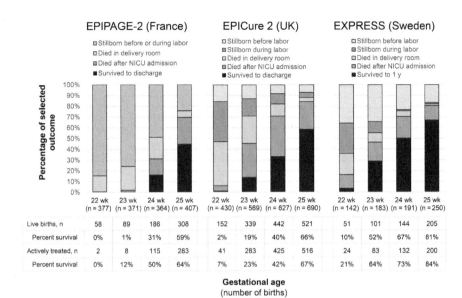

Fig. 4. Periviable birth outcomes by gestational age in population-based studies. Data from population-based studies in France,[15,56] the United Kingdom,[14,82] and Sweden[83] evaluating outcomes of live births and stillbirths are shown in **Table 1**. Pregnancies with termination are not included. Active treatment definitions vary by study but include measures of delivery room intervention or admission for neonatal care.

In addition, differences in case mix among cohorts studied can lead to biased comparisons of risk-adjusted mortality due to the Simpson paradox, which occurs when populations differing in case mix are grouped together and can lead to reversal of an association demonstrated when groups are compared separately.[31] This paradox has been demonstrated in studies using risk adjustment to compare standardized mortality ratios among different populations.[32,33]

Place of Birth

As previously discussed, country of birth has a large impact on the probability of survival.[34] Take, for example, the nearly universal death of infants born alive at 23 weeks of gestation in France compared with the approximately 50% reported survival among live births in Sweden (see **Fig. 2**). Some of this variation may be accounted for by national guideline statements and cultural preferences regarding perinatal care of periviable births,[35] as previously discussed. However, even within countries, there is substantial variation in survival among live births.

The level, volume, and quality of neonatal care provided at a given center or hospital has potential impacts on extremely preterm survival. Variation in neonatal care and outcomes by center,[10,36,37] region,[38] and country[39] has been well documented, and the level and volume of neonatal care provided has been associated with a center's rate of death or serious morbidity.[40,41] However, the level of neonatal care is not necessarily associated with some aspects of quality care, as demonstrated in a recent study of 134 California NICUs.[42] Within limits, greater availability of neonatal intensive care, measured by the number of neonatologists working in a given region, is associated with a decreased neonatal mortality rate.[43] However, the potential benefits of increased availability of neonatal intensive care may be offset by the associated de-regionalization of care that can occur as the number of NICUs increase, with a greater proportion of high-risk births occurring in lower volume centers.[44] In addition, hospital recognition for nursing excellence, a surrogate measure of quality of nursing care, is associated with a lower risk of early mortality in the first 7 days of life for VLBW infants, but not mortality before discharge.[45]

Variation in the Provision of Active Treatment

Intensive care is necessary for neonatal survival at periviable gestational ages. In the United States, the American Academy of Pediatrics statement on antenatal counseling recommends that decision making in the delivery room be individualized and family centered for births at 22 to 24 weeks of gestation, taking into account known fetal and maternal conditions and parental beliefs.[46] However, individual attitudes and biases of providers may impact shared decision making with families about whether to initiate or withhold active treatment. In a UK study that evaluated attitudes of 25 neonatologists toward resuscitation and care of extremely preterm infants, providers were grouped as having 1 of 3 types of attitudes toward decision making: (1) treatments should not be limited based on gestational age and technology should be used to help improve treatment of suffering and disability; (2) treatment should be provided based primarily on gestational age; and (3) treatment should be withheld or withdrawn based on quality-of-life principles to prevent disability.[47] Understanding these attitudes and biases, and minimizing them when discussing outcome data regarding survival with parents are important aspects of counseling about the outcomes of periviable birth.[48]

Biases affect decisions about care, and they may also affect the presentation of information for family counseling. One example of the latter is framing bias, which involves only discussing the probability of survival or the probability of mortality instead of presenting both potential outcomes.[49] Another example is misestimation of the probability of adverse outcomes. This was highlighted in a study in Victoria, Australia, where obstetric and neonatal provider estimates of survival and disability were compared with actual outcome rates within the same region and found to overestimate poor outcomes.[50] This is consistent with findings from a prior US study.[51] The use of model-based outcome estimates based on systematically collected data from multiple centers and incorporating several maternal and infant factors, including whether infants received active treatment, may be useful in decreasing these types of biases, as we discuss later in this article.[52]

Effect of Obstetric and Neonatal Active Treatment

Active treatment of fetuses and liveborn infants is one of the most important determinants of early survival for periviable births. In a multicenter study of 24 academically affiliated hospitals in the NICHD NRN, the proportion of live births receiving active treatment at 22 and 23 weeks of gestation ranged from 0% to 100% and 25% to 100%, respectively, among individual hospitals.[37] The variation in hospital rate of active treatment accounted for 78% of the observed differences in-hospital survival rates for infants born at 22 or 23 weeks of gestation. In contrast, only 22% and 1% of the differences in survival rates at 24 and 25 weeks of gestation, respectively, could be explained by variation in the hospital rate of active treatment. At some of the hospitals, most infants born at 22 weeks of gestation received active treatment whereas at others no infants born at 22 weeks did, a difference that may be reflective of institutional policies, clinician attitudes, or parental preferences.

In a national study in Sweden, regional rates of obstetric and neonatal active treatment were used to estimate the effects on survival among fetuses alive at the mother's admission.[53] The proportion of key obstetric interventions (birth at a level 3 unit, antenatal corticosteroids, cesarean delivery, and tocolysis) and neonatal interventions (surfactant administration, neonatologist present for delivery, intubation after birth, and NICU referral) were used to estimate the intensity of perinatal care and associate this intensity with the risk of stillbirth, death within 12 hours of birth, and death before 1 year of age. The range of activity scores, reflecting the intensity of active treatment, were 72 to 100. For each 5-point increase in activity score, the risk of stillbirth (adjusted odds ratio [OR] 0.90; 95% CI 0.83–0.97), death within 12 hours (0.75; 0.68–0.86), and death before 1 year (0.83; 0.75–0.91) all decreased significantly after accounting for several other characteristics known to affect fetal and infant outcomes. Regions of Sweden providing a high intensity of active treatment at 22 to 24 weeks of gestation (activity score 96–100) had a mortality rate of 35%, compared with a mortality rate of 59% among regions providing a low intensity of active treatment (activity score 74–80).

Importantly, active treatment occurs both before and after birth. In another study of live births before 27 weeks of gestation in Sweden, the effect of individual components of active obstetric treatment on death within 24 hours after live birth were estimated.[54] The risk of death decreased with each additional week of gestation (adjusted OR 0.3; 95% CI 0.2–0.4) after adjusting for differences in pregnancy and delivery characteristics; this decrease in risk of early mortality was similar to that seen with 2 components of obstetric active treatment: administration of antenatal corticosteroids (adjusted OR 0.3; 95% CI 0.1–0.6) and cesarean delivery (adjusted OR 0.4; 95% CI 0.2–0.9). In addition, observational studies have consistently demonstrated a lower risk of death among neonates born at less than 24 weeks of gestation exposed to antenatal corticosteroids.[55] In a population-based study of infants at 22 to 26 weeks of gestation in France, 96% of those infants who had neonatal intensive care withheld or withdrawn died in the delivery room compared with 1% of those who received intensive treatment, including oxygen therapy and endotracheal intubation.[56] At 22 weeks and 23 weeks of gestation, 96% and 91% of live births, respectively, had intensive care withheld or withdrawn and the limitation in active treatment mirrored the 96% and 92% of live births at these gestational ages who died in the delivery room. In the previously discussed study evaluating the effects of active treatment in a cohort of academically affiliated hospitals in the United States, overall survival rates at 22 weeks of gestation increased fourfold when restricting the denominator of analysis from all live births to those receiving active treatment, from 5% (95% CI 3–8) to 23% (95% CI 14–34), highlighting the importance of this factor to the survival estimate.[37] All infants born alive at 22 to 25 weeks of gestation who did not receive active treatment died before hospital discharge, with nearly all (97%–100% depending on gestational age at birth) dying within 12 hours of birth and all dying within 24 hours of birth. In contrast, among those who received active treatment, 41% of infants born alive at 22 weeks of gestation, and 20% of infants born alive at 23 weeks of gestation died within 12 hours of birth, with a much smaller proportion (2%–8%) dying within the first 12 hours at 24 and 26 weeks of gestation.[37] Therefore, recent recommendations emphasize the importance of stratifying outcomes by those infants who do and do not receive active treatment.[29]

A clearer understanding of decisions surrounding active treatment for periviable infants may facilitate better parental counseling and decision making. Large, systematic cohort studies that measure key characteristics and outcomes of periviable infants receiving intensive care versus those receiving comfort care may be used to estimate the benefits of and burdens of intensive care. One such analysis is described later in this article.[52] A strength of this analysis is the avoidance of a "self-fulfilling prophecy" for infants not given intensive care by estimating the proportion of additional infants who would have survived had such care been provided (the "maximum potential survival rate"). This method assumes that infants who died without receiving intensive care would have the same potential survival rate as infants given intensive care had they received it, which may be an overestimate. Therefore, the true survival rate had all periviable infants been given intensive care will likely be between the observed mortality rate and the maximum estimated survival rate.

Antenatal Factors

Beyond the gestational age at birth and provision of active treatment, which are often correlated, a number of other factors influence the likelihood of survival. Important antenatal factors that influence the prognosis of survival include estimated fetal weight, sex, plurality, and receipt of antenatal corticosteroids, with higher estimated fetal weight, female sex, singleton gestation, and receipt of antenatal corticosteroids associated with higher probability of survival.[52] As mentioned previously, these factors can be used in antenatal counseling to predict the probability of survival if intensive care is provided (available at https://www.nichd.nih.gov/about/org/der/branches/ppb/programs/epbo/Pages/index.aspx). Importantly, although the NICHD NRN extremely preterm birth outcome estimator has been externally validated across large populations including California, in the United States, and Victoria, in Australia,[57–60] individual centers may have better or worse outcomes.[61] Additionally, after birth, other factors, such as a the level of respiratory support and other clinical variables discussed later in this article, increase in prognostic value for prediction of survival, whereas the prognostic value of baseline characteristics, such as gestational age, decrease.[62]

Delivery Room Factors

In the delivery room, the Apgar score, traditionally associated with neonatal survival,[63] may be influenced by the provision or withholding of active treatment. The receipt of chest compressions or epinephrine in the delivery room is associated with a higher risk of mortality,[64] although this effect may vary by gestational age.[65] The visual assessment of extremely preterm neonates less than 26 weeks of gestation in the first seconds to minutes after birth by neonatal providers is a poor predictor of survival[66] and should not be used as a reliable prognostic characteristic to determine whether to provide or withhold resuscitative efforts.

Factors Beyond the Delivery Room

On the day of birth, variables such as receipt of surfactant and mechanical ventilation, outborn versus inborn status, and illness severity, which may be represented by the Score for Neonatal Acute Physiology version 2,[67] in addition to baseline factors, including gestational age, small for gestational age, gender, and exposure to antenatal corticosteroids, are important factors that can predict survival with and without morbidity of extremely preterm infants.[21] Beyond the first week of life through 28 days of age, the type of respiratory support (high-frequency ventilation, conventional ventilation, continuous positive airway pressure, nasal cannula, or none) and the highest fraction of inspired oxygen that an infant receives become the most significant predictors of survival, while the prognostic value of birth weight and gestational age decreases.[62,68] At 28 days of age, the highest fraction of inspired oxygen, the number of episodes of late-onset culture-negative infection, days of parenteral nutrition and days of continuous positive airway pressure are all independent negative predictors of survival to hospital discharge, with the highest fraction of inspired oxygen carrying the most weight.[62]

The timing of death varies by gestational age and, as an infant survives beyond the first few days of life, the probability of survival increases substantially[69] and continues to increase thereafter until 90 postnatal days (**Fig. 5**).[20] For infants born at 22 weeks of gestation between 2000 and 2011, 90% of all in-hospital deaths occurred within 12 hours of life and 1.4% occurred after 28 days of age, based on data from a multicenter study from the NICHD NRN.[12] The high frequency of early mortality likely reflects the frequent approach of comfort care for these infants. The proportion of deaths within 12 hours of birth among those infants with in-hospital death continues to decrease with each additional week of gestation, from 56% at 23 weeks to 26% at 24 weeks, and 18% at 25 weeks of gestation. Similarly, the proportion of deaths occurring after 28 days of age increases, from 8% at 23 weeks to 21% at 24 weeks, and 27% at 25 weeks. Important aspects of care during this period include fluid administration, nutrition, cardiorespiratory support, and prevention of intraventricular hemorrhage (IVH),[70] although randomized trials that include periviable infants are needed to identify additional interventions to improve outcomes in this population.

Racial and Social Associations with Survival

Among women in high-income countries, an adverse socioeconomic background is associated with twice the risk of stillbirth compared with women who are not from a

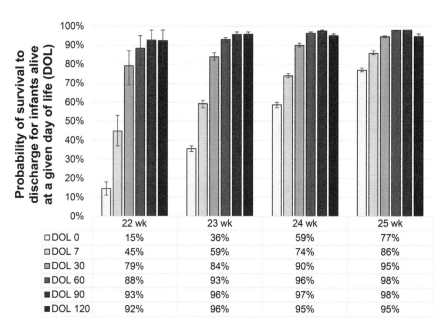

	22 wk	23 wk	24 wk	25 wk
□ DOL 0	15%	36%	59%	77%
□ DOL 7	45%	59%	74%	86%
▦ DOL 30	79%	84%	90%	95%
▪ DOL 60	88%	93%	96%	98%
▪ DOL 90	93%	96%	97%	98%
▪ DOL 120	92%	96%	95%	95%

Gestational age

Fig. 5. Changes in probability of survival to discharge among infants alive at a given day of life. Figure denotes changes in probability of survival to hospital discharge for infants who survive to 7 days of life (DOL) and beyond from a cohort of 64,896 infants in 362 US NICUs. Whisker bars indicate 95% CIs calculated with the Clopper-Pearson method. (*Data from* Hornik CP, Sherwood AL, Cotten CM, et al. Daily mortality of infants born at less than 30 weeks' gestation. Early Hum Dev 2016;96:27–30.)

disadvantaged background. Access to neonatal intensive care is one important mediator of the racial and social disparity in birth outcomes and is influenced by race, insurance status, and whether a woman received early prenatal care.[71] In addition, black race has been consistently linked with a higher overall risk of adverse birth outcomes,[72,73] although not gestational age–specific mortality at less than 32 weeks of gestation,[74] and is a risk factor for death after discharge from the NICU among ELBW infants.[75] However, one study, from the NICHD NRN, found that rehospitalization of ELBW infants was not associated with race/ethnicity after controlling for low family income, type of insurance, center, and other potential confounding variables.[76]

Withdrawal of Life-Sustaining Treatment

Approaches to withdrawal of life-sustaining treatment, which results in most deaths after infants are admitted to the NICU,[77,78] can explain some of the variation in reported rates of survival. Variation in the percentage of deaths following end-of-life decisions among European population-based cohorts varied significantly, with 81% of deaths following end-of-life decisions at ≤24 weeks of gestation in France compared with 55% at ≤25 weeks of gestation in the United Kingdom.[79] In a prospective observational study of 19 NICUs in Canada, 84% of all deaths occurred following a discussion of withdrawal of life-sustaining support and 41% were due to a prognosis of poor quality of life in the event of survival, whereas 35% were due to inevitability of death in the short-term and 24% to prevent prolonged suffering with death likely.[80] Neurologic complications of prematurity, particularly the presence of severe IVH (grade 3 or 4) or periventricular leukomalacia were common indications for withdrawal of life-sustaining treatment, although the proportion of infants with neurologic injury who underwent discussions varied from 10% to 86% across centers and 65% of the withdrawal of care was due to concerns regarding quality of life if the infant survived. The prognostic value accorded to indicators such as evidence for neurologic injury on an early cranial ultrasound may differ in clinical practice, as many infants who survive with either severe IVH or cystic periventricular leukomalacia on early cranial ultrasound are found to have no or mild impairment (51%) compared with those with a composite measure of neurodevelopmental impairment (28%).[81]

SUMMARY

In conclusion, survival among periviable births has improved since the 1950s, including over the past decade. There is wide variation in survival of periviable live births across developed countries and across different NICUs in the same country, although estimates of gestational age–specific survival are influenced by a number of factors that limit unbiased comparisons. Provision of active treatment, particularly at 22 and 23 weeks of gestation, varies widely among hospitals and developed nations, and this has a significant impact on reported survival rates. However, many other factors affect outcomes for infants born at periviable gestations. Improved reporting of outcomes following periviable birth may yield better understanding of the effects of obstetric and neonatal care in this area.

ACKNOWLEDGMENTS

The review was supported, in part, by the National Institutes of Health under award K23 HL128942 (R.M. Patel). The authors would like to acknowledge the NICHD Neonatal Research Network, including Rosemary Higgins, MD, Abhik Das, PhD, and the GDB subcommittee, for graciously providing recent data on periviable survival.

REFERENCES

1. Raju TN, Mercer BM, Burchfield DJ, et al. Periviable birth: executive summary of a joint workshop by the Eunice Kennedy Shriver National Institute of Child Health and Human Development, Society for Maternal-Fetal Medicine, American Academy of Pediatrics, and American College of Obstetricians and Gynecologists. Obstet Gynecol 2014;123(5):1083–96.
2. American College of Obstetricians and Gynecologists, Society for Maternal-Fetal Medicine, Ecker JL, Kaimal A, et al. Periviable birth: interim update. Am J Obstet Gynecol 2016;215(2):B2–12.
3. Stewart AL, Reynolds EO, Lipscomb AP. Outcome for infants of very low birth-weight: survey of world literature. Lancet 1981;1(8228):1038–40.
4. Rawlings G, Stewart A, Reynolds EO, et al. Changing prognosis for infants of very low birth weight. Lancet 1971;1(7698):516–9.
5. Bhat R, Raju TN, Vidyasagar D. Immediate and long-term outcome of infants less than 1000 grams. Crit Care Med 1978;6(3):147–50.
6. Paneth N, Kiely JL, Wallenstein S, et al. Newborn intensive care and neonatal mortality in low-birth-weight infants: a population study. N Engl J Med 1982; 307(3):149–55.
7. Gordon RR. Neonatal and "perinatal" mortality rates by birth weight. Br Med J 1977;2(6096):1202–4.
8. Hack M, Wright LL, Shankaran S, et al. Very-low-birth-weight outcomes of the National Institute of Child Health and Human Development Neonatal Network, November 1989 to October 1990. Am J Obstet Gynecol 1995;172(2 Pt 1):457–64.
9. Costeloe K, Hennessy E, Gibson AT, et al. The EPICure study: outcomes to discharge from hospital for infants born at the threshold of viability. Pediatrics 2000;106(4):659–71.
10. Stoll BJ, Hansen NI, Bell EF, et al. Neonatal outcomes of extremely preterm infants from the NICHD Neonatal Research Network. Pediatrics 2010;126(3):443–56.
11. Stoll BJ, Hansen NI, Bell EF, et al. Trends in care practices, morbidity, and mortality of extremely preterm neonates, 1993-2012. JAMA 2015;314(10):1039–51.
12. Patel RM, Kandefer S, Walsh MC, et al. Causes and timing of death in extremely premature infants from 2000 through 2011. N Engl J Med 2015;372(4):331–40.
13. Horbar JD, Carpenter JH, Badger GJ, et al. Mortality and neonatal morbidity among infants 501 to 1500 grams from 2000 to 2009. Pediatrics 2012;129(6): 1019–26.
14. Costeloe KL, Hennessy EM, Haider S, et al. Short term outcomes after extreme preterm birth in England: comparison of two birth cohorts in 1995 and 2006 (the EPICure studies). BMJ 2012;345:e7976.
15. Ancel PY, Goffinet F, Group E-W, et al. Survival and morbidity of preterm children born at 22 through 34 weeks' gestation in France in 2011: results of the EPIPAGE-2 cohort study. JAMA Pediatr 2015;169(3):230–8.
16. Shah PS, Sankaran K, Aziz K, et al. Outcomes of preterm infants <29 weeks gestation over 10-year period in Canada: a cause for concern? J Perinatol 2012;32(2):132–8.
17. Kusuda S, Fujimura M, Uchiyama A, et al, Japan Neonatal Research Network. Trends in morbidity and mortality among very-low-birth-weight infants from 2003 to 2008 in Japan. Pediatr Res 2012;72(5):531–8.
18. Ishii N, Kono Y, Yonemoto N, et al, Japan Neonatal Research Network. Outcomes of infants born at 22 and 23 weeks' gestation. Pediatrics 2013;132(1):62–71.

19. Su BH, Hsieh WS, Hsu CH, et al. Neonatal outcomes of extremely preterm infants from Taiwan: comparison with Canada, Japan, and the USA. Pediatr Neonatol 2015;56(1):46–52.
20. Hornik CP, Sherwood AL, Cotten CM, et al. Daily mortality of infants born at less than 30 weeks' gestation. Early Hum Dev 2016;96:27–30.
21. Ge WJ, Mirea L, Yang J, et al. Prediction of neonatal outcomes in extremely preterm neonates. Pediatrics 2013;132(4):e876–85.
22. Guinsburg R, Branco de Almeida MF, Dos Santos Rodrigues Sadeck L, et al. Proactive management of extreme prematurity: disagreement between obstetricians and neonatologists. J Perinatol 2012;32(12):913–9.
23. Serenius F, Kallen K, Blennow M, et al. Neurodevelopmental outcome in extremely preterm infants at 2.5 years after active perinatal care in Sweden. JAMA 2013;309(17):1810–20.
24. Chen F, Bajwa NM, Rimensberger PC, et al, Swiss Neonatal Network. Thirteen-year mortality and morbidity in preterm infants in Switzerland. Arch Dis Child Fetal Neonatal Ed 2016;101(5):F377–83.
25. Zegers MJ, Hukkelhoven CW, Uiterwaal CS, et al. Changing Dutch approach and trends in short-term outcome of periviable preterms. Arch Dis Child Fetal Neonatal Ed 2016;101(5):F391–6.
26. Agarwal P, Sriram B, Rajadurai VS. Neonatal outcome of extremely preterm Asian infants 28 weeks over a decade in the new millennium. J Perinatol 2015;35(4):297–303.
27. Boland RA, Davis PG, Dawson JA, et al. Outcomes of infants born at 22-27 weeks' gestation in Victoria according to outborn/inborn birth status. Arch Dis Child Fetal Neonatal Ed 2017;102(2):F153–61.
28. Guillen U, DeMauro S, Ma L, et al. Survival rates in extremely low birthweight infants depend on the denominator: avoiding potential for bias by specifying denominators. Am J Obstet Gynecol 2011;205(4):329.e1-7.
29. Rysavy MA, Marlow N, Doyle LW, et al. Reporting outcomes of extremely preterm births. Pediatrics 2016;138(3):1–7.
30. Guillen U, Weiss EM, Munson D, et al. Guidelines for the management of extremely premature deliveries: a systematic review. Pediatrics 2015;136(2):343–50.
31. Hernan MA, Clayton D, Keiding N. The Simpson's paradox unraveled. Int J Epidemiol 2011;40(3):780–5.
32. Marang-van de Mheen PJ, Shojania KG. Simpson's paradox: how performance measurement can fail even with perfect risk adjustment. BMJ Qual Saf 2014;23(9):701–5.
33. Manktelow BN, Evans TA, Draper ES. Differences in case-mix can influence the comparison of standardised mortality ratios even with optimal risk adjustment: an analysis of data from paediatric intensive care. BMJ Qual Saf 2014;23(9):782–8.
34. Patel RM, Rysavy MA. Global variation in neonatal intensive care: does it matter? J Pediatr 2016;177:6–7.
35. Janvier A, Lantos J. Delivery room practices for extremely preterm infants: the harms of the gestational age label. Arch Dis Child Fetal Neonatal Ed 2016;101(5):F375–6.
36. Horbar JD, Badger GJ, Lewit EM, et al. Hospital and patient characteristics associated with variation in 28-day mortality rates for very low birth weight infants. Vermont Oxford Network. Pediatrics 1997;99(2):149–56.

37. Rysavy MA, Li L, Bell EF, et al. Between-hospital variation in treatment and outcomes in extremely preterm infants. N Engl J Med 2015;372(19):1801–11.
38. Smith L, Draper ES, Manktelow BN, et al. Comparing regional infant death rates: the influence of preterm births <24 weeks of gestation. Arch Dis Child Fetal Neonatal Ed 2013;98(2):F103–7.
39. Shah PS, Lui K, Sjors G, et al. Neonatal outcomes of very low birth weight and very preterm neonates: an international comparison. J Pediatr 2016;177: 144–52.e6.
40. Lapcharoensap W, Gage SC, Kan P, et al. Hospital variation and risk factors for bronchopulmonary dysplasia in a population-based cohort. JAMA Pediatr 2015;169(2):e143676.
41. Jensen EA, Lorch SA. Effects of a birth hospital's neonatal intensive care unit level and annual volume of very low-birth-weight infant deliveries on morbidity and mortality. JAMA Pediatr 2015;169(8):e151906.
42. Profit J, Gould JB, Bennett M, et al. The association of level of care with NICU quality. Pediatrics 2016;137(3):e20144210.
43. Goodman DC, Fisher ES, Little GA, et al. The relation between the availability of neonatal intensive care and neonatal mortality. N Engl J Med 2002;346(20): 1538–44.
44. Holmstrom ST, Phibbs CS. Regionalization and mortality in neonatal intensive care. Pediatr Clin North Am 2009;56(3):617–30.
45. Lake ET, Staiger D, Horbar J, et al. Association between hospital recognition for nursing excellence and outcomes of very low-birth-weight infants. JAMA 2012; 307(16):1709–16.
46. Cummings J, Committee on Fetus and Newborn. Antenatal counseling regarding resuscitation and intensive care before 25 weeks of gestation. Pediatrics 2015; 136(3):588–95.
47. Gallagher K, Aladangady N, Marlow N. The attitudes of neonatologists towards extremely preterm infants: a Q methodological study. Arch Dis Child Fetal Neonatal Ed 2016;101(1):F31–6.
48. Kim UO, Basir MA. Informing and educating parents about the risks and outcomes of prematurity. Clin Perinatol 2014;41(4):979–91.
49. Haward MF, Murphy RO, Lorenz JM. Message framing and perinatal decisions. Pediatrics 2008;122(1):109–18.
50. Boland RA, Davis PG, Dawson JA, et al. What are we telling the parents of extremely preterm babies? Aust N Z J Obstet Gynaecol 2016;56(3):274–81.
51. Morse SB, Haywood JL, Goldenberg RL, et al. Estimation of neonatal outcome and perinatal therapy use. Pediatrics 2000;105(5):1046–50.
52. Tyson JE, Parikh NA, Langer J, et al. Intensive care for extreme prematurity–moving beyond gestational age. N Engl J Med 2008;358(16):1672–81.
53. Serenius F, Blennow M, Marsal K, et al. Intensity of perinatal care for extremely preterm infants: outcomes at 2.5 years. Pediatrics 2015;135(5):e1163–72.
54. Kallen K, Serenius F, Westgren M, et al. Impact of obstetric factors on outcome of extremely preterm births in Sweden: prospective population-based observational study (EXPRESS). Acta Obstet Gynecol Scand 2015;94(11):1203–14.
55. Park CK, Isayama T, McDonald SD. Antenatal corticosteroid therapy before 24 weeks of gestation: a systematic review and meta-analysis. Obstet Gynecol 2016;127(4):715–25.
56. Perlbarg J, Ancel PY, Khoshnood B, et al. Delivery room management of extremely preterm infants: the EPIPAGE-2 study. Arch Dis Child Fetal Neonatal Ed 2016;101(5):F384–90.

57. Lee HC, Green C, Hintz SR, et al. Prediction of death for extremely premature infants in a population-based cohort. Pediatrics 2010;126(3):e644–50.

58. Marrs CC, Pedroza C, Mendez-Figueroa H, et al. Infant outcomes after periviable birth: external validation of the Neonatal Research Network estimator with the BEAM trial. Am J Perinatol 2016;33(6):569–76.

59. Boland RA, Davis PG, Dawson JA, et al, Victorian Infant Collaborative Study Group. Predicting death or major neurodevelopmental disability in extremely preterm infants born in Australia. Arch Dis Child Fetal Neonatal Ed 2013;98(3): F201–4.

60. Ethridge JK Jr, Louis JM, Mercer BM. Accuracy of fetal weight estimation by ultrasound in periviable deliveries. J Matern Fetal Neonatal Med 2014;27(6): 557–60.

61. Alleman BW, Bell EF, Li L, et al. Individual and center-level factors affecting mortality among extremely low birth weight infants. Pediatrics 2013;132(1):e175–84.

62. Ambalavanan N, Carlo WA, Tyson JE, et al. Outcome trajectories in extremely preterm infants. Pediatrics 2012;130(1):e115–25.

63. Casey BM, McIntire DD, Leveno KJ. The continuing value of the Apgar score for the assessment of newborn infants. N Engl J Med 2001;344(7):467–71.

64. Wyckoff MH, Salhab WA, Heyne RJ, et al. Outcome of extremely low birth weight infants who received delivery room cardiopulmonary resuscitation. J Pediatr 2012;160(2):239–44.e2.

65. Handley SC, Sun Y, Wyckoff MH, et al. Outcomes of extremely preterm infants after delivery room cardiopulmonary resuscitation in a population-based cohort. J Perinatol 2015;35(5):379–83.

66. Manley BJ, Dawson JA, Kamlin CO, et al. Clinical assessment of extremely premature infants in the delivery room is a poor predictor of survival. Pediatrics 2010; 125(3):e559–64.

67. Richardson DK, Corcoran JD, Escobar GJ, et al. SNAP-II and SNAPPE-II: simplified newborn illness severity and mortality risk scores. J Pediatr 2001;138(1): 92–100.

68. Laughon MM, Langer JC, Bose CL, et al. Prediction of bronchopulmonary dysplasia by postnatal age in extremely premature infants. Am J Respir Crit Care Med 2011;183(12):1715–22.

69. Abdel-Latif ME, Kecskes Z, Bajuk B, Nsw and the ACT Neonatal Intensive Care Audit Group. Actuarial day-by-day survival rates of preterm infants admitted to neonatal intensive care in New South Wales and the Australian Capital Territory. Arch Dis Child Fetal Neonatal Ed 2013;98(3):F212–7.

70. Barrington KJ. Management during the first 72 h of age of the periviable infant: an evidence-based review. Semin Perinatol 2014;38(1):17–24.

71. Bronstein JM, Capilouto E, Carlo WA, et al. Access to neonatal intensive care for low-birthweight infants: the role of maternal characteristics. Am J Public Health 1995;85(3):357–61.

72. DeFranco EA, Hall ES, Muglia LJ. Racial disparity in previable birth. Am J Obstet Gynecol 2016;214(3):394.e1-7.

73. Schempf AH, Branum AM, Lukacs SL, et al. The contribution of preterm birth to the Black-White infant mortality gap, 1990 and 2000. Am J Public Health 2007; 97(7):1255–60.

74. MacDorman MF, Mathews TJ. Understanding racial and ethnic disparities in U.S. infant mortality rates. NCHS Data Brief 2011;(74):1–8.

75. De Jesus LC, Pappas A, Shankaran S, et al. Risk factors for post-neonatal intensive care unit discharge mortality among extremely low birth weight infants. J Pediatr 2012;161(1):70–4.e1-2.
76. Morris BH, Gard CC, Kennedy K, et al. Rehospitalization of extremely low birth weight (ELBW) infants: are there racial/ethnic disparities? J Perinatol 2005; 25(10):656–63.
77. Verhagen AA, Janvier A, Leuthner SR, et al. Categorizing neonatal deaths: a cross-cultural study in the United States, Canada, and The Netherlands. J Pediatr 2010;156(1):33–7.
78. Weiner J, Sharma J, Lantos J, et al. How infants die in the neonatal intensive care unit: trends from 1999 through 2008. Arch Pediatr Adolesc Med 2011;165(7): 630–4.
79. Pignotti MS, Berni R. Extremely preterm births: end-of-life decisions in European countries. Arch Dis Child Fetal Neonatal Ed 2010;95(4):F273–6.
80. Hellmann J, Knighton R, Lee SK, et al, Canadian Neonatal Network End of Life Study Group. Neonatal deaths: prospective exploration of the causes and process of end-of-life decisions. Arch Dis Child Fetal Neonatal Ed 2016;101(2): F102–7.
81. Hintz SR, Barnes PD, Bulas D, et al. Neuroimaging and neurodevelopmental outcome in extremely preterm infants. Pediatrics 2015;135(1):e32–42.
82. Moore T, Hennessy EM, Myles J, et al. Neurological and developmental outcome in extremely preterm children born in England in 1995 and 2006: the EPICure studies. BMJ 2012;345:e7961.
83. EXPRESS Group, Fellman V, Hellstrom-Westas L, et al. One-year survival of extremely preterm infants after active perinatal care in Sweden. JAMA 2009; 301(21):2225–33.

Long-Term Impact of Preterm Birth

Neurodevelopmental and Physical Health Outcomes

Thuy Mai Luu, MD, MSc[a],*,
Muhammad Oneeb Rehman Mian, PhD[b],
Anne Monique Nuyt, MD[a]

KEYWORDS

- Preterm birth • Neurodevelopment • Chronic health diseases
- Cardiovascular diseases • Obstructive lung diseases

KEY POINTS

- Among preterm-born school-age children and adolescents, 35% to 50% have neurodevelopmental deficits that warrant special educational services.
- Increased blood pressure, impaired vascular growth, signs of increased peripheral vascular resistance, and cardiac remodeling can be observed in early childhood in preterm-born children.
- Preterm-born children, especially those with intrauterine growth restriction and neonatal acute kidney injury, may be at risk for chronic kidney disease.
- Preterm-born children have reduced insulin sensitivity and higher risk for markers of metabolic syndrome in those with excessive childhood weight gain.
- Significant chronic airway obstruction occurs after preterm birth.

INTRODUCTION

What the early years hide is uncovered with time. Severe classic sequelae of preterm birth, such as cerebral palsy, significant intellectual disability, blindness, and deafness, are usually diagnosed during the first 2 years of life. Yet minor to moderate neurodevelopmental consequences of prematurity, including learning disabilities and behavioral problems, only become apparent as the child ages.[1] As modern

Disclosure Statement: The authors have nothing to disclose.
a Department of Pediatrics, Research Center, Centre Hospitalier Universitaire Sainte-Justine, 3175 Côte-Ste-Catherine, Montreal, Quebec H3T 1C5, Canada; b Department of Biomedical Sciences, Fetomaternal and Neonatal Pathologies Axis, Research Center, Centre Hospitalier Universitaire Sainte-Justine, University of Montreal, 3175 Côte-Ste-Catherine, Montreal, Quebec H3T 1C5, Canada
* Corresponding author.
E-mail address: thuy.mai.luu@umontreal.ca

Clin Perinatol 44 (2017) 305–314
http://dx.doi.org/10.1016/j.clp.2017.01.003

neonatology allows the first generations of survivors of extreme prematurity to reach adulthood, studies are now uncovering the long-term effects of preterm birth on other organ systems. Mortality in young adulthood is 40% higher in this population due to congenital, respiratory, endocrine, and cardiovascular defects.[2] Evidence suggests that in their 20s, that is, during the years of peak performance, individuals born preterm have reduced physiologic functional capacity compared with their term counterparts. As early as during school years, preterm-born children begin to exhibit mild dysfunction of 1 or more organ systems, which may evolve into early onset of overt chronic diseases and premature age-related decline in health. The paucity of longitudinal data has limited understanding, however, of whether preterm birth accelerates functional decline, with conflicting reports on the matter.[3,4]

There is an inverse relationship between gestational age and risk of neurodevelopmental impairment[5,6] and cardiovascular, metabolic, and pulmonary diseases. Consequently, children born very preterm display higher rates of dysfunction than those born late preterm.[7,8] This review focuses on the subgroup of children born very preterm.

NEURODEVELOPMENTAL OUTCOMES

Neonatal follow-up programs rightfully continue to focus on neurodevelopmental impairment, which affects 35% to 50% of school-age children born very preterm and, therefore, highlight the significant requirement for special educational support.[9–11] Very preterm children achieve cognitive scores that are on average 11 points to 12 points lower than term peers.[5,6] This cognitive deficit persists into adulthood, with IQ scores remaining fairly stable from ages 5 years to 6 years onward.[12,13] Furthermore, despite exhibiting IQ scores in the normal range, very preterm children remain vulnerable to a spectrum of neurodevelopmental deficits in expressive and receptive language, fine and gross motor abilities, processing speed, executive function (including verbal fluency, working memory, cognitive flexibility, inhibition, and planning), selective and sustained attention, visual and perceptual skills, and basic academic abilities in reading, spelling, and mathematics.[14,15] **Table 1** summarizes the findings from several meta-analyses. As the level of complexity of a task increases (ie, higher cognitive workload), the performance of a very preterm child often decreases.[16,17]

Beyond neuropsychological and motor functions, studies indicate that individuals born preterm tend to exhibit atypical psychosocial patterns. Johnson and Wolke[18] recently described a "preterm behavioral phenotype" that is characterized by inattention, introversion, anxiety, rigidity, and lower tendency for risk taking.[18,19] Autistic spectrum symptoms, notably in the domains of communication and social interactions, are also more prevalent in children born preterm compared with term controls.[20] Together these features may pose a significant risk for development of a global socially withdrawn personality during adulthood.[19]

The neuropsychological and behavioral-emotional deficits observed after preterm birth have a direct impact on learning and interpersonal relationships, contributing to the challenges faced by children born preterm during school years and beyond. Therefore, adequate support from the family and the community, especially at school, is crucial to promote resiliency and improve long-term well-being of these children.

HYPERTENSION AND CARDIOVASCULAR HEALTH

The first manifestations of hypertension and cardiovascular abnormalities as a consequence of premature birth appear during childhood. As early as 2.5 years of age, children born at less than 28 weeks display higher systolic and diastolic blood

Table 1
Summary of meta-analyses of neurodevelopmental outcomes after preterm birth

Neurodevelopmental Domains	Effect Size (SD Units) and 95% CI
Language[17,61]	Expressive language: −0.71 (−0.86, −0.55) Receptive language: −0.83 (−0.97, −0.69) Simple language function: −0.45 (−0.59, −0.30) Complex language function: −0.62 (−0.82, −0.43)
Motor[62]	Balance, manual dexterity, ball skills: −0.65 (−0.70, −0.60) Fine motor skills: −0.57 (−0.99, −0.73) Gross motor skills: −0.53 (−0.60, −0.46)
Visual motor integration[63]	−0.69 (−0.80, −0.58)
Attention[64,65]	Selective attention: −0.58 (−0.74, −0.43) Sustained attention: −0.67 (−1.03, −0.31)
Executive function[64,65]	Verbal fluency: −0.57 (−0.82, −0.32) Working memory: −0.36 (−0.47, −0.20) Cognitive flexibility: −0.49 (−0.66, −0.33) Inhibition: −0.50 (−0.89, −0.10) Planning: −0.69 (−0.88, −0.50)
Academic achievement[64]	Reading: −0.48 (−0.60, −0.34) Spelling: −0.76 (−1.13, −0.40) Mathematics: −0.60 (−0.74, −0.46)

Reference group: term-born controls.
 Effect size expressed in SD units: 0.2, small effect size; 0.5, moderate effect size; 0.8, large effect size.
 Simple language function refers to receptive vocabulary whereas complex language function represents total language score.

pressures.[21] Meta-analyses show that from childhood to young adulthood, individuals born preterm exhibit a 3.8 mm Hg to 4.6 mm Hg increase in resting systolic blood pressure and a 2.6 mm Hg increase in diastolic blood pressure, with an inverse relationship between systolic blood pressure and gestational age.[22–24] To put this into perspective, a 4 mm Hg rise in blood pressure has been associated with 20% increase in stroke mortality and 15% higher mortality from other vascular diseases.[25]

At the vascular level, preterm birth and related perinatal interventions may affect vessel size, capillary density, arterial stiffness, and endothelial function, although results in childhood and adolescence are sometimes contradictory (**Table 2**).[24] In general, vascular growth is impaired after preterm birth, resulting in reduced caliber of small and large arterial conduits[24,26,27] and capillary rarefaction.[28,29] Smaller resistance vessels seem to be more impacted compared with larger conduits, such as the aorta. Aortic pulse wave velocity, a classic index of aortic stiffness, is similar in preterm-born and term-born children.[24,26,27,30] On the contrary, augmentation index, which measures arterial pressure wave reflections, is higher in preterm children born at less than 26 weeks' gestational age or who are small for gestational age, suggesting increased peripheral vascular resistance.[30,31] Similarly, although there is no difference in endothelial function measured at the level of the brachial artery,[24,26,27] impairment is observed in smaller vessels of preterm-born adolescents.[32]

Few studies have examined long-term cardiac changes after preterm birth. Decreased left ventricular diameter along with increased interventricular septum thickness was described in 5-year-old very preterm children.[33] Reduced dimensions of the left ventricle also have been shown at 18 years (<28 weeks and/or <1000 g),[27] but no difference in function has been detected during the pediatric period.[27,33,34] Further

Table 2
Effect of preterm birth on the vascular tree and the heart in childhood and adolescence

	Measurement Method	Effect of Preterm Birth
Arterial size	Ultrasound imaging	• Narrower aorta • Narrower brachial artery • No difference in carotid intima-media thickness
Capillary density	Videomicroscopy (finger skin) Ocular fundus photography	• ↓ Dermal capillary density • ↓ Retinal vascularization
Arterial stiffness[a]	Aorta • Pulse wave velocity • Augmentation index Peripheral (brachial or radial) artery • Pulse wave velocity • Augmentation index	• No difference • No difference, but ↑ in those born <26 wk • No difference, but ↑ in those born SGA • No difference, but ↑ in those born <26 wk or SGA
Endothelial function[b]	Brachial flow-mediated dilatation Reactive hyperemia of the finger	• No difference • ↓ Microcirculatory response
Cardiac shape and function	Cardiac ultrasound imaging	• No difference in left and right ventricular function at rest and after hypoxic challenge • ↓ Left ventricular diameter and mass • ↑ Interventricular septum thickness

Abbreviation: SGA, small for gestational age.
[a] With increased arterial stiffness, pulse wave velocity and augmentation index are increased.
[b] With decreased endothelial function, flow-mediated dilatation is decreased.

investigation is warranted to fully characterize the development and progression of cardiac structural and functional alterations in preterm-born individuals.

Mechanisms mediating developmental programming of hypertension and cardiovascular disease after preterm birth likely involve multiple organ systems, including the vessels, the heart, the kidneys, and the sympathetic nervous system.[35] Together, these findings suggest that preterm birth impairs vascular growth and cardiomyocyte development. As a consequence, increased peripheral vascular resistance and cardiac remodeling may occur,[36,37] both of which can adversely modify future cardiovascular risk either independently or when compounded together.

RENAL HEALTH

Nephron number is an important determinant in blood pressure regulation and is reduced after preterm birth.[38] The long-term consequences of prematurity on renal health, however, remain to be investigated. In school-age children, extremely low birth weight (<1000 g) and neonatal acute kidney injury have been associated with smaller kidneys.[39–41] Markers of renal dysfunction, such as low glomerular filtration rate, have also been observed in children born preterm[42] and, most importantly, in those with intrauterine growth restriction.[31] These findings of reduced renal volume or function, however, have not been systematically confirmed in all studies.[42–44] Nevertheless, it has been advocated that individualized risk assessment for chronic kidney disease be done in preterm children, looking specifically for history of acute kidney injury, growth restriction, and ultrasonographic structural abnormalities, and that routine monitoring of blood pressure be performed during pediatric follow-up.[45]

METABOLIC OUTCOMES

Adverse metabolic changes contributing to the increase risk of cardiovascular events and diabetes have been related to preterm birth, independently of intrauterine growth restriction.[46,47] A recent systematic review indicated that individuals born preterm exhibit reduced insulin sensitivity from as early as infancy through to adulthood,[48] although fat mass seemed to become a stronger determinant with increased age.[23] In a cohort of preterm children born less than or equal to 34 weeks, Embelton and colleagues[49] examined more specifically the growth pattern from birth to early adolescence, comparing those with rapid catch-up weight gain (ie, upward weight percentile crossing) and those without any catch-up in relation to markers of metabolic syndrome. Predischarge (from birth to term-equivalent age) and early postdischarge (term-equivalent to 12 weeks) weight change was not strongly associated with metabolic alterations in adolescence. From 1 year to 9 to 12 years of age, however, preterm born children with excessive weight gain had greater percentage fat mass and waist circumference, decreased insulin sensitivity, decreased high-density lipoprotein, and higher blood pressure. Recent population-based studies on very preterm children or extremely preterm children with birth weight appropriate for gestational age or small for gestational age suggest no neurodevelopmental or cognitive advantage in excessive catch-up weight growth compared with following growth curve between birth and 24 months.[50,51] The most critical factor is catch-up head circumference growth.[52] Therefore, nutritional and lifestyle interventions to avoid excessive weight gain are warranted to optimize metabolic health in preterm-born individuals.

LONG-TERM PULMONARY FUNCTION: IS IT ASTHMA?

Preterm birth survivors with and without bronchopulmonary dysplasia (BPD) have life-long impairment of respiratory function, characterized by airflow limitation[53] that manifests with chronic cough and recurrent wheezing.[54] Pulmonary function tests in preterm school-aged children reveal reduced forced expiratory flows and volumes at the level of the proximal and more distal airways, decreased gas transfer at the alveolar-capillary junction, ventilation inhomogeneity, and air trapping compared with term-born peers.[55–58] Not surprisingly, pulmonary abnormalities are more pronounced in preterm children with moderate to severe BPD. These children also have impaired exercise capacity and 42% display significant airway obstruction (Tiffeneau index <75%).[3,58,59]

The clinical symptoms and signs of respiratory distress (discussed previously) in preterm-born children fit a pattern of obstructive lung disease that resembles asthma. Indeed, 20% to 25% of these children use bronchodilators and/or inhaled corticosteroids.[8,54,58] Whether this is truly asthma and should be treated as such remains open for debate. Airway hyper-responsiveness is more frequent in children born extremely preterm than in term controls.[57] As opposed to children with asthma, however, approximately 70% of preterm children do not respond to a bronchodilator.[54,56,60] Moreover, exhaled nitric oxide, an indirect measure of eosinophilic airway inflammation, is not increased[60] and prevalence of atopy is similar to term-born children.[56,57] Therefore, the pathophysiologic mechanisms of airway obstruction in preterm children likely differs from that of asthma.

Nevertheless, neonatal and postdischarge interventions to improve long-term pulmonary function are crucial to halt progression toward what is speculated could evolve into chronic obstructive pulmonary disease in adulthood.

PERSPECTIVES

Preterm birth induces structural and functional remodeling of multiple organ systems during a critical period of development. These alterations may have lasting adverse effects on health throughout the lifespan of prematurely born individuals. Whereas subtle dysfunctions may not become apparent at earlier ages, these may evolve with time to become neurodevelopmental disorders or other chronic diseases, conditions that may have a significant impact on well-being not least by imposing physical or neuropsychological and behavioral-emotional limitations. Despite ample evidence linking prematurity to adverse health outcomes, preterm birth remains under-recognized by the medical community as a significant risk factor and may contribute disproportionally to the burden of underdiagnosed and untreated chronic illnesses. Further investigations are crucial to understand pathophysiologic mechanisms underlying the developmental programming of health after preterm birth and to delineate potential

---

Summary of school-age and adolescent outcomes after preterm birth

Brain
- Deficits in cognition, language, fine and gross motor skills, visual-motor integration, attention, and executive function
- Specific learning difficulties in reading, spelling, and mathematics
- Preterm behavioral phenotype with anxiety, inattention, and social withdrawal

Long-term implications: lower educational attainment, interference with romantic and peer relationship, risk for mental health diseases

Heart and vessels
- Increased systolic and diastolic blood pressure
- Reduced vessel size and density
- Arterial stiffness[a]
- Endothelial dysfunction[a]
- Decreased left ventricular diameter and increased interventricular septum thickness

Long-term implications: risk for hypertension and cardiovascular diseases

Kidneys
- Decreased renal volume[a]
- Reduced glomerular filtration rate[a]

Long-term implications: risk for hypertension and chronic kidney diseases

Metabolism
- Decreased insulin sensitivity

Long-term implications: risk for type 2 diabetes mellitus

Lungs
- Airflow limitation
- Decreased alveolar gas transfer
- Air trapping
- Increased airway hyperresponsiveness
- Impaired exercise capacity

Long-term implications: risk for chronic obstructive pulmonary diseases

[a]Indicates inconsistent findings.

recovery pathways that inform on prospective future therapies. In the meantime, knowledge of risk factors and targeted screening to detect the earliest manifestations of dysfunctional organ systems is important to (1) improve neurodevelopmental outcomes via prompt referrals to early intervention services and (2) prevent chronic diseases through promotion of healthy lifestyle habits.

REFERENCES

1. Aylward GP. Neurodevelopmental outcomes of infants born prematurely. J Dev Behav Pediatr 2005;26(6):427–40.
2. Crump C, Sundquist K, Sundquist J, et al. Gestational age at birth and mortality in young adulthood. JAMA 2011;306(11):1233–40.
3. Doyle LW, Faber B, Callanan C, et al. Bronchopulmonary dysplasia in very low birth weight subjects and lung function in late adolescence. Pediatrics 2006; 118(1):108–13.
4. Clemm HH, Vollsaeter M, Roksund OD, et al. Exercise capacity after extremely preterm birth. Development from adolescence to adulthood. Ann Am Thorac Soc 2014;11(4):537–45.
5. Bhutta AT, Cleves MA, Casey PH, et al. Cognitive and behavioral outcomes of school-aged children who were born preterm: a meta-analysis. JAMA 2002; 288(6):728–37.
6. Kerr-Wilson CO, Mackay DF, Smith GC, et al. Meta-analysis of the association between preterm delivery and intelligence. J Public Health 2012;34(2):209–16.
7. Crump C, Winkleby MA, Sundquist K, et al. Risk of hypertension among young adults who were born preterm: a Swedish national study of 636,000 births. Am J Epidemiol 2011;173(7):797–803.
8. Crump C, Winkleby MA, Sundquist J, et al. Risk of asthma in young adults who were born preterm: a Swedish national cohort study. Pediatrics 2011;127(4): e913–20.
9. Luu TM, Ment LR, Schneider KC, et al. Lasting effects of preterm birth and neonatal brain hemorrhage at 12 years of age. Pediatrics 2009;123(3):1037–44.
10. Pinto-Martin J, Whitaker A, Feldman J, et al. Special education services and school performance in a regional cohort of low-birthweight infants at age nine. Paediatr Perinat Epidemiol 2004;18(2):120–9.
11. Johnson S, Hennessy E, Smith R, et al. Academic attainment and special educational needs in extremely preterm children at 11 years of age: the EPICure study. Arch Dis Child Fetal Neonatal Ed 2009;94(4):F283–9.
12. Breeman LD, Jaekel J, Baumann N, et al. Preterm cognitive function into adulthood. Pediatrics 2015;136(3):415–23.
13. Doyle LW, Cheong JL, Burnett A, et al. Biological and social influences on outcomes of extreme-preterm/low-birth weight adolescents. Pediatrics 2015; 136(6):e1513–20.
14. Anderson PJ. Neuropsychological outcomes of children born very preterm. Semin Fetal Neonatal Med 2014;19(2):90–6.
15. Msall ME, Park JJ. The spectrum of behavioral outcomes after extreme prematurity: regulatory, attention, social, and adaptive dimensions. Semin Perinatol 2008; 32(1):42–50.
16. Jaekel J, Baumann N, Wolke D. Effects of gestational age at birth on cognitive performance: a function of cognitive workload demands. PLoS One 2013;8(5): e65219.

17. van Noort-van der Spek IL, Franken MC, Weisglas-Kuperus N. Language functions in preterm-born children: a systematic review and meta-analysis. Pediatrics 2012;129(4):745–54.
18. Johnson S, Wolke D. Behavioural outcomes and psychopathology during adolescence. Early Hum Dev 2013;89(4):199–207.
19. Eryigit-Madzwamuse S, Strauss V, Baumann N, et al. Personality of adults who were born very preterm. Arch Dis Child Fetal Neonatal Ed 2015;100(6):F524–9.
20. Johnson S, Hollis C, Kochhar P, et al. Autism spectrum disorders in extremely preterm children. J Pediatr 2010;156(4):525–31.e522.
21. Bonamy AK, Kallen K, Norman M. High blood pressure in 2.5-year-old children born extremely preterm. Pediatrics 2012;129(5):e1199–204.
22. de Jong F, Monuteaux MC, van Elburg RM, et al. Systematic review and meta-analysis of preterm birth and later systolic blood pressure. Hypertension 2012; 59(2):226–34.
23. Parkinson JR, Hyde MJ, Gale C, et al. Preterm birth and the metabolic syndrome in adult life: a systematic review and meta-analysis. Pediatrics 2013;131(4): e1240–63.
24. Edwards MO, Watkins WJ, Kotecha SJ, et al. Higher systolic blood pressure with normal vascular function measurements in preterm-born children. Acta Paediatr 2014;103(9):904–12.
25. Prospective Studies Collaboration. Age-specific relevance of usual blood pressure to vascular mortality: a meta-analysis of individual data for one million adults in 61 prospective studies. Lancet 2002;360(9349):1903–13.
26. Bonamy AK, Bendito A, Martin H, et al. Preterm birth contributes to increased vascular resistance and higher blood pressure in adolescent girls. Pediatr Res 2005;58(5):845–9.
27. Kowalski RR, Beare R, Doyle LW, et al. Elevated blood pressure with reduced left ventricular and aortic dimensions in adolescents born extremely preterm. J Pediatr 2016;172:75–80.e72.
28. Bonamy AK, Martin H, Jorneskog G, et al. Lower skin capillary density, normal endothelial function and higher blood pressure in children born preterm. J Intern Med 2007;262(6):635–42.
29. Hellstrom A, Hard AL, Niklasson A, et al. Abnormal retinal vascularisation in preterm children as a general vascular phenomenon. Lancet 1998;352(9143):1827.
30. McEniery CM, Bolton CE, Fawke J, et al. Cardiovascular consequences of extreme prematurity: the EPICure study. J Hypertens 2011;29(7):1367–73.
31. Chan PY, Morris JM, Leslie GI, et al. The long-term effects of prematurity and intrauterine growth restriction on cardiovascular, renal, and metabolic function. Int J Pediatr 2010;2010:280402.
32. Singhal A, Kattenhorn M, Cole TJ, et al. Preterm birth, vascular function, and risk factors for atherosclerosis. Lancet 2001;358(9288):1159–60.
33. Mikkola K, Leipälä J, Boldt T, et al. Fetal growth restriction in preterm infants and cardiovascular function at five years of age. J Pediatr 2007;151(5):494–9, 499.e491–492.
34. Joshi S, Wilson DG, Kotecha S, et al. Cardiovascular function in children who had chronic lung disease of prematurity. Arch Dis Child Fetal Neonatal Ed 2014;99(5): F373–9.
35. Asztalos E. Antenatal corticosteroids: a risk factor for the development of chronic disease. J Nutr Metab 2012;2012:930591.

36. Lewandowski AJ, Davis EF, Yu G, et al. Elevated blood pressure in preterm-born offspring associates with a distinct antiangiogenic state and microvascular abnormalities in adult life. Hypertension 2015;65(3):607–14.
37. Lewandowski AJ, Augustine D, Lamata P, et al. Preterm heart in adult life: cardiovascular magnetic resonance reveals distinct differences in left ventricular mass, geometry, and function. Circulation 2013;127(2):197–206.
38. Sutherland MR, Bertagnolli M, Lukaszewski MA, et al. Preterm birth and hypertension risk: the oxidative stress paradigm. Hypertension 2014;63(1):12–8.
39. Bruel A, Rozé J-C, Quere M-P, et al. Renal outcome in children born preterm with neonatal acute renal failure: IRENEO-a prospective controlled study. Pediatr Nephrol 2016;31(12):2365–73.
40. Zaffanello M, Brugnara M, Bruno C, et al. Renal function and volume of infants born with a very low birth-weight: a preliminary cross-sectional study. Acta Paediatr 2010;99(8):1192–8.
41. Kwinta P, Klimek M, Drozdz D, et al. Assessment of long-term renal complications in extremely low birth weight children. Pediatr Nephrol 2011;26(7):1095–103.
42. Rodriguez-Soriano J, Aguirre M, Oliveros R, et al. Long-term renal follow-up of extremely low birth weight infants. Pediatr Nephrol 2005;20(5):579–84.
43. Rakow A, Johansson S, Legnevall L, et al. Renal volume and function in school-age children born preterm or small for gestational age. Pediatr Nephrol 2008; 23(8):1309–15.
44. Iacobelli S, Loprieno S, Bonsante F, et al. Renal function in early childhood in very low birthweight infants. Am J Perinatol 2007;24(10):587–92.
45. Carmody JB, Charlton JR. Short-term gestation, long-term risk: prematurity and chronic kidney disease. Pediatrics 2013;131(6):1168–79.
46. Hofman PL, Regan F, Jackson WE, et al. Premature birth and later insulin resistance. N Engl J Med 2004;351(21):2179–86.
47. Kistner A, Rakow A, Legnevall L, et al. Differences in insulin resistance markers between children born small for gestational age or born preterm appropriate for gestational age. Acta Paediatr 2012;101(12):1217–24.
48. Tinnion R, Gillone J, Cheetham T, et al. Preterm birth and subsequent insulin sensitivity: a systematic review. Arch Dis Child 2014;99(4):362–8.
49. Embleton ND, Korada M, Wood CL, et al. Catch-up growth and metabolic outcomes in adolescents born preterm. Arch Dis Child 2016;101:1026–31.
50. Belfort MB, Kuban KC, O'Shea TM, et al. Weight status in the first 2 years of life and neurodevelopmental impairment in extremely low gestational age newborns. J Pediatr 2016;168:30–5.e32.
51. Guellec I, Lapillonne A, Marret S, et al. Effect of intra- and extrauterine growth on long-term neurologic outcomes of very preterm infants. J Pediatr 2016;175: 93–9.e91.
52. Leppanen M, Lapinleimu H, Lind A, et al. Antenatal and postnatal growth and 5-year cognitive outcome in very preterm infants. Pediatrics 2014;133(1):63–70.
53. Baraldi E, Carraro S, Filippone M. Bronchopulmonary dysplasia: definitions and long-term respiratory outcome. Early Hum Dev 2009;85(10 Suppl):S1–3.
54. Fawke J, Lum S, Kirkby J, et al. Lung function and respiratory symptoms at 11 years in children born extremely preterm: the EPICure study. Am J Respir Crit Care Med 2010;182(2):237–45.
55. Gibson AM, Doyle LW. Respiratory outcomes for the tiniest or most immature infants. Semin Fetal Neonatal Med 2014;19(2):105–11.

56. Ronkainen E, Dunder T, Peltoniemi O, et al. New BPD predicts lung function at school age: follow-up study and meta-analysis. Pediatr Pulmonol 2015;50(11):1090–8.
57. Lum S, Kirkby J, Welsh L, et al. Nature and severity of lung function abnormalities in extremely pre-term children at 11 years of age. Eur Respir J 2011;37(5):1199–207.
58. MacLean JE, DeHaan K, Fuhr D, et al. Altered breathing mechanics and ventilatory response during exercise in children born extremely preterm. Thorax 2016;71(11):1012–9.
59. Welsh L, Kirkby J, Lum S, et al. The EPICure study: maximal exercise and physical activity in school children born extremely preterm. Thorax 2010;65(2):165–72.
60. Baraldi E, Bonetto G, Zacchello F, et al. Low exhaled nitric oxide in school-age children with bronchopulmonary dysplasia and airflow limitation. Am J Respir Crit Care Med 2005;171(1):68–72.
61. Barre N, Morgan A, Doyle LW, et al. Language abilities in children who were very preterm and/or very low birth weight: a meta-analysis. J Pediatr 2011;158(5):766–74.e761.
62. de Kieviet JF, Piek JP, Aarnoudse-Moens CS, et al. Motor development in very preterm and very low-birth-weight children from birth to adolescence: a meta-analysis. JAMA 2009;302(20):2235–42.
63. Geldof CJ, van Wassenaer AG, de Kieviet JF, et al. Visual perception and visual-motor integration in very preterm and/or very low birth weight children: a meta-analysis. Res Dev Disabil 2012;33(2):726–36.
64. Aarnoudse-Moens CS, Weisglas-Kuperus N, van Goudoever JB, et al. Meta-analysis of neurobehavioral outcomes in very preterm and/or very low birth weight children. Pediatrics 2009;124(2):717–28.
65. Mulder H, Pitchford NJ, Hagger MS, et al. Development of executive function and attention in preterm children: a systematic review. Dev Neuropsychol 2009;34(4):393–421.

Adult Consequences of Extremely Preterm Birth

Cardiovascular and Metabolic Diseases Risk Factors, Mechanisms, and Prevention Avenues

Anne Monique Nuyt, MD[a],*, Jean-Claude Lavoie, PhD[a,b],
Ibrahim Mohamed, MD, MSc[a], Katryn Paquette, MD[a],
Thuy Mai Luu, MD, MSc[c]

KEYWORDS

- Preterm birth • Developmental origin of adult health and diseases
- Cardiovascular diseases • Metabolic syndrome • Hypertension • Inflammation
- Oxygen • Parenteral nutrition

KEY POINTS

- Extremely preterm birth occurs at a time of active vasculogenesis and organogenesis.
- Incidence of risk factors for chronic cardiovascular and metabolic diseases is higher in young adults born extremely preterm, such as high blood pressure, modified arterial structure, smaller kidneys, impaired glucose tolerance, gestational hypertension and diabetes, and preeclampsia.
- Understanding the role of altered organogenesis and of altered organ function should allow targeted preventive and therapeutic strategies to minimize development of chronic disease-related morbidity in preterm born adults.

INTRODUCTION

Many chronic adult diseases have their onset during development, from fetus to childhood. Preterm birth, affecting nearly 12% of US children each year, is the main cause of neonatal mortality and morbidity. With the major advances in perinatal and neonatal

The authors have nothing to disclose.
[a] Division of Neonatology, Department of Pediatrics, Faculty of Medicine, Research Center, Centre Hospitalier Universitaire Sainte-Justine, Université de Montréal, 3175 chemin de la Côte-Sainte-Catherine, Montreal, Quebec H3T 1C5, Canada; [b] Department of Nutrition, Faculty of Medicine, Research Center, Centre Hospitalier Universitaire Sainte-Justine, Université de Montréal, 3175 chemin de la Côte-Sainte-Catherine, Montreal, Quebec H3T 1C5, Canada; [c] Division of General Pediatrics, Department of Pediatrics, Faculty of Medicine, Research Center, Centre Hospitalier Universitaire Sainte-Justine, Université de Montréal, 3175 chemin de la Côte-Sainte-Catherine, Montreal, Quebec H3T 1C5, Canada
* Corresponding author.
E-mail address: anne-monique.nuyt@recherche-ste-justine.qc.ca

Clin Perinatol 44 (2017) 315–332
http://dx.doi.org/10.1016/j.clp.2017.01.010
0095-5108/17/© 2017 Elsevier Inc. All rights reserved.

medicine over the last 30 years, most preterm and extremely preterm infants now survive. The first generations of these extremely preterm infants are reaching young adulthood, and their numbers are increasing. Beyond their well-studied neurodevelopment, other health consequences associated with preterm birth are being found now that these infants we cared for are entering active work life and having their own families.[1]

Childhood and adolescent studies have been reviewed in Thuy Mai Luu and colleagues' article, "Long-Term Impact of Preterm Birth: Neurodevelopmental and Physical Health Outcomes," in this issue; this report focuses on adult cardiovascular, renal, and metabolic health of individuals born extremely preterm. Evidence from clinical and from preclinical experimental studies of preterm birth and preterm birth–related neonatal conditions are presented, and the possible role of specific neonatal factors on the pathophysiology of organ structural and functional maladaptive changes is reviewed.

WHY ARE PRETERM INFANTS MORE VULNERABLE?

Preterm birth, especially extremely preterm birth, occurs at a critical stage of organ development (**Fig. 1**). The brain is in a rapidly expanding phase of neuronal migration and establishment of gyri and sophisticated connectivity, all of which are exquisitely sensitive to external perturbation. Lungs are in the late canalicular stage, during which

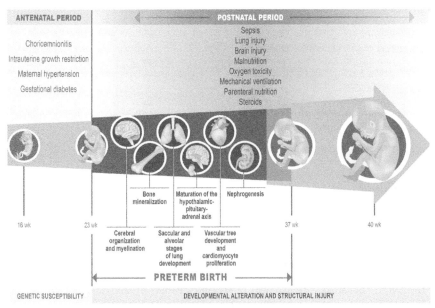

Fig. 1. Preterm birth, and especially extremely preterm birth, occurs at critical stages of organ development. Adverse intrauterine conditions that may lead to preterm birth and impact programming of long term health and diseases include chorioamnionitis, fetal growth restriction, maternal hypertension and gestational diabetes. Prematurity-related complications such as sepsis, lung and brain injury, or malnutrition and their treatments (oxygen, parenteral nutrition, steroids) can further alter organ system development. (*From* Luu TM, Katz SL, Leeson P, et al. Preterm birth: risk factor for early-onset chronic diseases. CMAJ 2016;188:737; with permission. This work is protected by copyright and the making of this copy was with the permission of the Canadian Medical Association Journal (http://www.cmaj.ca/) and Access Copyright. Any alteration of its content or further copying in any form whatsoever is strictly prohibited unless otherwise permitted by law.)

epithelial differentiation from type I to type II cells occurs, and distal airways and air-blood interface are formed. Extremely preterm birth therefore disrupts the normal sequence of lung development, resulting in an arrest in alveolar and pulmonary vascular growth.[2] Retinal vascularization, critical for choroidal oxygen supply, is nearly absent and is programmed to be completed only around term. Beyond these key organs associated with well-known major short-term complications of extremely preterm birth, important disturbances at the level of other actively developing organs are now becoming evident because their clinical manifestations appear much later in life.[3]

Two common mechanisms during intrauterine and neonatal life can contribute to increased risk of chronic adult diseases. First, *maladaptation* refers to the adverse consequences of the process through which the fetus or neonate adapt to face changes in the environment to enhance chance of survival. One such example is premature transition of the cardiovascular system to postnatal physiology, which will subsequently lead to altered heart and conduit vessel development. Second, direct injury from insults such as oxidative stress, sepsis, or poor perfusion can affect the kidneys, the myocardial cells, and the microvasculature of many organs including but not restricted to the eyes, brain, lungs, and muscles.

IMPACT OF PRETERM BIRTH ON ADULT CHRONIC CARDIOVASCULAR, RENAL, AND METABOLIC DISEASES
Cardiovascular Consequences

The link between preterm birth and higher blood pressure is clearly seen in several studies. A significant inverse correlation between systolic blood pressure and gestational age at birth has been consistently observed from childhood to adulthood in preterm-born individuals.[4–10] A recent large study confirmed a previous meta-analysis[11] and found that systolic and diastolic blood pressures in preterm young adults were an average of 3.4 mm Hg (95% confidence interval, 2.2–4.6 mm Hg) and 2.1 mm Hg (95% confidence interval, 1.3–3.0 mm Hg) higher, respectively, versus those in term young adults.[12] Considering that pregnancy is "an open window" to future cardiovascular health, a population-based study in Quebec found that women born preterm, particularly if born very preterm (<32 weeks of gestational age), had an increased risk of gestational hypertension and preeclampsia and an increased incidence of chronic hypertension compared with women born at term. The association between preterm birth and pregnancy hypertensive complications was independent of the women's birth weight being small for gestational age.[13] A large population-based Swedish cohort study found that as early as young adulthood, preterm individuals display a higher risk of cerebrovascular diseases and death from cardiovascular diseases.[14]

The increased risk of hypertension evidenced in individuals born preterm is likely to be multifactorial in origin, with preterm birth resulting in alterations to vascular, cardiac, and renal development/function and neural autonomic pathways.

Clinical and experimental studies show that factors associated with preterm birth disrupt vascular development resulting in adulthood structural changes in the macrovasculature (specifically narrower aorta and carotid) and impair angiogenesis leading to decreased microvessel density in the lungs and peripheral vasculature including striated muscles.[9,15–21] Retinal vascular caliber and density as well as cutaneous capillary density were decreased in young adults who were born at 29 to 30 weeks of gestational age, independently of a neonatal diagnosis of retinopathy of prematurity.[4,9] In preterm adults, decreased cutaneous microvascular density correlates with higher blood pressure and levels of circulating antiangiogenic factors (soluble endoglin and soluble fms-like tyrosine kinase-1).[15] However, studies examining the impact of preterm birth on arterial stiffness and on endothelial dysfunction, recognized as early predictors of cardiovascular diseases,[22,23] found inconsistent results.[24] Importantly, other conditions associated with preterm birth can also impact long-term organ development and function; antenatal exposure to maternal preeclampsia leads to a different pattern of vascular dysfunction in young adults born preterm, possibly through an inflammatory and antiangiogenic antenatal environment.[24–26] Antenatal steroids seem associated with decreased aortic distensibility and increased pulse wave velocity,[27] whereas neonatal intravenous lipid administration and associated elevation in infant cholesterol levels was associated with greater aortic stiffness in early adulthood.[28]

Preterm birth also has a direct effect on myocardial tissue.[29] Structural cardiac MRI studies in 20- to 39-year-old adults born preterm (mean gestational age, 30.3 weeks and birth weight 1300 g) found altered cardiac shape characterized by blood pressure–independent increase in left and right ventricular mass and reduced ventricular volumes.[30,31] Impaired systolic and diastolic function is also documented. However, in a cohort of younger adults (18 years old) born more prematurely (mean gestational age, 25.7 weeks; birth weight, 900 g), left ventricular mass was reduced.[32] Further studies are needed to determine whether developmental stage of cardiac tissue and gestational age (very preterm vs extremely preterm) have different impacts. Considering that cardiomyocytes proliferate actively until about 36 weeks of gestational age (after which maturation, differentiation, and growth by hypertrophy predominate),[33,34] deleterious neonatal conditions (hypoxia, hyperoxia, inflammation), as in very and extremely preterm birth, may have a significant impact on myocardial cells and tissue[35–37] and lead to impaired adult cardiac health. This finding is supported by results of animal studies. Adult rats exposed to hyperoxia or treated with dexamethasone during the first postnatal days—as models of prematurity-related conditions—show cardiomyocyte hypertrophy, fibrosis, and increased susceptibility to heart failure.[38,39] In a lamb model of preterm birth, Bensley and colleagues[40] showed cardiomyocyte hypertrophy, disrupted maturation (increased number of binucleated and trinucleated cardiomyocytes, and increased nuclear ploidy), and increased myocardial interstitial fibrosis in young adulthood. Overall, taking these studies into consideration, one may postulate that the heart of very preterm born individuals may display an enhanced susceptibility to the impact of blood pressure elevation and associated risk factors for heart disease naturally occurring with advancing age.

Interestingly, perinatal interventions can be effective at preventing the adverse cardiac changes associated with preterm birth. A recent substudy of a large cohort of young adults born very preterm found a protective role of neonatal nutrition with human milk (vs formula) on left ventricular structure and function.[41] Whereas postnatal dexamethasone seems deleterious, exposure to antenatal glucocorticoids (similar to the doses given in human preterm labor) resulted in increased maturation of the cardiomyocytes (more binuclear cells) and improved neonatal myocardial function in preterm piglets.[42]

Renal Consequences

Nephrogenesis proceeds well into the third trimester of pregnancy.[43] Although nephrogenesis continues postnatally after preterm birth, the process seems altered.[44,45]

Nephron number is an important indicator of renal functional capacity and strongly correlated with the development of high blood pressure.[46–48] Several studies have found an association between low birth weight and the development of renal conditions in adults, without, however, adjusting for the possible contribution of preterm birth.[49–52] More recent work shows that children and adults born preterm exhibit smaller kidneys (ultrasound scan measures) versus those born at term, with smaller kidneys correlating with lower gestational age.[53–57]

In most studies so far published, renal function does not seem to be significantly impacted by very preterm birth,[58] although reports suggest enhanced susceptibility to "second hits" (in addition to preterm birth–related conditions), such as neonatal acute kidney injury or obesity.[58,59] In the few adult studies published, glomerular filtration rate and the degree of albuminuria were similar between those born preterm (<32 weeks, <1500 g) and at full term.[55,60] More sensitive markers such as cystatin C[61] are slightly elevated in preterm-born toddlers[62] but have not been reported in preterm-born adults.

Experimentally, transient neonatal exposure of newborn rats to high oxygen (O_2) levels impairs nephrogenesis (which in rodents proceeds up to day 7 postnatal) resulting in 25% fewer nephrons in adults[17,63]; interestingly, despite marked reduction in nephron numbers, adult renal function only mildly differ between groups.[64] Other factors commonly encountered in neonatal intensive care units such as antibiotics and nonsteroidal anti-inflammatory molecules have been found in experimental studies to impair nephrogenesis.[65–71] The impact of nutrition was mostly studied in a rodent model of low-protein-fed dams, which found reduced nephron numbers in offspring.[72,73] Pathologic studies of preterm infants show that superimposed acute kidney injury sustained during neonatal intensive care unit stay can further decrease nephrogenesis.[45]

Studies suggest that preterm children and adults have smaller kidneys. Research on renal function, particularly in adults born extremely preterm (<29 weeks), remains limited but certainly much deserved. Taken together, reports of mild dysfunction, higher blood pressure, and reduced kidney size suggest that those born more preterm may be at higher risk of secondary injuries (hits) or progressive long-term kidney disease, a major cardiovascular risk factor. Optimal nutrition and minimizing the use of nephrotoxic drugs during the neonatal period should help minimize the impact of preterm birth on long-term renal health, but this remains formally unexplored.

Metabolic Consequences: Lipid and Glucose Metabolism

Adverse metabolic changes contributing to the increase risk of cardiovascular diseases and type 2 diabetes have been observed in adult survivors of prematurity. Studies have found higher fasting insulin levels and higher HOMA-IR indices (Homeostatic model assessment of insulin resistance) in adults born very preterm,[74–77] greater use of insulin or oral hypoglycemic agents,[78] and increased incidence of gestational diabetes and type 2 diabetes.[13,79]

Preterm versus term adults also display higher fasting low-density lipoprotein levels, although no differences were detected regarding high-density lipoproteins and triglycerides.[80] A link between preterm birth and obesity has not been found, and, in fact, findings indicate that preterm adults tend to have lower body mass index,[80] although one small report documented abdominal accumulation of fat in individuals born preterm with intrauterine growth restriction.[81] However, neonatal nutrition and growth of preterm infants impact later cardiovascular disease risk factors. Accelerated weight gain relative to length over the first months after term equivalent age is associated with higher fat percentage, waist circumference, serum triglycerides, and nonalcoholic fatty liver disease, a hepatic manifestation of the metabolic syndrome.[82,83]

The mechanisms leading to long-term dysregulation of metabolism after preterm birth remain unclear. Impaired glucose homeostasis can result from pancreatic β cell dysfunction with poor insulin secretion or insulin resistance. Pancreatic β cells are formed predominantly during the third trimester and then proliferate until about 2 years.[84] A maladaptive intrauterine or extrauterine environment (eg, preterm birth) could disrupt development of β-cell mass with subsequent low insulin secretion. In addition, nutritional deficits inherent to preterm birth,[85,86] exposure to antenatal steroids,[27] and rapid catch-up growth in infancy[83] may play a role through increased visceral adiposity,[87,88] which is associated with enhanced production of inflammatory cytokines and insulin resistance. Preterm birth is increasingly linked to impaired glucose homeostasis, but few studies have focused on extremely preterm birth. Moreover, contributions of other perinatal conditions (intrauterine growth restriction, maternal preeclampsia, obesity or diabetes), neonatal nutrition, family history, childhood growth patterns, physical activity levels, and other cardiovascular risk factors were not reported.

POSSIBLE CONTRIBUTORS TO INCREASED CHRONIC DISEASE RISK IN INDIVIDUALS BORN PRETERM

Many factors often inherent to the conditions surrounding extremely preterm birth can impact organ development and lead to adult health consequences. These include inflammation and oxidative stress through chorioamnionitis, preeclampsia, neonatal infections, oxygen-induced conditions, ventilation, parenteral nutrition, and medications including antibiotics, plastic-derived environmental contaminants, formula versus breast milk, lack of specific nutrients and vitamins (omega-3, vitamin D), and disruption of dark-light cycle and of circadian rhythm/sleep pattern. This review focuses on overall pathophysiology of oxidative stress and inflammation-related damage and parenteral nutrition.

Oxygen, Oxidative Stress, and Inflammation

Preterm birth reflects intrauterine disturbances that are often inherently pro-oxidant and proinflammatory in nature, such as preeclampsia, maternal diabetes and obesity, infection, and prolonged rupture of membranes.[89–97] Increased inflammatory cytokines such as tumor necrosis factor-α and interleuken-6 are reported in amniotic fluid and cord blood in pregnancies with preeclampsia and placental insufficiency and in animal models.[98,99] Intrauterine inflammation has repercussions in the infants as shown by postnatal increases in interleukin-6 and monocyte chemoattractant protein-1 in extremely preterm infants (25–26 weeks) born to mothers with chorioamnionitis.[100] Lipid peroxidation (oxLDL and 8-PGF2α), reduced antioxidant enzyme activity in cord blood, and increased markers of oxidative stress are reported in the placentas of pregnancies complicated by obesity, intrauterine growth restriction, or preterm labor.[101–105]

Antioxidant enzyme levels normally increase during the third trimester of pregnancy. The preterm newborn is thus relatively deficient in antioxidants at birth when confronted with a massive increase in partial pressure of oxygen (P_{O2}) in addition to several pro-oxidant molecules from parenteral nutrition (a significant source of hydrogen peroxide; see below), medications, and plastic derivatives.[106–108] Preterm newborns have lower levels of antioxidant enzymes, reduced induction capacity, and significantly increased levels of indices of oxidative stress.[109–116]

Further, much organ development, and the associated vasculogenesis, is driven by hypoxia inducible factor (HIF). Nephrogenesis is driven by HIF-derived growth factors, which is postulated to be inhibited in preterm infants given the dramatic increase in

P_{O_2} from fetal to newborn life. In the myocardium, HIF controls genes involved in prioritizing lipid versus glucose energy metabolism, and a failure to repress HIF-derived gene expression impairs myocardial neonatal adaptation in the transgenic mouse model.[18,117]

Epigenetic Changes

Antenatal and perinatal exposures (chorioamnionitis, preeclampsia, glucocorticoids, maternal diabetes, or depression) can lead to epigenetic changes in human cord blood cells and in specific organs in animal models (brain regions, lungs, kidneys, adrenals).[118,119] These epigenetic changes may be associated with stable phenotypic and behavioral alterations. Few studies have examined epigenetic changes in adult preterms. In a study of 12 very preterm (born at 26 weeks) versus 12 term subjects, whole-blood analysis found that DNA-methylation changes observed at birth had largely but not totally resolved by age 18.[120] One should not conclude that changes in epigenetic markers are not present in adults born preterm, but rather that this study underlines the importance of examining specific cell type, global DNA, and gene-specific changes in discreet regulatory regions, other epigenetic changes such as histone modification, and finely characterize the study subjects in terms of the disease of interest.

Parenteral Nutrition, Beyond Nutrition

The in vivo contribution of all nutrients included in parenteral nutrition is essential for the nutrition and growth of extremely preterm infants. However, the "in the bag" reactivity of some nutrients leads to generation of toxic inorganic (hydrogen peroxide [H_2O_2]) and organic peroxides (ie, ascorbylperoxide, lipid peroxides).[107,121–126] In addition, these reactions are amplified by ambient light through the photosensitive riboflavin, which catalyzes these reactions.[127]

In vivo, peroxides react with thiol functions of glutathione and proteins and may disrupt cell function.[128,129] Indeed, to preserve redox equilibrium and cellular homeostasis, reactive oxygen species such as peroxides are detoxified by a complex system of enzymes (superoxide dismutase, catalase), vitamins, and molecules such as the tripeptide glutathione (γ-Glu-Cys-Gly). Glutathione is a ubiquitous molecule that is key to antioxidant defense mechanisms. It is abundant and exists in dynamic equilibrium between its oxidized (GSSG) and reduced (GSH) states. The GSH/GSSG ratio is an important indicator of the redox environment[130] that regulates various biochemical processes involved in cell proliferation and survival.[131]

Oxidation of glutathione, shifting the redox potential value toward a more oxidized status, is associated with stimulation of tumor necrosis factor-α during inflammation[132] and was found to increase cell apoptosis,[131] resulting in a newborn animal model, in lung remodeling with reduced alveolar development.[133] Glutathione levels are directly related to gestational age and sex of the infant at birth; at less than 32 weeks, the level was only about 15% of full-term levels and was even lower in boys.[134,135] In infants born extremely preterm, lower neonatal glutathione levels, a more oxidized redox state, and high ascorbylperoxide in the urine correlated with bronchopulmonary dysplasia incidence, severity, or death.[136,137] Few studies have reported the long-term cardio-metabolic impact of parenteral nutrition; guinea pigs that received parenteral nutrition or H_2O_2 during the first week of life show at 3 months (adults) lower glucose tolerance and an energy deficiency phenotype.[106] Young adults exposed to intravenous parenteral lipids showed increased aortic rigidity and decreased left ventricular function.[28]

Epigenetic modifications could underlie the deleterious effects of oxidized redox state through inhibition of the methionine adenosyltransferase (MAT).[138] This enzyme transforms methionine into S-adenosylmethionine. S-adenosylmethionine is an essential cosubstrate for methylation of several molecules, including the methylation of DNA cytosine.[139] Thus, inhibition of MAT during the perinatal period could impact long-term health of the individual by an epigenetic modification of gene expression. In newborn guinea pigs, infusion of parenteral nutrition or H_2O_2 at similar concentrations to those measured in the parenteral nutrition led to a decreased DNA methylation level that persisted at least 2 months after cessation of infusion.[140]

In addition, MAT is also the first step in the transformation of methionine to cysteine. The cellular availability of cysteine is a well-known limiting step in glutathione synthesis. Indeed, inhibition of MAT by peroxides from parenteral nutrition is associated with a lower glutathione level and a more oxidized redox potential.[138] Oxidized thiols are normally recycled in their native state by glutaredoxin,[138,141] the activity of which also depends on the redox potential value of glutathione.[138] Therefore, in addition to peroxides from parenteral nutrition, oxidized redox state contributes to the inhibition of MAT[137] and to decreased DNA methylation.

Prevention of peroxide generation in parenteral nutrition

Currently, the only way to reduce the oxidation of nutrients is full photoprotection, which can reduce by half the peroxide concentration measured in parenteral nutrition infused at the bedside.[107,124] Photoprotection of parenteral nutrition in the neonatal intensive care unit is associated with lower triglyceridemia and blood glucose levels,[142] enhanced advancement of enteral nutrition tolerance,[143] more stable blood pressures in a selected population of critically ill female infants,[136] and a significant (25%) reduction of bronchopulmonary dysplasia documented in 2 randomized controlled unicenter studies.[124,144] Importantly, a recent meta-analysis (4 trials, 800 infants born at 26 ± 1–31 ± 2 weeks of gestation) found a significant reduction in mortality in infants receiving light-protected (vs light-exposed) parenteral nutrition.[145]

Unfortunately, full photoprotection of parenteral nutrition is challenging in daily clinical settings. Efficient photoprotection (bag and tubing) should block 300- to 500-nm wavelengths (riboflavin excitation) and should be uninterrupted from the parenteral nutrition compounding in the pharmacy until its infusion to the infant; a few minutes of ambient light is enough to cancel the beneficial effect of photoprotection.[146] It is already known that partial photoprotection adds no advantage while consuming valuable resources.[147] Furthermore, the concentration of peroxides in parenteral nutrition directly depends on the concentration of multivitamin preparation[107] (especially vitamin C[127]). Although photoprotection of parenteral nutrition containing 1% (vol/vol) standard multivitamin preparation can efficiently prevent excessive peroxide generation to observe health benefits, photoprotection is not sufficient for parenteral nutrition containing $\geq 2\%$ multivitamin preparation, which is the case for most extremely preterm infants. This fact may explain, at least in part, the failure of a recent multicenter study to show the beneficial impact of photoprotection on incidence of bronchopulmonary dysplasia in premature infants.[148]

Other possible interventions

Enhancing antioxidant capacity in the most vulnerable preterm infants could be another alternative. Experimentally, in newborn guinea pigs, supplementation of parenteral nutrition with glutathione normalized plasma glutathione and lung morphology.[149] Whether such a therapeutic avenue to counteract and quench the peroxides generated in parenteral nutrition would be effective at reducing short- and long-term complications in the most vulnerable infants remains to be evaluated.

SUMMARY

An increasing number of epidemiologic and clinical studies clearly show that preterm birth, and especially extremely preterm birth, is associated already in young adult life with risk factors for chronic cardiovascular and metabolic diseases such as higher blood pressure and glucose intolerance. Profound changes in physiologic demands to the developing organs that are associated with the premature transition to ex utero life can impact cell proliferation, organ growth, and function. More specifically for cardiovascular and metabolic diseases, hemodynamic changes are associated with reduced proliferation and accelerated maturation of cardiomyocytes and nephrons. Experimental data further bring arguments for a causal effect of elements characterizing preterm birth such as oxidative stress (through increased Po_2, exposure to oxygen, and parenteral nutrition combined with poor antioxidant capacity), an imbalance between nutrition (whether too little or too much) and cell metabolism, and growth, resulting in defective angiogenesis, altered organogenesis, and possible epigenetic modifications. Preterm birth may therefore bring an additional risk to familial history and genetic background for cardiovascular diseases and diabetes. Beyond the academic debate about whether adult dysfunctions are associated with or caused by conditions related to extremely preterm birth, it should now be recommended to specifically target this group for screening for cardiovascular disease risk factors, from childhood to adulthood, particularly women in their reproductive years. Further, special attention should be made to avoiding additional damages through second hits such as kidney injury and overweight.

In the neonatal intensive care unit, current studies support minimizing exposures to pro-oxidants and to nephrotoxic drugs, optimizing parenteral nutrition composition and its practical and effective photoprotection, promoting breast milk feeding, and optimizing nutrition. Nutrition factors include avoiding excessive fat accumulation, especially after term equivalent age, while allowing maximal healthy growth, which is essential for neurodevelopment. Future research should be designed to finely determine the mechanisms involved in adult consequences of extremely preterm birth, aiming at preventing thrifty organ (mal)development and implementing very early in life measures, which will allow recovery or at least healthy compensation in case of fixed organ damages. Finally, there is a clear need for increased awareness among health care providers, families, and now the preterm-born young adults themselves, as they are entering their active independent lives and having children.

Summary: adult cardiovascular and metabolic outcomes after very preterm birth

Heart and vessels

- Higher blood pressure, higher rates of hypertension including hypertensive complications of pregnancy, higher cerebrovascular diseases and rates of death from cardiovascular causes

- Changes in ventricle wall thickness, which may be related to degree of prematurity

Kidneys

- Smaller kidneys. Probable increased susceptibility to second hits. In young adulthood, no clinically significant impact on renal function is reported.

Metabolic: glucose and lipid metabolism

- Higher glucose intolerance, type 2 diabetes including gestational diabetes

- No major dyslipidemia in young adulthood

- Increased rates of nonalcoholic fatty liver disease and abdominal obesity

---

Best practices for preventing or decreasing long-term cardiovascular and metabolic outcomes

Neonatal and infant life

- Optimizing parenteral nutrition to decrease peroxide load; however, practical guidelines still require research
- Optimizing neonatal nutrition and promoting breast milk
- Optimizing infant growth, preventing excessive weight gain relative to length, especially after term equivalent age

Childhood and adulthood

- Avoiding second hits such as obesity, acute kidney injury
- Insure long-term health follow-up
- Involve families and preterm-born subjects in optimizing their long-term health.

REFERENCES

1. Saigal S. Preemie voices. Victoria (Canada): FriesenPress; 2014.
2. Jobe AH. The new bronchopulmonary dysplasia. Curr Opin Pediatr 2011;23: 167–72.
3. Luu TM, Katz SL, Leeson P, et al. Preterm birth: risk factor for early-onset chronic diseases. CMAJ 2016;188:736–46.
4. Kistner A, Jacobson L, Jacobson SH, et al. Low gestational age associated with abnormal retinal vascularization and increased blood pressure in adult women. Pediatr Res 2002;51:675–80.
5. Kistner A, Celsi G, Vanpee M, et al. Increased systolic daily ambulatory blood pressure in adult women born preterm. Pediatr Nephrol 2005;20:232–3.
6. Irving RJ, Belton NR, Elton RA, et al. Adult cardiovascular risk factors in premature babies. Lancet 2000;355:2135–6.
7. Hack M. Young adult outcomes of very-low-birth-weight children. Semin Fetal Neonatal Med 2006;11:127–37.
8. Bonamy AK, Bendito A, Martin H, et al. Preterm birth contributes to increased vascular resistance and higher blood pressure in adolescent girls. Pediatr Res 2005;58:845–9.
9. Bonamy AK, Martin H, Jorneskog G, et al. Lower skin capillary density, normal endothelial function and higher blood pressure in children born preterm. J Intern Med 2007;262:635–42.
10. Bonamy AK, Kallen K, Norman M. High blood pressure in 2.5-year-old children born extremely preterm. Pediatrics 2012;129:e1199–204.
11. de Jong F, Monuteaux MC, van Elburg RM, et al. Systematic review and meta-analysis of preterm birth and later systolic blood pressure. Hypertension 2012; 59:226–34.
12. Hovi P, Vohr B, Ment LR, et al. Blood pressure in young adults born at very low birth weight: adults born preterm international collaboration. Hypertension 2016; 68:880–7.
13. Boivin A, Luo ZC, Audibert F, et al. Pregnancy complications among women born preterm. CMAJ 2012;184:1777–84.
14. Ueda P, Cnattingius S, Stephansson O, et al. Cerebrovascular and ischemic heart disease in young adults born preterm: a population-based Swedish cohort study. Eur J Epidemiol 2014;29:253–60.

15. Lewandowski AJ, Davis EF, Yu G, et al. Elevated blood pressure in preterm-born offspring associates with a distinct antiangiogenic state and microvascular abnormalities in adult life. Hypertension 2015;65:607–14.

16. Thebaud B, Ladha F, Michelakis ED, et al. Vascular endothelial growth factor gene therapy increases survival, promotes lung angiogenesis, and prevents alveolar damage in hyperoxia-induced lung injury: evidence that angiogenesis participates in alveolarization. Circulation 2005;112:2477–86.

17. Yzydorczyk C, Comte B, Cambonie G, et al. Neonatal oxygen exposure in rats leads to cardiovascular and renal alterations in adulthood. Hypertension 2008; 52:889–95.

18. Sutherland MR, Bertagnolli M, Lukaszewski MA, et al. Preterm birth and hypertension risk: the oxidative stress paradigm. Hypertension 2014;63:12–8.

19. Boardman H, Birse K, Davis EF, et al. Comprehensive multi-modality assessment of regional and global arterial structure and function in adults born preterm. Hypertens Res 2016;39(1):39–45.

20. Bassareo PP, Fanos V, Puddu M, et al. Reduced brachial flow-mediated vasodilation in young adult ex extremely low birth weight preterm: a condition predictive of increased cardiovascular risk? J Matern Fetal Neonatal Med 2010; 23(Suppl 3):121–4.

21. Hovi P, Turanlahti M, Strang-Karlsson S, et al. Intima-media thickness and flow-mediated dilatation in the Helsinki study of very low birth weight adults. Pediatrics 2011;127:e304–11.

22. Brunner H, Cockcroft JR, Deanfield J, et al, Working Group on E and Endothelial Factors of the European Society of Hypertension. Endothelial function and dysfunction. Part II: association with cardiovascular risk factors and diseases. A statement by the Working Group on Endothelins and Endothelial Factors of the European Society of Hypertension. J Hypertens 2005;23:233–46.

23. Flammer AJ, Anderson T, Celermajer DS, et al. The assessment of endothelial function: from research into clinical practice. Circulation 2012;126:753–67.

24. Lewandowski AJ, Leeson P. Preeclampsia, prematurity and cardiovascular health in adult life. Early Hum Dev 2014;90:725–9.

25. Davis EF, Newton L, Lewandowski AJ, et al. Pre-eclampsia and offspring cardiovascular health: mechanistic insights from experimental studies. Clin Sci 2012; 123:53–72.

26. Lazdam M, de la Horra A, Pitcher A, et al. Elevated blood pressure in offspring born premature to hypertensive pregnancy: is endothelial dysfunction the underlying vascular mechanism? Hypertension 2010;56:159–65.

27. Kelly BA, Lewandowski AJ, Worton SA, et al. Antenatal glucocorticoid exposure and long-term alterations in aortic function and glucose metabolism. Pediatrics 2012;129:e1282–90.

28. Lewandowski AJ, Lazdam M, Davis E, et al. Short-term exposure to exogenous lipids in premature infants and long-term changes in aortic and cardiac function. Arterioscler Thromb Vasc Biol 2011;31:2125–35.

29. Zecca E, Romagnoli C, Vento G, et al. Left ventricle dimensions in preterm infants during the first month of life. Eur J Pediatr 2001;160:227–30.

30. Lewandowski AJ, Augustine D, Lamata P, et al. Preterm heart in adult life: cardiovascular magnetic resonance reveals distinct differences in left ventricular mass, geometry, and function. Circulation 2013;127:197–206.

31. Lewandowski AJ, Bradlow WM, Augustine D, et al. Right ventricular systolic dysfunction in young adults born preterm. Circulation 2013;128:713–20.

32. Kowalski RR, Beare R, Doyle LW, et al, Victorian Infant Collaborative Study Group. Elevated blood pressure with reduced left ventricular and aortic dimensions in adolescents born extremely preterm. J Pediatr 2016;172:75–80.e2.

33. Oparil S, Bishop S, Clubb FJ. Myocardial cell hypertrophy or hyperplasia. Hypertension 1984;6:III38–43.

34. Clubb FJ, Bishop S. Formation of binucleated myocardial cells in the neonatal rat. An index for growth hypertrophy. Lab Invest 1984;50:571–7.

35. Paradis AN, Gay MS, Wilson CG, et al. Newborn hypoxia/anoxia inhibits cardiomyocyte proliferation and decreases cardiomyocyte endowment in the developing heart: role of endothelin-1. PLoS One 2015;10:e0116600.

36. Tare M, Bensley JG, Moss TJ, et al. Exposure to intrauterine inflammation leads to impaired function and altered structure in the preterm heart of fetal sheep. Clin Sci 2014;127:559–69.

37. Velten M, Hutchinson KR, Gorr MW, et al. Systemic maternal inflammation and neonatal hyperoxia induces remodeling and left ventricular dysfunction in mice. PLoS One 2011;6:e24544.

38. Bal MP, de Vries WB, Steendijk P, et al. Histopathological changes of the heart after neonatal dexamethasone treatment: studies in 4-, 8-, and 50-week-old rats. Pediatr Res 2009;66:74–9.

39. Bertagnolli M, Huyard F, Cloutier A, et al. Transient neonatal high oxygen exposure leads to early adult cardiac dysfunction, remodeling and activation of the renin-angiotensin system. Hypertension 2014;63(1):143–50.

40. Bensley JG, Stacy VK, De Matteo R, et al. Cardiac remodelling as a result of preterm birth: implications for future cardiovascular disease. Eur Heart J 2010;31:2058–66.

41. Lewandowski AJ, Lamata P, Francis JM, et al. Breast milk consumption in preterm neonates and cardiac shape in adulthood. Pediatrics 2016. [Epub ahead of print].

42. Kim MY, Eiby YA, Lumbers ER, et al. Effects of glucocorticoid exposure on growth and structural maturation of the heart of the preterm piglet. PLoS One 2014;9:e93407.

43. Hinchliffe SA, Lynch MR, Sargent PH, et al. The effect of intrauterine growth retardation on the development of renal nephrons. Br J Obstet Gynaecol 1992;99:296–301.

44. Sutherland MR, Gubhaju L, Moore L, et al. Accelerated maturation and abnormal morphology in the preterm neonatal kidney. J Am Soc Nephrol 2011;22:1365–74.

45. Rodriguez MM, Gomez AH, Abitbol CL, et al. Histomorphometric analysis of postnatal glomerulogenesis in extremely preterm infants. Pediatr Dev Pathol 2004;7:17–25.

46. Ingelfinger JR, Woods LL. Perinatal programming, renal development, and adult renal function. Am J Hypertens 2002;15:46S–9S.

47. Mackenzie HS, Brenner BM. Fewer nephrons at birth: a missing link in the etiology of essential hypertension? Am J Kidney Dis 1995;26:91–8.

48. Keller G, Zimmer G, Mall G, et al. Nephron number in patients with primary hypertension. N Engl J Med 2003;348:101–8.

49. Hoy WE, Rees M, Kile E, et al. A new dimension to the Barker hypothesis: low birthweight and susceptibility to renal disease. Kidney Int 1999;56:1072–7.

50. Vikse BE, Irgens LM, Leivestad T, et al. Low birth weight increases risk for end-stage renal disease. J Am Soc Nephrol 2008;19:151–7.

51. White SL, Perkovic V, Cass A, et al. Is low birth weight an antecedent of CKD in later life? A systematic review of observational studies. Am J Kidney Dis 2009; 54:248–61.
52. Benz K, Amann K. Maternal nutrition, low nephron number and arterial hypertension in later life. Biochim Biophys Acta 2010;1802:1309–17.
53. Rakow A, Johansson S, Legnevall L, et al. Renal volume and function in school-age children born preterm or small for gestational age. Pediatr Nephrol 2008;23: 1309–15.
54. Kwinta P, Klimek M, Drozdz D, et al. Assessment of long-term renal complications in extremely low birth weight children. Pediatr Nephrol 2011;26:1095–103.
55. Keijzer-Veen MG, Kleinveld HA, Lequin MH, et al. Renal function and size at young adult age after intrauterine growth restriction and very premature birth. Am J Kidney Dis 2007;50:542–51.
56. Keijzer-Veen MG, Dulger A, Dekker FW, et al. Very preterm birth is a risk factor for increased systolic blood pressure at a young adult age. Pediatr Nephrol 2010;25:509–16.
57. Zaffanello M, Brugnara M, Bruno C, et al. Renal function and volume of infants born with a very low birth-weight: a preliminary cross-sectional study. Acta Paediatr 2010;99:1192–8.
58. Carmody JB, Charlton JR. Short-term gestation, long-term risk: prematurity and chronic kidney disease. Pediatrics 2013;131:1168–79.
59. Abitbol CL, Chandar J, Rodriguez MM, et al. Obesity and preterm birth: additive risks in the progression of kidney disease in children. Pediatr Nephrol 2009;24: 1363–70.
60. Kistner A, Celsi G, Vanpee M, et al. Increased blood pressure but normal renal function in adult women born preterm. Pediatr Nephrol 2000;15:215–20.
61. Ferguson MA, Waikar SS. Established and emerging markers of kidney function. Clin Chem 2012;58:680–9.
62. Carballo-Magdaleno D, Guizar-Mendoza JM, Amador-Licona N, et al. Renal function, renal volume, and blood pressure in infants with antecedent of antenatal steroids. Pediatr Nephrol 2011;26:1851–6.
63. Popescu CR, Sutherland MR, Cloutier A, et al. Hyperoxia exposure impairs nephrogenesis in the neonatal rat: role of HIF-1alpha. PloS One 2013;81(2): e82421.
64. Sutherland MR, Beland C, Lukaszewski MA, et al. Age- and sex-related changes in rat renal function and pathology following neonatal hyperoxia exposure. Physiol Rep 2016;4(15):e12887.
65. Bueters RR, Kusters LJ, Klaasen A, et al. Antibiotics and renal branching morphogenesis: comparison of toxicities. Pediatr Res 2014;76:508–14.
66. Gilbert T, Gaonach S, Moreau E, et al. Defect of nephrogenesis induced by gentamicin in rat metanephric organ culture. Lab Invest 1994;70:656–66.
67. Gilbert T, Lelievre-Pegorier M, Merlet-Benichou C. Immediate and long-term renal effects of fetal exposure to gentamicin. Pediatr Nephrol 1990;4:445–50.
68. Olliges A, Wimmer S, Nusing RM. Defects in mouse nephrogenesis induced by selective and non-selective cyclooxygenase-2 inhibitors. Br J Pharmacol 2011; 163:927–36.
69. Sutherland MR, Yoder BA, McCurnin D, et al. Effects of ibuprofen treatment on the developing preterm baboon kidney. Am J Physiol Renal Physiol 2012;302: F1286–92.
70. Frolich S, Olliges A, Kern N, et al. Temporal expression of the PGE2 synthetic system in the kidney is associated with the time frame of renal developmental

vulnerability to cyclooxygenase-2 inhibition. Am J Physiol Renal Physiol 2012; 303:F209–19.

71. Komhoff M, Wang JL, Cheng HF, et al. Cyclooxygenase-2-selective inhibitors impair glomerulogenesis and renal cortical development. Kidney Int 2000;57: 414–22.

72. Villar-Martini VC, Carvalho JJ, Neves MF, et al. Hypertension and kidney alterations in rat offspring from low protein pregnancies. J Hypertens Suppl 2009; 27:S47–51.

73. Brennan KA, Kaufman S, Reynolds SW, et al. Differential effects of maternal nutrient restriction through pregnancy on kidney development and later blood pressure control in the resulting offspring. Am J Physiol Regul Integr Comp Physiol 2008;295:R197–205.

74. Dalziel SR, Parag V, Rodgers A, et al. Cardiovascular risk factors at age 30 following pre-term birth. Int J Epidemiol 2007;36:907–15.

75. Mathai S, Cutfield WS, Derraik JG, et al. Insulin sensitivity and beta-cell function in adults born preterm and their children. Diabetes 2012;61:2479–83.

76. Rotteveel J, van Weissenbruch MM, Twisk JW, et al. Infant and childhood growth patterns, insulin sensitivity, and blood pressure in prematurely born young adults. Pediatrics 2008;122:313–21.

77. Hovi P, Andersson S, Eriksson JG, et al. Glucose regulation in young adults with very low birth weight. N Engl J Med 2007;356:2053–63.

78. Crump C, Winkleby MA, Sundquist K, et al. Risk of diabetes among young adults born preterm in Sweden. Diabetes Care 2011;34:1109–13.

79. Kaijser M, Bonamy AK, Akre O, et al. Perinatal risk factors for diabetes in later life. Diabetes 2009;58:523–6.

80. Parkinson JR, Hyde MJ, Gale C, et al. Preterm birth and the metabolic syndrome in adult life: a systematic review and meta-analysis. Pediatrics 2013;131: e1240–63.

81. Evensen KA, Steinshamn S, Tjonna AE, et al. Effects of preterm birth and fetal growth retardation on cardiovascular risk factors in young adulthood. Early Hum Dev 2009;85:239–45.

82. Breij LM, Kerkhof GF, Hokken-Koelega AC. Risk for nonalcoholic fatty liver disease in young adults born preterm. Horm Res Paediatr 2015;84:199–205.

83. Kerkhof GF, Willemsen RH, Leunissen RW, et al. Health profile of young adults born preterm: negative effects of rapid weight gain in early life. J Clin Endocrinol Metab 2012;97:4498–506.

84. Gregg BE, Moore PC, Demozay D, et al. Formation of a human beta-cell population within pancreatic islets is set early in life. J Clin Endocrinol Metab 2012;97: 3197–206.

85. Singhal A, Cole TJ, Fewtrell M, et al. Breastmilk feeding and lipoprotein profile in adolescents born preterm: follow-up of a prospective randomised study. Lancet 2004;363:1571–8.

86. Singhal A, Farooqi IS, O'Rahilly S, et al. Early nutrition and leptin concentrations in later life. Am J Clin Nutr 2002;75:993–9.

87. Greer FR. Long-term adverse outcomes of low birth weight, increased somatic growth rates, and alterations of body composition in the premature infant: review of the evidence. J Pediatr Gastroenterol Nutr 2007;45(Suppl 3):S147–51.

88. Rotteveel J, van Weissenbruch MM, Twisk JW, et al. Abnormal lipid profile and hyperinsulinaemia after a mixed meal: additional cardiovascular risk factors in young adults born preterm. Diabetologia 2008;51:1269–75.

89. Arguelles S, Machado MJ, Ayala A, et al. Correlation between circulating bio-markers of oxidative stress of maternal and umbilical cord blood at birth. Free Radic Res 2006;40:565–70.
90. Biri A, Onan A, Devrim E, et al. Oxidant status in maternal and cord plasma and placental tissue in gestational diabetes. Placenta 2006;27:327–32.
91. Gupta S, Agarwal A, Sharma RK. The role of placental oxidative stress and lipid peroxidation in preeclampsia. Obstet Gynecol Surv 2005;60:807–16.
92. Haynes RL, Baud O, Li J, et al. Oxidative and nitrative injury in periventricular leukomalacia: a review. Brain Pathol 2005;15:225–33.
93. Peuchant E, Brun JL, Rigalleau V, et al. Oxidative and antioxidative status in pregnant women with either gestational or type 1 diabetes. Clin Biochem 2004;37:293–8.
94. Redman CW, Sargent IL. Latest advances in understanding preeclampsia. Science 2005;308:1592–4.
95. Saugstad OD. Oxidative stress in the newborn–a 30-year perspective. Biol Neonate 2005;88:228–36.
96. Vincent HK, Taylor AG. Biomarkers and potential mechanisms of obesity-induced oxidant stress in humans. Int J Obes(lond) 2006;30:400–18.
97. Woods JR Jr. Reactive oxygen species and preterm premature rupture of membranes-a review. Placenta 2001;22(Suppl A):S38–44.
98. Heyborne KD, Witkin SS, McGregor JA. Tumor necrosis factor-alpha in mid-trimester amniotic fluid is associated with impaired intrauterine fetal growth. Am J Obstet Gynecol 1992;167:920–5.
99. Hahn-Zoric M, Hagberg H, Kjellmer I, et al. Aberrations in placental cytokine mRNA related to intrauterine growth retardation. Pediatr Res 2002;51:201–6.
100. Aghai ZH, Camacho J, Saslow JG, et al. Impact of histological chorioamnionitis on tracheal aspirate cytokines in premature infants. Am J Perinatol 2012;29: 567–72.
101. Leduc L, Delvin E, Ouellet A, et al. Oxidized low-density lipoproteins in cord blood from neonates with intra-uterine growth restriction. Eur J Obstet Gynecol Reprod Biol 2011;156:46–9.
102. Fujimaki A, Watanabe K, Mori T, et al. Placental oxidative DNA damage and its repair in preeclamptic women with fetal growth restriction. Placenta 2011;32: 367–72.
103. Mestan K, Matoba N, Arguelles L, et al. Cord blood 8-isoprostane in the preterm infant. Early Hum Dev 2012;88:683–9.
104. Negi R, Pande D, Kumar A, et al. In vivo oxidative DNA damage and lipid per-oxidation as a biomarker of oxidative stress in preterm low-birthweight infants. J Trop Pediatr 2012;58:326–8.
105. Weinberger B, Nisar S, Anwar M, et al. Lipid peroxidation in cord blood and neonatal outcome. Pediatr Int 2006;48:479–83.
106. Kleiber N, Chessex P, Rouleau T, et al. Neonatal exposure to oxidants induces later in life a metabolic response associated to a phenotype of energy defi-ciency in an animal model of total parenteral nutrition. Pediatr Res 2010;68: 188–92.
107. Lavoie JC, Belanger S, Spalinger M, et al. Admixture of a multivitamin prepara-tion to parenteral nutrition: the major contributor to in vitro generation of perox-ides. Pediatrics 1997;99:E6.
108. Lai TT, Bearer CF. Iatrogenic environmental hazards in the neonatal intensive care unit. Clin Perinatol 2008;35:163–81, ix.

109. Jankov RP, Negus A, Tanswell AK. Antioxidants as therapy in the newborn: some words of caution. Pediatr Res 2001;50:681–7.
110. Saik LA, Hsieh HL, Baricos WH, et al. Enzymatic and immunologic quantitation of erythrocyte superoxide dismutase in adults and in neonates of different gestational ages. Pediatr Res 1982;16:933–7.
111. Georgeson GD, Szony BJ, Streitman K, et al. Antioxidant enzyme activities are decreased in preterm infants and in neonates born via caesarean section. Eur J Obstet Gynecol Reprod Biol 2002;103:136–9.
112. Vento M, Moro M, Escrig R, et al. Preterm resuscitation with low oxygen causes less oxidative stress, inflammation, and chronic lung disease. Pediatrics 2009; 124(3):e439–49.
113. Vina J, Vento M, Garcia-Sala F, et al. L-cysteine and glutathione metabolism are impaired in premature infants due to cystathionase deficiency. Am J Clin Nutr 1995;61:1067–9.
114. Asikainen TM, White CW. Pulmonary antioxidant defenses in the preterm newborn with respiratory distress and bronchopulmonary dysplasia in evolution: implications for antioxidant therapy. Antioxid Redox Signal 2004;6:155–67.
115. Thibeault DW. The precarious antioxidant defenses of the preterm infant. Am J Perinatol 2000;17:167–81.
116. O'Donovan DJ, Fernandes CJ. Free radicals and diseases in premature infants. Antioxid Redox Signal 2004;6:169–76.
117. Breckenridge RA, Piotrowska I, Ng KE, et al. Hypoxic regulation of hand1 controls the fetal-neonatal switch in cardiac metabolism. PLoS Biol 2013;11: e1001666.
118. Joss-Moore LA, Lane RH, Albertine KH. Epigenetic contributions to the developmental origins of adult lung disease. Biochem Cell Biol 2015;93:119–27.
119. Crudo A, Petropoulos S, Moisiadis VG, et al. Prenatal synthetic glucocorticoid treatment changes DNA methylation states in male organ systems: multigenerational effects. Endocrinology 2012;153:3269–83.
120. Cruickshank MN, Oshlack A, Theda C, et al. Analysis of epigenetic changes in survivors of preterm birth reveals the effect of gestational age and evidence for a long term legacy. Genome Med 2013;5:96.
121. Neuzil J, Darlow BA, Inder TE, et al. Oxidation of parenteral lipid emulsion by ambient and phototherapy lights: potential toxicity of routine parenteral feeding. J Pediatr 1995;126:785–90.
122. Silvers KM, Darlow BA, Winterbourn CC. Lipid peroxide and hydrogen peroxide formation in parenteral nutrition solutions containing multivitamins. JPEN J Parenter Enteral Nutr 2001;25:14–7.
123. Knafo L, Chessex P, Rouleau T, et al. Association between hydrogen peroxide-dependent byproducts of ascorbic acid and increased hepatic acetyl-CoA carboxylase activity. Clin Chem 2005;51:1462–71.
124. Bassiouny MR, Almarsafawy H, Abdel-Hady H, et al. A randomized controlled trial on parenteral nutrition, oxidative stress, and chronic lung diseases in preterm infants. J Pediatr Gastroenterol Nutr 2009;48:363–9.
125. Maghdessian R, Cote F, Rouleau T, et al. Ascorbylperoxide contaminating parenteral nutrition perturbs the lipid metabolism in newborn Guinea pig. J Pharmacol Exp Ther 2010;334:278–84.
126. Miloudi K, Comte B, Rouleau T, et al. The mode of administration of total parenteral nutrition and nature of lipid content influence the generation of peroxides and aldehydes. Clin Nutr 2012;31:526–34.

127. Laborie S, Lavoie JC, Chessex P. Paradoxical role of ascorbic acid and ribo-flavin in solutions of total parenteral nutrition: implication in photoinduced peroxide generation. Pediatr Res 1998;43:601–6.
128. Brandes N, Schmitt S, Jakob U. Thiol-based redox switches in eukaryotic proteins. Antioxid Redox Signal 2009;11:997–1014.
129. Winterbourn CC. The biological chemistry of hydrogen peroxide. Methods Enzymol 2013;528:3–25.
130. Kemp M, Go YM, Jones DP. Nonequilibrium thermodynamics of thiol/disulfide redox systems: a perspective on redox systems biology. Free Radic Biol Med 2008;44:921–37.
131. Schafer FQ, Buettner GR. Redox environment of the cell as viewed through the redox state of the glutathione disulfide/glutathione couple. Free Radic Biol Med 2001;30:1191–212.
132. Suyavaran A, Ramamurthy C, Mareeswaran R, et al. TNF-alpha suppression by glutathione preconditioning attenuates hepatic ischemia reperfusion injury in young and aged rats. Inflamm Res 2015;64:71–81.
133. Elremaly W, Mohamed I, Mialet-Marty T, et al. Ascorbylperoxide from parenteral nutrition induces an increase of redox potential of glutathione and loss of alveoli in newborn Guinea pig lungs. Redox Biol 2014;2:725–31.
134. Kuster A, Tea I, Ferchaud-Roucher V, et al. Cord blood glutathione depletion in preterm infants: correlation with maternal cysteine depletion. PLoS One 2011;6: e27626.
135. Lavoie JC, Chessex P. Gender and maturation affect glutathione status in human neonatal tissues. Free Radic Biol Med 1997;23:648–57.
136. Chessex P, Watson C, Kaczala GW, et al. Determinants of oxidant stress in extremely low birth weight premature infants. Free Radic Biol Med 2010;49: 1380–6.
137. Mohamed I, Elremaly W, Rouleau T, et al. Ascorbylperoxide contaminating parenteral nutrition is associated with bronchopulmonary dysplasia or death in extremely preterm infants. JPEN J Parenter Enteral Nutr 2016. [Epub ahead of print].
138. Elremaly W, Rouleau T, Lavoie JC. Inhibition of hepatic methionine adenosyltransferase by peroxides contaminating parenteral nutrition leads to a lower level of glutathione in newborn Guinea pigs. Free Radic Biol Med 2012;53: 2250–5.
139. Mato JM, Lu SC. Role of S-adenosyl-L-methionine in liver health and injury. Hepatology 2007;45:1306–12.
140. Yara S, Levy E, Elremaly W, et al. Total parenteral nutrition induces sustained hypomethylation of DNA in newborn Guinea pigs. Pediatr Res 2013;73:592–5.
141. Peskin AV, Pace PE, Behring JB, et al. Glutathionylation of the active site cysteines of peroxiredoxin 2 and recycling by glutaredoxin. J Biol Chem 2016;291: 3053–62.
142. Khashu M, Harrison A, Lalari V, et al. Impact of shielding parenteral nutrition from light on routine monitoring of blood glucose and triglyceride levels in preterm neonates. Arch Dis Child Fetal Neonatal Ed 2009;94:F111–5.
143. Khashu M, Harrison A, Lalari V, et al. Photoprotection of parenteral nutrition enhances advancement of minimal enteral nutrition in preterm infants. Semin Perinatol 2006;30:139–45.
144. Chessex P, Harrison A, Khashu M, et al. In preterm neonates, is the risk of developing bronchopulmonary dysplasia influenced by the failure to protect total parenteral nutrition from exposure to ambient light? J Pediatr 2007;151:213–4.

145. Chessex P, Laborie S, Nasef N, et al. Shielding parenteral nutrition from light improves survival rate in premature infants: a meta-analysis. JPEN J Parenter Enteral Nutr 2015. [Epub ahead of print].
146. Friel J. Postnatal oxidative stress and the role of enteral and parenteral nutrition perinatal and prenatal disorders. New York: Springer; 2014. p. 343–70.
147. Sherlock R, Chessex P. Shielding parenteral nutrition from light: does the available evidence support a randomized, controlled trial? Pediatrics 2009;123: 1529–33.
148. Laborie S, Denis A, Dassieu G, et al. Shielding parenteral nutrition solutions from light: a randomized controlled trial. JPEN J Parenter Enteral Nutr 2015;39: 729–37.
149. Elremaly W, Mohamed I, Rouleau T, et al. Adding glutathione to parenteral nutrition prevents alveolar loss in newborn Guinea pig. Free Radic Biol Med 2015;87: 274–81.

Epidemiology of Periviable Births

The Impact and Neonatal Outcomes of Twin Pregnancy

Cande V. Ananth, PhD, MPH[a,b,*], Suneet P. Chauhan, MD[c]

KEYWORDS

- Neonatal morbidity • Neonatal mortality • Glucocorticosteroid • Limits of viability
- Periviable gestational age • Twins

KEY POINTS

- Periviable births (delivered at 20 to 25 weeks) occur in 0.4% of all births, but account for up to 40% of infant deaths in the United States.
- Among twins, 2.5% of births occur at periviable gestations.
- Neonatal mortality rates among twins delivered at 22 to 23 weeks declined between 2005 and 2013 and remained unchanged at other periviable gestations.
- Composite neonatal morbidity among twins increased substantially at 23 weeks between 2005 and 2013, and remained unchanged at other periviable gestations.
- Whether twins delivered at periviable gestations suffer from long-term consequences of neurodevelopmental and cognitive deficits remains unknown.

INTRODUCTION

Birth at the "threshold of viability" is a term that is sometimes used to classify newborns at the borderline of viability. This term introduces much ambiguity because it encompasses various definitions of perinatal end points based on gestational age at delivery and birthweight, and the cutoff changes with improvements in perinatal outcomes over time. It included deliveries from 20 to 28 weeks or newborns with

Disclosure: The authors have nothing to disclose.
[a] Department of Obstetrics and Gynecology, College of Physicians and Surgeons, Columbia University, 622 West 168 Street, New York, NY 10032, USA; [b] Department of Epidemiology, Joseph L. Mailman School of Public Health, Columbia University, 722 West 168 Street, New York, NY 10032, USA; [c] Department of Obstetrics, Gynecology, and Reproductive Sciences, McGovern Medical School, University of Texas, 6432 Fannin Street, MSB 3.286, Houston, TX 77030, USA
* Corresponding author. Department of Obstetrics and Gynecology, College of Physicians and Surgeons, Columbia University, 622 West 168th Street, New York, NY 10032.
E-mail address: cande.ananth@columbia.edu

birthweight of 400 g to 1500 g.[1] Gestational age cutoffs to define threshold of viability have included very preterm (22–27 weeks), extremely preterm (22–28 weeks), born before 28 weeks, preterm (<37 weeks), and extreme preterm delivery.[1] Based on birthweight, newborns are described as very low birthweight (<1500 g), or extremely low birthweight (<1000 g).

A recent 2014 workshop, sponsored by the Eunice Kennedy Shriver National Institute of Child Health and Human Development, Society for Maternal–Fetal Medicine, the Section on Perinatal Pediatrics of the American Academy of Pediatrics, and the American Congress of Obstetricians and Gynecologists, reached the consensus that periviable birth is the preferred term, and it includes deliveries at $20^{0/6}$ to $25^{6/7}$ weeks, regardless of the birthweight. Although births within this gestational age range occur in 0.4% of all deliveries in the United States, they account for about 40% of all infant deaths.[2] Among survivors these newborns are at substantial risk for neonatal morbidity, and long-term sequelae including cerebral palsy, microcephaly, attention-deficit/hyperactivity disorder, and asthma.[1]

The 2016 obstetric care consensus[2] laconically describes neonatal outcomes after periviable birth; provides current evidence and recommendations regarding use antenatal corticosteroids, tocolytics, magnesium sulfate for neuroprotection, and antibiotics in the setting of preterm premature rupture of membranes or for group B streptococci; and indications for possible cesarean delivery. The guideline also addresses the issue of family counseling with the goal of incorporating informed patient preferences.[2] This national guideline, however, does not provide epidemiologic data on periviable births among twins. As a matter of fact, the word "twin" does not appear in the document.

For clinicians and researchers alike, population-based data on periviable live births among twins is important for at least four reasons. First, the frequency of twin births, which had previously plateaued, is now increasing.[3–6] The twinning rate (births in twin deliveries per 1000 total births) increased by 76% between 1980 and 2009 (from 18.9 to 33.2 per 1000), remained stable from 2009 through 2012, and rose 2% between 2012 and 2013.[5] Second, about 20% to 24% of all births delivered at periviable gestational ages are from a multiple gestation.[5] Third, neonatal morbidity and mortality after delivery at periviable gestations may differ sufficiently between singleton and twin newborns, warranting modifications in counseling of women and in obstetric management.[7–10] Fourth, population-based publications on twins and periviable birth may be an impetus for researchers.

We designed this study to describe temporal changes in the prevalence of twin live births at the periviable gestational ages in the United States over 9 years (2005–2013). We describe the epidemiologic characteristics of women who deliver twin live births at periviable gestational ages (ie, 20–25 weeks), and contrast neonatal mortality and morbidity among twins born at the periviable gestations with those who are born later.

MATERIAL AND METHODS

This study involved twin births in the United States between 2005 and 2013, the data for which were derived from the US vital statistics data of live births linked to infant deaths. These data were assembled by the National Center for Health Statistics of the Centers for Disease Control and Prevention. We restricted the study to states that implemented the 2003 revision of birth certificates. Therefore, the number of states (and the total number of births) gradually increased with advancing years, beginning with 12 states in 2005,[11] 21 states in 2006, 23 states in 2007, 28 states in 2009 (66% of all births), 33 states in 2010 (76% of all births), 36 states in 2011

(83% of all births), 38 states in 2012 (86% of all births), and 41 states and the District of Columbia in 2013 (90% of all births).[12] These data are deidentified, and publically available, so they do not qualify as human subjects research. Therefore, we did not seek ethics approval from a human subjects committee.

Gestational age in this cohort (reported in completed weeks) was based on the best obstetric estimate, completed by the attendant at delivery based on the best available prenatal dating method, primarily ultrasound.

Neonatal Outcomes

The primary outcomes included neonatal mortality and a composite neonatal morbidity. Neonatal mortality was defined as a live-born twin that died within the first 27 days. The composite neonatal morbidity included newborns with one or more of the following conditions or diagnoses: neonatal seizures, assisted ventilation (<30 minutes and $\geq$6 hours), significant birth injury, neonatal intensive care unit admission, and 5-minute Apgar score less than 4. Significant birth injury included skeletal fractures, peripheral nerve injury, or soft tissue or solid organ hemorrhage.

Cohort Composition

Between 2005 and 2013, there were 805,972 twin live births in the study cohort. Of these, we sequentially excluded twins with missing gestational age (n = 18,387), gestational age less than 20 weeks (n = 1850), or gestational age 43 weeks or more (n = 56). We further excluded twins that were diagnosed with a chromosomal anomaly or major malformation (n = 2924), and those that were delivered outside of a hospital (n = 2440). After all exclusions, 780,315 nonmalformed twin live births remained for analysis.

Statistical Analysis

We examined the distribution of twin live births at each gestation week in the periviable period (20, 21, 22, 23, 24, and 25 weeks), and later in gestation (26–27, 28–33, 34–36, and 37–42 weeks). We then examined neonatal mortality and a composite neonatal morbidity among twin live births, overall and by each gestation week in the periviable period. This analysis was followed by an examination of gestational age-specific changes in rates of adverse neonatal outcomes between 2005 and 2013.

We fit log-linear regression analyses to estimate the relative risk and 95% confidence interval based on log-binomial models. These models were fit to examine changes in rates of adverse neonatal outcomes between 2005 and 2013 overall, and changes in outcomes at each gestation week in the periviable period, and later, with births at greater than or equal to 37 weeks as the reference. We also estimated the risk difference (with 95% confidence interval) as a measure of effect that provides an assessment of the excess risk of the outcome among the exposed (say, in 2013) over the baseline (in 2005).

All analyses were adjusted for the confounding effects of several covariates. These included maternal age, primiparity, maternal race/ethnicity, single marital status, highest education, and smoking 3 months before pregnancy.

RESULTS

Overall, of the 780,315 nonmalformed twin live births, 2.5% were delivered at 20 to 25 weeks. The distribution of maternal and infant characteristics among twin live births in 2005 and 2013 and the change in distributions are shown in **Table 1**. The proportion of women less than 20 years that delivered twins declined by almost half between

Table 1
Maternal and neonatal characteristics among twin live births overall, and at periviable gestational ages (20–25 wk): United States, 2005 to 2013

	All Twin Live Births, %			Twin Live Births at Periviable Gestations, %	
	2005–2013 (n = 780,315)	2005 (n = 38,866)	2013 (n = 118,324)	2005 (n = 997)	2013 (n = 3032)
Maternal Characteristics					
Maternal age (y)					
<20	4.4	6.1	3.2	12.6	6.5
20–24	16.9	18.9	15.5	24.6	21.5
25–29	26.3	26.6	26.3	27.2	26.2
30–34	29.4	28.1	31.3	21.6	28.5
35–39	17.2	16.1	17.6	11.6	13.5
≥40	5.8	4.2	6.1	2.4	4.0
Primiparity	19.3	18.1	19.3	20.4	24.0
Single marital status	32.0	30.6	32.1	50.1	44.0
Race/ethnicity					
White	65.0	64.9	65.3	50.4	52.3
African-American	15.8	15.7	17.1	30.2	31.3
Hispanic	18.0	18.9	16.4	18.2	14.8
Other	1.2	0.5	1.2	1.3	1.6
Highest education					
≤8 y	3.0	3.9	2.3	3.4	1.7
High school	31.9	36.9	28.6	50.4	35.9
Some college	50.3	48.1	52.4	38.9	50.6
Beyond college	14.8	11.1	16.7	7.3	11.9

Prepregnancy smoking	8.0	10.8	7.1	14.5	9.7
Labor induction	10.8	11.2	11.8	5.2	4.4
Cesarean delivery	75.2	73.3	75.1	47.7	50.9
Neonatal characteristics					
Gestational age (wk)					
20	0.2	0.3	0.2	9.9	7.5
21	0.2	0.3	0.2	9.7	9.4
22	0.4	0.3	0.4	13.4	14.9
23	0.5	0.5	0.5	17.9	18.6
24	0.6	0.6	0.6	22.2	25.2
25	0.6	0.7	0.6	26.9	24.4
26–27	1.7	1.9	1.6	—	—
28–33	25.3	27.0	24.7	—	—
34–36	30.9	32.6	29.8	—	—
≥37	39.6	36.0	41.4	—	—
Birthweight, g (%)					
<400	0.4	0.5	0.4	19.2	16.6
400–499	0.4	0.5	0.5	16.2	16.4
500–599	0.6	0.7	0.6	20.1	20.3
600–699	0.6	0.7	0.6	18.7	19.5
700–799	0.7	0.8	0.6	14.9	15.4
800–899	0.7	0.7	0.7	5.6	6.8
900–999	0.8	0.8	0.7	2.5	2.4
1000–1499	5.6	5.8	5.5	2.3	1.6
≥1500	90.2	89.5	90.4	0.6	1.1
Glucocorticosteroid use	8.9	7.7	10.6	18.3	24.4

2005 (6.1%) and 2013 (3.2%), whereas the proportion of women aged 40 years or more increased by 45% (from 4.2% to 6.1%). The proportion of women with higher education increased over the study period, whereas smoking prevalence rates declined from 8.0% in 2005 to 7.1% in 2013. Although about 5% of periviable twins were induced in 2005 and 2013, almost half underwent cesarean delivery. Changes in maternal and neonatal characteristics of twin live-borns delivered at periviable gestations (20–25 weeks) between 2005 and 2013 are also shown in **Table 1**. Most of the changes in maternal and neonatal characteristics seen for the whole cohort were also evident in the analysis restricted to mothers who delivered twins at periviable gestations. In particular, steroid use increased from 18.3% to 24.4% between 2005 and 2013.

The distribution of twin live births between 2005 and 2013 at the periviable gestational ages are shown in **Fig. 1**. Twin live births delivered at 20 weeks declined by 32% (from 0.25% in 2005 to 0.19% in 2013), whereas births at 22 to 24 weeks increased by 11%, 4%, and 11%, respectively. Twin live births declined by 11% between 2005 (0.69%) and 2013 (0.63%) **(Fig. 2)**.

The risks of twin neonatal and infant mortality, and composite neonatal morbidity across gestational age are shown in **Fig. 1**. Neonatal mortality among twin live births declined sharply with advancing gestational age, beginning at 22 weeks. In contrast, composite neonatal morbidity began to decline starting at 28 weeks of gestation. Twin mortality and composite neonatal morbidity revealed no clinically appreciable differences at 28 weeks and beyond between 2005 and 2013 (data not shown).

Twin neonatal mortality and composite morbidity between 2005 and 2013 are shown in **Table 2**. At 22 and 23 weeks gestation, neonatal mortality rates among twin live births were lower by 11.9% and 13.8%, respectively, in 2013 than in 2005. Over the same period, twin neonatal mortality rates declined by 35% (relative risk, 0.65; 95% confidence interval, 0.49–0.84) and 21% (relative risk, 0.79; 95% confidence interval, 0.70–0.91) at 22 and 23 weeks, respectively. Neonatal mortality at other periviable gestational ages and beyond remained stable between 2005 and 2013. In contrast, composite neonatal morbidity rates among twin live births at 23 weeks increased substantially between 2005 and 2013 (from 904.5 to 959.2 per 1000) **(Table 3)**.

DISCUSSION
Main Findings

Virtually all previous studies of births at periviable gestational ages have been restricted to singleton births or have combined twins with singleton births. The epidemiology of twin live births at periviable gestations, and their survival and morbidity remain virtually unknown. An important finding of this analysis is that, compared with 2005, the neonatal mortality for twins delivered at 23 and 24 weeks was lower in 2013. After adjustment for confounding factors, neonatal mortality was 12% lower in 2013 than 2005 for twins delivered at 23 weeks; and 14% lower for twins delivered at 24 weeks. The improvement in mortality was not seen for deliveries at 20 to 22 weeks or for those born at 25 weeks (or later). Concomitant with the improvement in survival over time, there is a significant increased likelihood of neonatal morbidity at 23 weeks, although not at 24 weeks.

Interpretation of Findings

The potential reasons for the improvement in mortality at 23 and 24 weeks are improved counseling about the neonatal outcomes with periviable births, use of antenatal corticosteroids, use of antibiotics for ruptured membranes or group B

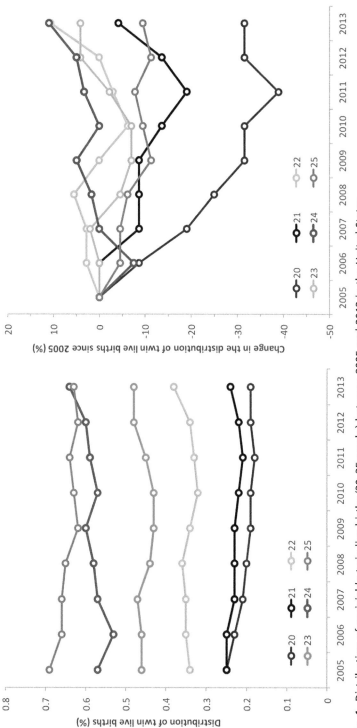

Fig. 1. Distribution of periviable twin live births (20–25 weeks) between 2005 and 2013 in the United States.

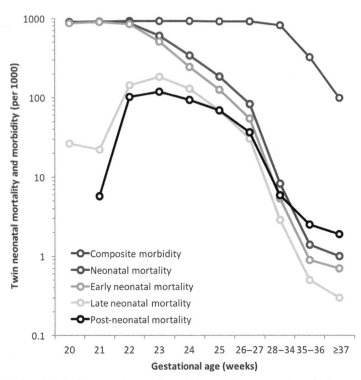

Fig. 2. Risk (per 1000) of neonatal mortality and composite neonatal morbidity among twin periviable live births (20–25 weeks), and at later gestational ages between 2005 and 2013 in the United States.

streptococci, provider's willingness to perform a cesarean delivery for fetal benefit at these periviable gestational ages, continuous electronic fetal monitoring during labor, active intensive treatment of the newborn vis-à-vis neonatal resuscitation, and management in an intensive care unit at the threshold of viability.[13–18] However, the improved neonatal survival at 22 and 23 weeks gestation seems to have resulted in an unintended consequence of increasing the risk of neonatal morbidity (at 23 weeks). This analysis provides granular data about periviable twin births, which was not available at the time when the obstetric care consensus on the topic was published.[2]

Neonatal survival and morbidity data at periviable gestations are strongly influenced by birth registration practices.[19,20] At the population level, variations in birth registration laws can potentially bias international rankings and comparisons of mortality and morbidity statistics.[21] Another reason for the large variability in the frequency of births and neonatal mortality at periviable gestations includes large variation in stillbirth ratios, especially at very early preterm gestations.[21] Even within the United States, variations in practice patterns in the care of twin pregnancies across states, especially delivery at periviable gestations and the care of the severely preterm twin newborns, are likely to have affected these findings.

Indeed, the lower neonatal mortality rates among twin live-borns at 23 and 24 weeks in 2013 compared with 2005 is the unexpected increase in neonatal morbidity rates at 24 weeks. Similar findings have been reported among singleton gestations.[22] Furthermore, preliminary evidence shows increased rates of moderate to severe disability at 2 years of 100%, 44.4%, 33.3%, and 30.4%, respectively, among singleton

Table 2
Risk (per 1000) of neonatal mortality and morbidity in 2005 and 2013 among twins at the borderline of viability: Unites States twin live births

Neonatal Outcomes Among Twin Live Births	Gestational Age at Delivery											
	20 wk		21 wk		22 wk		23 wk		24 wk		25 wk	
	2005	2013	2005	2013	2005	2013	2005	2013	2005	2013	2005	2013
Number of twin live births	99	227	97	286	134	451	178	564	221	763	268	741
Neonatal mortality	858.6	876.7	917.5	930.1	835.8	873.6	736.0	590.4	457.0	321.1	227.6	168.7
Early neonatal mortality	848.5	872.2	917.5	930.1	828.4	855.9	691.0	503.5	307.7	216.3	160.4	108.0
Late neonatal mortality	66.7[a]	34.5[a]	—	—	43.5[a]	123.1	145.5	175.0	215.7	133.8	80.0	68.1
Postneonatal mortality	—	—	—	—	181.8	105.3	191.5	116.9	75.0	90.7	115.9	55.2
Composite neonatal morbidity	848.5	919.9	948.5	898.6	917.9	933.5	904.5	959.2	932.1	935.8	929.1	924.4
Neonatal seizures	—	—	—	—	—	—	—	7.1[a]	4.5[a]	—	—	—
Assisted ventilation <30 min	61.9	22.5	161.3	14.3[a]	219.7	116.3	445.1	462.5	522.7	514.6	615.7	494.6
Assisted ventilation ≥6 h	51.5[a]	4.5[a]	64.5	10.7[a]	90.9	64.9	260.1	292.9	340.9	350.0	380.6	341.0
Significant birth injury	20.6[a]	—	—	—	—	—	—	—	—	2.6[a]	14.9[a]	4.1[a]
NICU admission	195.5	107.6	247.3	92.9	386.4	308.7	589.6	676.8	827.3	861.1	880.6	887.2
5-min Apgar score <4	888.9	939.0	957.0	932.8	754.0	877.9	479.3	494.6	215.6	221.2	158.3	156.9

Abbreviation: NICU, neonatal intensive care unit.
[a] Indicates that the number of cases is too few (<5) for stable estimates of risk.

infants born at 21 to 23, 24, 25, and 26 weeks gestation. At 5 years, moderate to severe disability rates were 16.7%, 22.2%, and 14.3%, respectively, for those born at 24, 25, and 26 weeks gestation.[23] Despite the benefits of surfactant and glucocorticosteroids (almost one-fourth of twin live births in 2013 were administered steroids before birth) to improve survival of extremely preterm infants,[24,25] it is reasonable to speculate that clinicians' opinions and attitudes about providing neonatal intensive care to sick twin newborns[26] may have partly contributed to the observed prevalence estimates of adverse outcomes. Another complicating factor regarding the very high mortality of infants at these extremely low gestational ages concerns ethical end-of-life decisions.[27]

Limitations of the Data

A few limitations of the study merit discussion. First, the possibility of registering a live-born twin at the borderline of viability as a stillborn has been reported in a few states in the United States.[28] This practice is to avoid having to complete two certificates (first a live birth, and then an infant death) instead of a single certificate of stillbirth. If this is true, then a small fraction of twins recorded as twin stillbirths in this cohort may

Table 3
Changes in neonatal mortality and morbidity between 2005 and 2013 among births at the borderline of viability: Unites States twin live births

Gestational Age (wk)	Neonatal Mortality		Composite Neonatal Morbidity	
	Adjusted Risk Difference (95% CI)	Adjusted Risk Ratio (95% CI)	Adjusted Risk Difference (95% CI)	Adjusted Risk Ratio (95% CI)
20	2.7 (−7.5 to 12.9)	0.96 (0.87 to 1.05)	5.9 (−7.8 to 19.5)	0.92 (0.84 to 1.01)
21	0.8 (−9.1 to 10.7)	0.99 (0.92 to 1.08)	4.6 (−15.6 to 6.5)	1.05 (0.98 to 1.12)
22	3.1 (−4.2 to 10.4)	1.27 (0.83 to 1.92)	2.3 (−3.7 to 8.2)	1.25 (0.63 to 2.44)
23	−11.9 (−19.5 to −4.3)	0.65 (0.49 to 0.84)	4.7 (−1.9 to 11.3)	2.22 (1.18 to 4.17)
24	−13.8 (−21.2 to −6.4)	0.79 (0.70 to 0.91)	0.8 (−6.0 to 7.6)	1.27 (0.73 to 2.22)
25	−5.7 (−11.9 to 0.6)	—[a]	0.2 (−6.1 to 6.4)	0.94 (0.57 to 1.56)
26–27	−2.0 (−4.4 to 0.4)	0.98 (0.95 to 1.01)	−1.0 (−3.7 to 1.6)	0.93 (0.69 to 1.27)
28–33	−0.3 (−0.5 to 0.0)	1.00 (0.99 to 1.01)	7.3 (−6.4 to 8.2)	1.54 (1.47 to 1.61)
34–36	−0.5 (−1.5 to 0.6)	—[a]	3.6 (−2.6 to 4.5)	1.05 (1.04 to 1.06)
≥37	0.0 (−1.0 to 0.1)	—[a]	−1.7 (−2.3 to −1.1)	0.98 (0.97 to 1.00)

Risk difference and risk ratios were adjusted for the confounding effects of maternal age, primiparity, maternal education, race/ethnicity, maternal education, and smoking before pregnancy.

Abbreviation: CI, confidence interval.

[a] The models did not converge.

have been erroneously excluded. Therefore, the risks of adverse neonatal outcomes among twins that we report are likely conservative. The possibility of transcriptional errors in recording gestational age may have affected the findings to some extent. Because the database does not link the two twins to the same mother, the possibility of the variance estimates being imprecise from ignoring the intracluster correlation cannot be discounted.[29,30] Finally, this study is based on states that implemented the 2003 revision of birth certificates, so the analysis does not include data on all twin live births in the United States. The extent to which any systematic differences in the composition of women that delivered twin live births in this study contrasted against all twin live births in the United States remains unknown.

Strengths of the Study

Gestational age in this study was based on the best obstetric estimate, and this is superior to either the clinical estimate or one based on menstrual dating alone. In fact, best obstetric estimate of gestational age dating is now being adopted for all standard reporting of vital statistics data by the National Center for Health Statistics.[31] The sheer volume of twin live births, at the borderline of viability (20–25 weeks) and beyond, offers generalizability of findings.

SUMMARY

This study based on data on a large cohort of twin live births in the United States shows that 2.5% of twin live-born infants are delivered at periviable gestational ages. Between 2005 and 2013, there seems to have been an improvement in twin neonatal survival rates at 23 and 24 weeks gestational age, but at the expense of an untoward increase in twin neonatal morbidity rates at 23 weeks. These observations notwithstanding, this study underscores the acute need for large multicenter studies on twins to evaluate the short- and long-term consequences of infant and childhood survival, and neurodevelopmental and cognitive deficits, if any, among those delivered at periviable gestational ages.

REFERENCES

1. Chauhan SP, Ananth CV. Periviable births: epidemiology and obstetrical antecedents. Semin Perinatol 2013;37:382–8.
2. Obstetric care consensus No. 4: periviable birth. Obstet Gynecol 2016;127: e157–69.
3. Ananth CV, Chauhan SP. Epidemiology of twinning in developed countries. Semin Perinatol 2012;36:156–61.
4. Chauhan SP, Scardo JA, Hayes E, et al. Twins: prevalence, problems, and preterm births. Am J Obstet Gynecol 2010;203:305–15.
5. Hamilton BE, Martin JA, Osterman MJ, et al. Births: final data for 2014. Natl Vital Stat Rep 2015;64:1–64.
6. Bateni ZH, Clark SL, Sangi-Haghpeykar H, et al. Trends in the delivery route of twin pregnancies in the United States, 2006-2013. Eur J Obstet Gynecol Reprod Biol 2016;205:120–6.
7. Misra DP, Ananth CV. Infant mortality among singletons and twins in the United States during 2 decades: effects of maternal age. Pediatrics 2002;110:1163–8.
8. Joseph K, Liu S, Demissie K, et al. A parsimonious explanation for intersecting perinatal mortality curves: understanding the effect of plurality and of parity. BMC Pregnancy Childbirth 2003;3:3.

9. Louwen F, Antwerpen I, Ernst T, et al. Outcome in single and twin pregnancies at 20 to 24 weeks gestation: ten years experience in one perinatal center. Clin Exp Obstet Gynecol 2013;40:342–4.

10. Petit N, Cammu H, Martens G, et al. Perinatal outcome of twins compared to singletons of the same gestational age: a case-control study. Twin Res Hum Genet 2011;14:88–93.

11. Martin JA, Hamilton BE, Sutton PD, et al. Births: final data for 2005. Natl Vital Stat Rep 2007;56:1–103.

12. Martin JA, Hamilton BE, Osterman MJ, et al. Births: final data for 2013. Natl Vital Stat Rep 2015;64:1–65.

13. Litmanovitz I, Reichman B, Arnon S, et al. Perinatal factors associated with active intensive treatment at the border of viability: a population-based study. J Perinatol 2015;35:705–11.

14. Salihu HM, Salinas-Miranda AA, Hill L, et al. Survival of pre-viable preterm infants in the United States: a systematic review and meta-analysis. Semin Perinatol 2013;37:389–400.

15. Stokes TA, Watson KL, Boss RD. Teaching antenatal counseling skills to neonatal providers. Semin Perinatol 2014;38:47–51.

16. Tucker Edmonds B, McKenzie F, Macheras M, et al. Morbidity and mortality associated with mode of delivery for breech periviable deliveries. Am J Obstet Gynecol 2015;213:70.e1–12.

17. Tucker Edmonds B, McKenzie F, Panoch JE, et al. Comparing neonatal morbidity and mortality estimates across specialty in periviable counseling. J Matern Fetal Neonatal Med 2015;28:2145–9.

18. Wapner RJ. Antenatal corticosteroids for periviable birth. Semin Perinatol 2013; 37:410–3.

19. Kramer MS, Platt RW, Yang H, et al. Registration artifacts in international comparisons of infant mortality. Paediatr Perinat Epidemiol 2002;16:16–22.

20. Joseph KS, Liu S, Rouleau J, et al. Influence of definition based versus pragmatic birth registration on international comparisons of perinatal and infant mortality: population based retrospective study. BMJ 2012;344:e746.

21. Deb-Rinker P, Leon JA, Gilbert NL, et al. Differences in perinatal and infant mortality in high-income countries: artifacts of birth registration or evidence of true differences? BMC Pediatr 2015;15:112.

22. Thompson K, Gardiner J, Resnick S. Outcome of outborn infants at the borderline of viability in Western Australia: a retrospective cohort study. J Paediatr Child Health 2016;52:728–33.

23. Poon WB, Ho SK, Yeo CL. Short- and long-term outcomes at 2, 5 and 8 years old for neonates at borderline viability: an 11-year experience. Ann Acad Med Singapore 2013;42:7–17.

24. Allen MC, Donohue PK, Dusman AE. The limit of viability–neonatal outcome of infants born at 22 to 25 weeks' gestation. N Engl J Med 1993;329:1597–601.

25. Stevens TP, Blennow M, Soll RF. Early surfactant administration with brief ventilation vs selective surfactant and continued mechanical ventilation for preterm infants with or at risk for RDS. Cochrane Database Syst Rev 2002;(4):CD003063.

26. Ananth CV, Liu S, Joseph KS, et al. A comparison of foetal and infant mortality in the United States and Canada. Int J Epidemiol 2009;38:480–9.

27. Kelly J, Welch E. Ethical decision-making regarding infant viability. Nurs Ethics 2016. 969733016677869. [Epub ahead of print].

28. Ehrenthal DB, Wingate MS, Kirby RS. Variation by state in outcomes classification for deliveries less than 500 g in the United States. Matern Child Health J 2011;15:42–8.
29. Ananth CV, Platt RW, Savitz DA. Regression models for clustered binary responses: implications of ignoring the intracluster correlation in an analysis of perinatal mortality in twin gestations. Ann Epidemiol 2005;15:293–301.
30. Louis GB, Dukic V, Heagerty PJ, et al. Analysis of repeated pregnancy outcomes. Stat Methods Med Res 2006;15:103–26.
31. Martin JA, Osterman MJ, Kirmeyer SE, et al. Measuring gestational age in vital statistics data: transitioning to the obstetric estimate. Natl Vital Stat Rep 2015; 64:1–20.

Medical and Surgical Interventions Available Before a Periviable Birth

Edward K. Chien, MD, MBA[a,b],*, Kelly S. Gibson, MD[a,b]

KEYWORDS

- Periviable birth • Progesterone • Antenatal corticosteroids • Magnesium sulfate
- Cerclage • Amniocentesis

KEY POINTS

- Periviable deliveries are a small proportion of all deliveries, but contribute greatly to long-term morbidities.
- Few studies exist on interventions in the periviable period.
- Limited data suggest that antenatal corticosteroids and magnesium sulfate may be beneficial and tocolysis may help achieve latency for these therapies.
- Prophylactic progesterone or cerclage are associated with a reduction in preterm deliveries.
- Amniocentesis may help guide therapy when there is a suspicion of intrauterine infection.

INTRODUCTION

Last year the preterm birthrate decreased to 9.67% in the United States with approximately 1 out of every 145 live born infants (0.69%) delivered before 28 weeks of gestation.[1] Neonates born at this early gestation face higher rates of morbidity and mortality, in the initial resuscitation and among the long-term survivors than do infants born later in the preterm period.[2,3] Those delivered between 22 0/7 weeks and 25 6/7 weeks are considered periviable. The earliest consistently reported survival is for those born after 22 weeks, thus the small group of infants born between 22 and 26 weeks face disproportionately high rates of mortality and morbidity, including pulmonary, infectious, and neurologic sequelae and developmental delay.[4,5]

The authors have nothing to disclose.
[a] Department of Reproductive Biology, Case Western Reserve University, 10900 Euclid Avenue, Cleveland, OH 44106, USA; [b] Division of Maternal Fetal Medicine, Department of Obstetrics and Gynecology, Metrohealth Medical Center, 2500 Metrohealth Drive, Suite G237, Cleveland, OH 44109, USA
* Corresponding author. Division of Maternal Fetal Medicine, Department of Obstetrics and Gynecology, Metrohealth Medical Center, 2500 Metrohealth Drive, Suite G237, Cleveland, OH 44109.
E-mail address: echien@metrohealth.org

Many risk factors have been described that identify individuals at risk for preterm birth with prior history of spontaneous preterm birth and a short cervix in the mid-trimester having the greatest sensitivity and specificity.[6] In the past decade, prophylactic therapy has focused on these primary risk factors. However, the ability to identify individuals who will deliver preterm is poor. More than half of women delivering preterm do not have an antecedent risk factor for preterm delivery, such as a prior preterm birth, pregnancy loss, or a short cervix.[7] Women with periviable birth often present with preterm labor or preterm premature rupture of membranes. Therefore interventions that may improve outcome can be gleaned from studies related to preterm labor. These strategies are primarily focused on either delaying delivery or preparing the fetus for an early delivery. The available interventions include medical and surgical evaluation (**Box 1**). Tocolysis, progesterone, and cerclage may help prolong a pregnancy. Simultaneously, magnesium sulfate and antenatal corticosteroids may be administered for newborn benefit.

Most preterm birth research and intervention has focused on reduction of preterm birth before 34, 36, or 37 weeks of gestation.[8–10] Some of these studies report outcomes by stratifying results at 28 weeks of gestation. However, because early preterm birth is not typically the primary outcome these studies are insufficiently powered to identify the impact of the study intervention at earlier gestational ages. Not surprisingly outcomes for the periviable period between 22 and 26 weeks of gestation are also not typically available. Interventions are often restricted to those considered potentially viable, and even in recent years those at 23 to 24 weeks of gestation were excluded from many studies. Interventions that prolong gestation by even a few days within the periviable period may significantly decrease mortality and morbidity. Thus, an improved understanding of the efficacy and available interventions within this time period is critical.

Other factors also have been shown to contribute to outcomes in the periviable period. Variations in practices between hospitals and among providers for the resuscitation and care given in the periviable period are some of the factors that contribute to variability in outcomes.[11,12] Factors that may contribute to differences in local practices include resource availability, provider experience, or other biases. This variation compounds the difficulty in data interpretation because a periviable death at one institution that provides only comfort care should not be viewed similarly to a periviable death after a full and aggressive resuscitation at another. Determining the "denominator" for whom resuscitation was planned is an important factor in understanding the outcomes related to the periviable period.

Box 1
Interventions

Surgical Interventions

Cerclage

Amniocentesis

Medical Interventions

Progesterone

Corticosteroids

Magnesium sulfate

Tocolysis

Given these limitations we discuss the potential role of medical and surgical interventions on outcomes based on what can be gleaned from larger studies targeted at reducing preterm birth. The focus is on the following medical interventions: tocolysis, progesterone, magnesium sulfate, and corticosteroids. We also discuss the role of two primary procedural interventions in the management of periviable birth, amniocentesis and cervical cerclage.

SURGICAL INTERVENTIONS
Cerclage

The use of prophylactic cerclage remains controversial,[13] but of all the interventions being discussed, the cerclage may have the greatest impact specific to periviable outcomes. The indications for cerclage are categorized into (1) history-indicated cerclage, (2) ultrasound-indicated cerclage, and (3) physical examination–indicated cerclage (**Box 2**). Well-performed randomized clinical trials evaluating the efficacy of cerclage are limited. The use of a cerclage based on obstetric history is generally referred to as a prophylactic cerclage and has been prescribed for those with prior history of a second trimester pregnancy loss often associated with painless cervical dilation. Ultrasound-indicated cerclage has become a more frequent event in this era of transvaginal cervical length assessment. A short cervical length with or without a history of preterm birth is recognized as a risk for preterm birth. The physical examination–indicated cerclage is performed when the cervix is dilated with the fetal membranes protruding into the cervical canal past the internal cervical os or hourglassing into the vagina. The data to support these procedures for reducing periviable birth are discussed. The technical aspects of cerclage placement and perioperative management are outside the scope of this article. The use of single versus double suture, tocolytics, antibiotics, and suture material are not discussed but may impact surgical success and are found elsewhere.

The biologic basis for cervical insufficiency/incompetence is still limited. The causes for cervical insufficiency are believed to be multifactorial. Cervical competence refers to the ability to maintain the fetus in utero through gestation. The mechanical properties are influenced by a variety of factors including subclinical infection, inflammation, hormonal environment, genetic predisposition, and mechanical environment.[14] The placement of a cerclage is believed to reinforce the mechanical properties of the cervix to prevent early or progressive deformation of the cervix[15] but it may improve outcome through other mechanisms, such as enhancing the barrier function by reducing access to bacteria. The cerclage does not necessarily reverse or inhibit the mechanisms responsible for the loss of tissue resistance that can occur because of infection or inflammation, and this may limit potential benefits a cerclage can provide.

In general, evidence to support prophylactic cerclage placement is lacking. In the most recent Cochrane review evaluating the use of cerclage in singleton pregnancies, the authors concluded that there was insufficient evidence for a cerclage to improve

---

Box 2
Cerclage indications

History indicated (prophylactic)

Ultrasound indicated

Physical examination indicated

perinatal outcomes.[16] This conclusion was based on a meta-analysis of three trials, with one study from the United Kingdom's Medical Research Council contributing 82% of participants.[17] The Medical Research Council study determined that the number needed to treat to reduce one preterm birth was 25 and concluded that a prophylactic cerclage is most warranted in individuals with three prior preterm deliveries.[17] The Cochrane review noted there was no reduction in births before 28 weeks when comparing cerclage with no cerclage. The use of prophylactic cerclage is less likely to impact the incidence of periviable births but may reduce preterm delivery before 37 weeks.

The association of transvaginal cervical length in the mid-trimester and preterm birth has led to what is referred to as an ultrasound-indicated cervical cerclage. In the past two decades several trials have been performed to evaluate the benefit of cerclage in women with a short cervical length. One large multicentered trial did not find a significant reduction in preterm birth before 35 weeks.[9] A planned secondary analysis did demonstrate a reduction in previable birth (<24 weeks) with a reduction in perinatal mortality after cerclage placement in women at high risk of preterm birth because of cervical shortening to 25 mm or less.[9] A subsequent patient-level meta-analysis of five trials, including this study, evaluated the benefit of cerclage in reducing preterm birth, perinatal mortality, and morbidity.[18] This meta-analysis demonstrated reductions in preterm birth before 24, 28, 32, and 37 weeks of gestation suggesting that ultrasound-indicated cerclage may reduce periviable births. For individuals with a cervical length less than 16 mm, the benefit of cerclage was less clear for reducing births before 24 weeks (relative risk [RR], 0.53; 95% confidence interval [CI], 0.24–1.16). This patient-level meta-analysis suggests the primary benefit of ultrasound-indicated cerclage was in high-risk women with a cervical length between 15 and 25 mm with respect to periviable birth, but was unable to identify reductions in morbidities with this intervention.[18,19] The use of an ultrasound-indicated cerclage for women without a prior history of spontaneous preterm birth and a short cervix has yet to be demonstrated.

Examination-indicated cerclage (rescue cerclage) has been well described in the literature, although only one small randomized controlled trial has been performed.[20] Several observational studies have described individuals receiving a cerclage and compared them with others managed expectantly.[21–23] In a systematic review and meta-analysis performed to evaluate the benefit of an examination-indicated cerclage, 10 studies involving 757 women with sufficient information for analysis were identified.[24] The authors found a significant benefit in those undergoing a cerclage, with an average prolongation of 34 days accompanied by reductions in newborn morbidity and mortality. The average prolongation of pregnancy after the identification of cervical dilation and prolapsing membranes was 14 days in the expectant management group. Physical examination–indicated cerclage reduced the preterm birth rate between 24 and 28 weeks of gestation. The authors reported several differences between the cerclage and expectant management groups including the gestational age at enrollment. Cerclage placement based on ultrasound-identified cervical shortening or because of early cervical dilation is associated with complications including membrane rupture and increased rates of cervical lacerations.[25] Reported rates of rupture vary but are as frequent as 1%. Cervical laceration rates of 7% have also been reported. In the absence of a randomized clinical trial it seems that an examination–indicated cerclage is of potential clinical benefit for reducing periviable births.

Amniocentesis

Amniocentesis has been advocated as a method to evaluate for intrauterine infection in those presenting with contractions in the periviable period. When a patient presents in labor or with a short cervix but intact membranes, infection is a common finding in the periviable period.[26] In patients where the diagnosis of infection is possible but not clinically obvious, amniocentesis is used to sample the amniotic fluid and evaluate for infection by performing a Gram stain, evaluating analytes/biomarkers, and for culture. In individuals with prolapsing membranes amniocentesis for amnio reduction has been described to reduce the degree of prolapse in advance of cerclage placement, although other techniques are also available.

The amniotic fluid levels of glucose and a variety of inflammatory markers have been associated with preterm delivery caused by infection. Glucose values greater than 20 mg/dL are considered normal, whereas values less than 5 mg/dL have a positive amniotic fluid culture in 90% of cases.[27,28] Interleukin-6 has also been consistently shown to be elevated in cases with intra-amniotic infection and risk for preterm delivery but is generally not available for clinical use.[28] A recent meta-analysis found that women who delivered preterm had significantly higher amniotic fluid interleukin-6 and matrix metalloproteinase-8 levels, and a significantly lower glucose level than those delivering at term (interleukin-6: difference in means = 0.32; 95% CI, 0.22–0.43; P<.001; matrix metalloproteinase-8: difference in means = 4.47; 95% CI, 0.83–8.11; P = .016; glucose: difference in means = −5.22; 95% CI, −8.19 to −2.26; P = .001).[29] Despite the utility of these markers to identify inflammation, the sensitivity and specificity for identifying culture-positive intra-amniotic infection remains poor. A small trial that compared the outcomes of neonates whose mothers were randomized to amniocentesis or observation after presenting in preterm labor without clinical suspicion of infection reported no benefit to amniocentesis.[30] Thus, although amniocentesis is a useful tool in those at risk for infection, it does not seem to improve outcomes in other instances of preterm labor.

In women with symptoms of chorioamnionitis, amniocentesis offers an option to gather information about an infectious cause that is used to guide management. Infection is one of the few antenatal indicators outside of gestational age at delivery that identify individuals at greater risk for poor neurologic outcome. The additional information provided by amniocentesis can help to guide decisions during the periviable period. Management decisions, such as when to administer antenatal corticosteroids or magnesium sulfate or whether to tocolyze or place a cerclage, depend on the understanding of why a particular patient is at risk for preterm delivery.

MEDICAL INTERVENTIONS
Progesterone

Progesterone has become the single most common intervention for preterm birth prevention in individuals identified at high risk. Various formulations of progesterone have been advocated based on clinical findings and published research studies. The mechanism of action in reducing preterm birth is still unclear. Progesterone has been shown to inhibit myometrial activity, reduce collagen turnover, and alter cervical mucous, which are all plausible explanations for its efficacy.[31–33] Intramuscular 17-hydroxyprogesterone caproate (17-OHPC), when used for prophylaxis, has been shown to reduce preterm birth in individuals with a prior spontaneous preterm delivery but not in nulliparous women with a short cervix.[34,35] Berghella and coworkers[36] analyzed a subset of individuals from the original Maternal Fetal Medicine Unit Network trial evaluating 17-OHPC in individuals with prior preterm birth and a short cervix.[34] This study demonstrated a significant reduction in births before 24 weeks in individuals receiving intramuscular 17-OHPC and having a short cervix, from 20% to 2%. The total preterm birth rate before 37 weeks was no different. This suggests that 17-OHPC may reduce periviable births in individuals with a short cervix and a prior history of preterm birth but not necessarily reduce the overall number of preterm births before 37 weeks.

The use of intravaginal progesterone has been advocated for individuals with a short cervical length in the mid-trimester of pregnancy based on several randomized clinical trials.[36,37] Secondary analysis of these progesterone intervention trials suggested a potential benefit of progesterone on reducing periviable birth without having a significant impact on the preterm birth rate.[36,37] The recently published OPPTIMUM trial evaluated a heterogeneous population at risk for preterm birth including a short cervical length and found no difference in preterm birth rates.[38] Although not powered specifically to evaluate a short cervical length there was a trend toward reduced preterm birth rates in individuals receiving vaginal progesterone with a cervical length of 25 mm or less.[38] There did not seem to be a reduction in preterm births before 25 weeks of gestation. Although intravaginal progesterone may reduce preterm birth, the long-term benefits remain unclear. Unfortunately, most individuals destined to have a periviable birth have no identifiable risk factor or a prior spontaneous preterm birth.[11] With the widespread use of cervical length evaluation, individuals without a history of spontaneous preterm birth are being identified with a short cervix. Vaginal progesterone has been advocated in this group of patients including by the American College of Obstetrics and Gynecology.[39]

The utility of vaginal progesterone for prevention of periviable birth is unknown. The PROMISE study evaluate the utility of vaginal progesterone in women with recurrent miscarriages.[40] In this multicenter international trial, women with recurrent miscarriages were randomized to vaginal progesterone or placebo. The preterm birth and live birth rates after 24 weeks were not different. Given this information vaginal progesterone is unlikely to have clinical benefit for reducing periviable birth without a short cervix and may have only marginal, if any, benefit for individuals with a short cervix but without other risk factors.

Most women destined to have a periviable birth are not under treatment with progesterone. This has led to multiple investigations to determine the efficacy of progesterone on the acute management of spontaneous preterm labor. A systematic review and meta-analysis performed by Suhag and coworkers[41] addressed the issue of maintenance progesterone therapy after arrested preterm labor. The authors identified five randomized trials that included 441 singleton gestations and found a reduction in preterm birth less than 37 weeks. However, they concluded that vaginal progesterone could not be advocated because of the poor quality of the published studies. The earliest gestational age included in these studies was 24 weeks, limiting the ability to address the impact on the entire periviable period. Although studies have suggested a slight prolongation of gestation, progesterone has not been demonstrated to be an effective tocolytic or to improve perinatal outcomes.[32] The use of progesterone in combination with other agents has also not been shown to be beneficial.[42] These studies suggest that progesterone is unlikely to be beneficial during periviable period for maintenance therapy.

Vaginal progesterone and 17-OHPC are being used clinically in different populations for varying indications. Data to support the clinical benefit for either of these treatments in reducing periviable birth are limited. Further study is warranted to understand the impact of these agents on the periviable period.

Antenatal Corticosteroids

In 1972 Liggins and Howie[43] published their sentinel work demonstrating a reduction in respiratory distress in neonates who were exposed to antenatal corticosteroids. Two decades later the National Institutes of Health concluded that there was strong evidence that glucocorticoids reduce adverse neonatal outcomes, including death, the respiratory distress syndrome, and other complications when administered for fetuses between 24 and 34 weeks of gestation.[44] This period of gestation includes the saccular phase of lung development, and steroid administration induces the type II pneumocytes to increase surfactant production.[45]

The periviable period encompasses the cannicular phase of lung development when type II pneumocytes are beginning to flatten and line the alveoli. Most randomized trials on the use of antenatal corticosteroids excluded this gestational age. Additionally, most studies use respiratory distress as a primary outcome, and essentially all periviable neonates develop respiratory distress because of the absence of alveolar development in their lungs. Recent studies have therefore evaluated other outcomes for infants exposed to steroids in the periviable period to assess whether there is any benefit at these gestational ages.

The only studies reporting on the early periviable period are retrospective cohort studies. **Table 1** includes the summary of these studies. Carlo and colleagues[46] reviewed neonates born at hospitals in the Eunice Kennedy Shriver National Institute of Child Health and Human Development Neonatal Research Network from 1993 to 2009 and reported a significantly benefit at 23 weeks and older with antenatal corticosteroids. A significant reduction in death and neurodevelopmental impairment at 18 months for infants whose mothers had received antenatal corticosteroids was demonstrated (83.4% vs 90.5% at 23 weeks, 68.4% vs 80.3% at 24 weeks, and 52.7% vs 67.9% at 25 weeks). At 22 weeks of gestation there was a nonsignificant trend toward benefit because of small numbers (90.2% vs 93.1%; n = 383).[45] Similarly, Mori and colleagues[47] found a significant survival benefit even at 22 to 23 weeks in neonates at 87 tertiary centers in Japan.

Other studies reporting on outcomes of periviable neonates have consistently shown antenatal corticosteroid administration to be of benefit with an adjusted odds ratio for death with steroids versus without around 0.6.[48-50] Based on those data, Wapner[51] estimated that seven to nine infants needed to be treated to prevent one death. In a single center where resuscitation was routine, antenatal corticosteroid administration was strongly associated with increased survival (odds ratio, 5.27) with a number needed to treat of only 2.4 to prevent a single death.[52,53] These various nonrandomized cohorts suggest a benefit for antenatal corticosteroids in the 22-to-23-week gestational window.

Table 1 Adjusted odds ratio of neonatal morbidity and mortality by week of gestation antenatal corticosteroids				
	Death	Chronic Lung Disease	Intraventricular Hemorrhage	Major Disability or Death at 18 mo
Carlo et al,[46] 2011; United States				
22 wk	0.61 (0.34–1.07)	1.33 (0.51–3.45)	0.94 (0.20–4.49)	0.80 (0.29–2.21)
23 wk	0.49 (0.39–0.61)	0.83 (0.57–1.21)	0.59 (0.40–0.87)	0.58 (0.42–0.80)
24 wk	0.64 (0.54–0.76)	1.69 (1.30–2.20)	0.81 (0.61–1.08)	0.62 (0.49–0.78)
25 wk	0.57 (0.48–0.69)	1.33 (1.06–1.67)	0.56 (0.44–0.72)	0.61 (0.50–0.74)
Mori et al,[47] 2011; Japan				
22–23 wk	0.72 (0.53–0.97)	0.71 (0.34–1.42)	1.13 (0.79–1.60)	—
24–25 wk	0.65 (0.50–0.86)	1.01 (0.75–1.36)	0.64 (0.51–0.79)	—

Data presented as adjusted odds ratio (95% CI).

Magnesium Sulfate

Although antenatal corticosteroids have been associated with a reduction of intraventricular hemorrhage, periventricular leukomalacia, and death, the risk of cerebral palsy for those born during the periviable period remains high at 8% to 12%.[46] Cerebral palsy describes a group of disorders of development involving movement and posture, causing activity limitation. These disorders are attributed to nonprogressive disturbances that occurred in the developing fetal or infant brain.[52] Approximately half of cerebral palsy is attributed to preterm birth.[2]

The potential benefit of magnesium sulfate on neurodevelopmental outcome was recognized in a study evaluating magnesium sulfate for seizure prophylaxis in individuals with preeclampsia, the MAGPIE trial.[54] Infants of women exposed to magnesium sulfate were observed to have a reduction in cerebral palsy, possibly as a result of a reduction in intraventricular hemorrhage in very preterm neonates.[55-57] These observations, which held biologic plausibility via reduction in reperfusion injury and free radical damage, led to several large clinical trials.[58-62]

Clinical trials evaluating the impact of magnesium sulfate on neurodevelopment outcome have conflicting results. Although two initial trials did not show a significant benefit of magnesium sulfate treatment,[58,59] three larger studies have suggested a benefit to magnesium sulfate therapy. In 2003, the ActoMgSO4 trial studied 1062 Australian women at risk of delivery before 30 weeks. The combined outcome of stillbirth or death before the age of 2 was less frequent among the children of women randomized to magnesium sulfate than among those who received placebo (13.8% vs 17.1%; RR, 0.83; 95% CI, 0.64–1.09). Substantial gross motor dysfunction was significantly less common among children treated with magnesium sulfate (3.4% vs 6.6%; RR, 0.51 [0.29–0.91]).[59] The PREMAG trial, conducted in France and including a 2-year follow-up, found no benefit for cerebral palsy (16.1% vs 20.2%; adjusted odds ratio, 0.65 [0.42–1.03]) but did find an improvement in gross motor dysfunction (25.6% vs 30.8%; 0.62 [0.41–0.93]).[61] Finally, the National Institute of Child Health and Human Development Maternal Fetal Medicine Units network conducted a trial in the United States and found no difference in the primary outcome of cerebral palsy or death (11.3% vs 11.7%; RR, 0.97 [0.77–1.23]), but did find a significant reduction in cerebral palsy alone (1.9% vs 3.5%; 0.55 [0.32–0.95]).[62] The primary benefit was in infants born before 28 weeks. Combining these studies in a systemic review, magnesium sulfate was associated with a significant reduction in the combined outcome of cerebral palsy or fetal/infant death (RR, 0.85 [0.74–0.98]).[63]

Overall, maternal treatment with magnesium sulfate seems to improve neurologic outcomes when administered before a preterm birth as early as 24 weeks (number needed to treat is 63).[64] The clinical benefit seems to be in those born at earlier gestational ages. Although not all periviable gestational ages were included in the studies presented, given the high risk for adverse neurologic outcomes and potential benefit at the earlier gestational age windows, this therapy may provide significant benefit in the periviable period when delivery is imminent.

Tocolysis

The use of tocolytic therapy continues to evolve with preferences that are often institutionally dependent. A variety of agents have been investigated over the past four decades; the most common include beta-mimetics, magnesium sulfate, oxytocin receptor antagonists, calcium channel blockers, and cyclooxygenase inhibitors. Among these agents the evidence to support their efficacy varies, and none have specifically addressed the periviable period. When compared with placebo, most of these agents have been shown to delay delivery from 48 hours to 7 days[65–69] in the setting of preterm labor with intact membranes but evidence to support newborn benefit is lacking. Tocolytic trials rarely enroll participants before 24 weeks of gestation and older studies often used higher gestational age limits for enrollment.[68] The mean gestational age of enrolled participants often runs from 28 to 32 weeks.[68] These limitations prevent evidence-based recommendations concerning the use of tocolysis in the periviable period.

The periviable period is associated with rapidly increasing rates of survival from 22 to 26 weeks with significant declines in perinatal morbidity. The potential benefit of tocolytics with a delay of a few days could substantially improve outcome. Despite this the use of tocolysis should be evaluated with caution. In the presence of preterm premature rupture of membranes tocolysis has been associated with prolongation of gestation but also higher rates of perinatal mortality because of increased rates of infectious morbidity.[70] Tocolytics are commonly used in conjunction with the placement of cervical cerclage. No randomized clinical studies have been performed specifically evaluating the benefit of tocolysis on outcomes in conjunction with cerclage placement.

Systematic reviews of the most commonly prescribed agents have been performed. Based on these reviews the evidence to support a prolongation of gestation for magnesium sulfate and the oxytocin receptor antagonist Atosiban is lacking.[65,66] The APOSTEL III trial comparing Atosiban to nifedipine failed to show a significant difference in outcomes with the median time to delivery of 4 days for Atosiban and 7 days for nifedipine.[71] There is evidence to support the use of magnesium sulfate for neuroprotection,[63] although it has not been shown to be an effective tocolytic agent. Ritodrine, the only medication approved by the Food and Drug Administration for tocolysis (beta-mimetic), has been shown to delay delivery up to 48 hours, but it is no longer commercially available. Other beta-mimetics seem to have similar efficacy for pregnancy prolongation. Nifedipine (calcium channel blocker) and indomethacin (cyclooxygenase inhibitor) are effective at inhibiting contractions thereby delaying delivery.[67,68] Indomethacin has been shown to reduce rates of preterm delivery before 37 weeks and reduce the rate of delivery within 48 hours of initiation.[67] Nifedipine seems to have the greatest inhibitory effect with lower preterm birth rates before 37 and 34 weeks when compared with any other tocolytic agent.[68] The use of nifedipine is also associated with a lower rate of births within 7 days of therapy initiation compared with other tocolytic agents.[68] A single trial compared nifedipine with indomethacin and found a lower rate of preterm births in individuals exposed to nifedipine.[72] These trials did not include pregnancies in the periviable period limiting generalizability.

Tocolytic therapy has been shown to delay delivery an average of 48 to 72 hours for the general preterm population. There is no reason to believe that these agents would be less effective at delaying delivery during the periviable period from 22 to 26 weeks. However, evidence supporting an improvement in newborn outcomes is lacking and warrants further study. The potential benefit of a few additional days in utero could substantially reduce the risk of mortality and morbidity in the periviable period. Of the agents with the most promise, nifedipine and indomethacin therapy would be good candidates for evaluation based on their mechanism of action and risk-benefit profile.

SUMMARY/DISCUSSION

Periviable birth is a major contributor to perinatal morbidity and mortality. Interventions to improve perinatal outcome related to periviable birth have not been specifically studied. Survivors born during the periviable period are at high risk for having developmental delays and major physical disabilities. The interventions discussed prolong pregnancy from nonviability into the periviable period placing the fetus at risk for significant disabilities. The parents of the fetus should be carefully counseled on the potential outcomes before embarking on many of these interventions given the potential social and economic impact a severely impaired infant may have on the family unit.

Of all the interventions reviewed, ultrasound-indicated and examination-indicated cerclage have the greatest evidence for reducing periviable birth. Progesterone therapy has been demonstrated to be effective at reducing recurrent preterm birth and therefore may improve or reduce the incidence of periviable birth. Several randomized trials have suggested a clinical benefit of magnesium sulfate on neurologic outcomes in very preterm birth but the benefit for gestations before 24 weeks has not been tested. Given the high morbidity related to gestations before 24 weeks the clinical benefit likely outweighs any risk. Cohort studies strongly suggest a benefit of antenatal corticosteroids for improving outcomes for infants born at 22 and 23 weeks of gestation. In the absence of additional data where intervention is planned antenatal corticosteroids should be administered when possible. Tocolytics have not been evaluated in randomized clinical trials for gestations at 22 or 23 weeks. Tocolytic agents have been shown to be effective in delaying delivery for 48 hours. Given that during the periviable period the change in mortality for each day of gestation may improve a few percentage points it is a reasonable intervention that should be considered. Research is needed to better clarify the benefit of these interventions on outcome before 24 weeks of gestation, a period that has not been studied.

REFERENCES

1. Hamilton BE, Martin JA, Osterman MJK, et al. no 12. Births: final data for 2014. National vital statistics reports, vol. 64. Hyattsville (MD): National Center for Health Statistics; 2015.
2. Wood NS, Marlow N, Costeloe K, et al. Neurologic and developmental disability after extremely preterm birth. EPICure Study Group. N Engl J Med 2000;343(6): 378–84.
3. Tucker J, McGuire W. Epidemiology of preterm birth. BMJ 2004;329(7467): 675–8.
4. Raju TN, Mercer BM, Burchfield DJ, et al. Periviable birth: executive summary of a joint workshop by the Eunice Kennedy Shriver National Institute of Child Health and Human Development, Society for Maternal-Fetal Medicine, American Academy of Pediatrics, and American College of Obstetricians and Gynecologists. Am J Obstet Gynecol 2014;210(5):406–17.
5. Lau C, Ambalavanan N, Chakraborty H, et al. Extremely low birth weight and infant mortality rates in the United States. Pediatrics 2013;151:855–60.
6. Goldenberg RL, Iams JD, Mercer BM, et al. The preterm prediction study: the value of new vs standard risk factors in predicting early and all spontaneous preterm births. NICHD MFMU Network. Am J Public Health 1998;88(2):233–8.
7. Mercer B, Milluzzi C, Collin M. Periviable birth at 20 to 26 weeks of gestation: proximate causes, previous obstetric history and recurrence risk. Am J Obstet Gynecol 2005;193(3 Pt 2):1175–80.
8. Romero R, Nicolaides KH, Conde-Agudelo A, et al. Vaginal progesterone decreases preterm birth ≤ 34 weeks of gestation in women with a singleton pregnancy and a short cervix: an updated meta-analysis including data from the OPPTIMUM study. Ultrasound Obstet Gynecol 2016;48(3):308–17.

9. Owen J, Hankins G, Iams JD, et al. Multicenter randomized trial of cerclage for preterm birth prevention in high-risk women with shortened midtrimester cervical length. Am J Obstet Gynecol 2009;201:375.e1-8.

10. Haas DM, Caldwell DM, Kirkpatrick P, et al. Tocolytic therapy for preterm delivery: systematic review and network meta-analysis. BMJ 2012;345:e6226.

11. Rysavy MA, Li L, Bell EF, et al. Between-hospital variation in treatment and outcomes in extremely preterm infants. N Engl J Med 2015;372(19):1801–11.

12. Tomlinson MW, Kaempf JW, Ferguson LA, et al. Caring for the pregnant woman presenting at periviable gestations: acknowledging the ambiguity and uncertainty. Am J Obstet Gynecol 2010;202:529.e1-6.

13. Rand L, Norwitz E. Current controversies in cervical cerclage. Semin Perinatol 2003;27(1):73–85.

14. Mahendroo M. Cervical remodeling in term and preterm birth: insights from an animal model. Reproduction 2012;143:429–38.

15. House M, Socrate S. The cervix as a biomechanical structure. Ultrasound Obstet Gynecol 2006;28:745–9.

16. Alfirevic Z, Stampalija T, Roberts D, et al. Cervical stitch (cerclage) for preventing preterm birth in singleton pregnancy. Cochrane Database Syst Rev 2012;(4):CD008991.

17. Quinn M. Final report of the MRC/RCOG randomised controlled trial of cervical cerclage. Br J Obstet Gynaecol 1993;100(12):1154–5.

18. Berghella V, Rafael TJ, Szychowski JM, et al. Cerclage for short cervix on ultrasonography in women with singleton gestations and previous preterm birth: a meta-analysis. Obstet Gynecol 2011;117:663–71.

19. Szychowski JM, Owen J, Hankins G, et al. Vaginal Ultrasound Trial Consortium. Can the optimal cervical length for placing ultrasound-indicated cerclage be identified? Ultrasound Obstet Gynecol 2016;48(1):43–7.

20. Althuisius SM, Dekker GA, Hummel P, et al. Cervical incompetence prevention randomized cerclage trial: emergency cerclage with bed rest versus bed rest alone. Am J Obstet Gynecol 2003;189:907–10.

21. Stupin JH, David M, Siedentopf JP, et al. Emergency cerclage versus bed rest for amniotic sac prolapse before 27 gestational weeks: a retrospective, comparative study of 161 women. Eur J Obstet Gynecol Reprod Biol 2008;139:32–7.

22. Debby A, Sadan O, Glezerman M, et al. Favorable outcome following emergency second trimester cerclage. Int J Gynaecol Obstet 2007;96:16–9.

23. Daskalakis G, Papantoniou N, Mesogitis S, et al. Management of cervical insufficiency and bulging fetal membranes. Obstet Gynecol 2006;107:221–6.

24. Ehsanipoor RM, Seligman NS, Saccone G, et al. Physical examination-indicated cerclage: a systematic review and meta-analysis. Obstet Gynecol 2015;126(1):125–35.

25. Dahlke JD, Sperling JD, Chauhan SP, et al. Cervical cerclage during periviability: can we stabilize a moving target? Obstet Gynecol 2016;127(5):934–40.

26. Hillier SL, Martins J, Krohn M, et al. A case-control study of chorioamnionic infection and histologic chorioamnionitis in prematurity. N Engl J Med 1988;319:972–8.

27. Romero R, Brody DT, Oyarzun E, et al. Infection and labor: III. Interleukin-1—a signal for the onset of parturition. Am J Obstet Gynecol 1989;160:1117–23.

28. Kiltz RJ, Burke MS, Porreco RP. Amniotic fluid glucose concentration as a marker for intra-amniotic infection. Am J Obstet Gynecol 1991;78:619.

29. Romero R, Yoon BH, Mazor M, et al. The diagnostic and prognostic value of amniotic fluid white blood cell count, glucose, interleukin-6, and Gram stain in

patients with preterm labor and intact membranes. Am J Obstet Gynecol 1993; 169:805.

30. Maki Y, Furukawa S, Kodama Y, et al. Amniocentesis for threatened preterm labor with intact membranes and the impact on adverse outcome in infants born at 22 to 28 weeks of gestation. Early Hum Dev 2015;91(5):333–7.

31. Anderson L, Martin W, Higgins C, et al. The effect of progesterone on myometrial contractility, potassium channels, and tocolytic efficacy. Reprod Sci 2009;16(11): 1052–61.

32. Su LL, Samue M, Chong YS. Progestational agents for treating threatened or established preterm labour. Cochrane Database Syst Rev 2010;(1):CD006770.

33. Dodd JM, Flenady V, Cincotta R, et al. Prenatal administration of progesterone for preventing preterm birth in women considered to be at risk of preterm birth. Cochrane Database Syst Rev 2006;(1):CD004947.

34. Meis PJ, Klebanoff M, Thom E, et al. Prevention of recurrent preterm delivery by 17 alpha-hydroxyprogesterone caproate. N Engl J Med 2003;348(24):2379–85.

35. Grobman WA, Thom EA, Spong CY, et al, Eunice Kennedy Shriver National Institute of Child Health and Human Development Maternal-Fetal Medicine Units (MFMU) Network. 17 alpha-hydroxyprogesterone caproate to prevent prematurity in nulliparas with cervical length less than 30 mm. Am J Obstet Gynecol 2012; 207(5):390.e1-8.

36. Berghella V, Figueroa D, Szychowski JM, et al, Vaginal Ultrasound Trial Consortium. 17-alpha-hydroxyprogesterone caproate for the prevention of preterm birth in women with prior preterm birth and a short cervical length. Am J Obstet Gynecol 2010;202(4):351.e1-6.

37. Hassan SS, Romero R, Vidyadhari D, et al. Vaginal progesterone reduces the rate of preterm birth in women with a sonographic short cervix: a multicenter, randomized, double-blind, placebo-controlled trial. Ultrasound Obstet Gynecol 2011; 38(1):18–31.

38. Marlow N, Messow CM, Shennan A, et al, OPPTIMUM Study Group. Vaginal progesterone prophylaxis for preterm birth (the OPPTIMUM study): a multicentre, randomised, double-blind trial. Lancet 2016;387(10033):2106–16.

39. American College of Obstetrics & Gynecology. ACOG practice bulletin no. 130: prediction and prevention of preterm birth. Obstet Gynecol 2012;120(4):964–73.

40. Coomarasamy A, Williams H, Truchanowicz E, et al. A randomized trial of progesterone in women with recurrent miscarriages. N Engl J Med 2015;373(22): 2141–8.

41. Suhag A, Saccone G, Berghella V. Vaginal progesterone for maintenance tocolysis: a systematic review and metaanalysis of randomized trials. Am J Obstet Gynecol 2015;213(4):479–87.

42. Rozenberg P, Chauveaud A, Deruelle P, et al, Groupe De Recherche En Obstétrique et Gynécologie. Prevention of preterm delivery after successful tocolysis in preterm labor by 17 alpha-hydroxyprogesterone caproate: a randomized controlled trial. Arch Gynecol Obstet 2012;285(3):585–90.

43. Liggins GC, Howie RN. A controlled trial of antepartum glucocorticoid treatment for prevention of the respiratory distress syndrome in premature infants. Pediatrics 1972;50(4):515–25.

44. Effect of corticosteroids for fetal maturation on perinatal outcomes. NIH Consens Statement 1994;12(2):1–24.

45. Gonzales LW, Ballard PL, Ertsey R, et al. Glucocorticoids and thyroid hormones stimulate biochemical and morphological differentiation of human fetal lung in organ culture. J Clin Endocrinol Metab 1986;62:678–91.

46. Carlo WA, McDonald SA, Fanaroff AA, et al. Association of antenatal corticosteroids with mortality and neurodevelopmental outcomes among infants born at 22 to 25 weeks' gestation. Eunice Kennedy Shriver National Institute of Child Health and Human Development Neonatal Research Network. JAMA 2011;306:2348–58.
47. Mori R, Kusuda S, Fujimura M. Antenatal corticosteroids promote survival of extremely preterm infants born at 22 to 23 weeks of gestation. Neonatal Research Network Japan. J Pediatr 2011;159:110–4.e1.
48. Tyson J, Parikh N, Langer J, et al. Intensive care for extreme prematurity: moving beyond gestational age. N Engl J Med 2008;358(16):1672–81.
49. Hayes E, Paul D, Stahl G, et al. Effect of antenatal corticosteroids on survival for neonates born at 23 weeks of gestation. Obstet Gynecol 2008;111(4):921–6.
50. Bader D, Kugelman A, Boyko V, et al. Risk factors and estimation tool for death among extremely premature infants: a national study. Pediatrics 2010;125(4):696–703.
51. Wapner RJ. Antenatal corticosteroids for periviable birth. Semin Perinatol 2013;37(6):410–3.
52. Kyser KL, Morriss FH Jr, Bell EF, et al. Improving survival of extremely preterm infants born between 22 and 25 weeks of gestation. Obstet Gynecol 2012;119(4):795–800.
53. Bax M, Goldstein M, Rosenbaum P, et al, Executive Committed for the Definition of Cerebral Palsy. Proposed definition and classification of cerebral palsy, April 2005. Dev Med Child Neurol 2005;47:571–6.
54. Altman D, Carroli G, Duley L, et al, Magpie Trial Collaboration Group. Do women with pre-eclampsia, and their babies, benefit from magnesium sulphate? The Magpie Trial: a randomized placebo-controlled trial. Lancet 2002;359:1877–90.
55. Van de Bor M, Verloove-Vanhorick SP, Brand R, et al. Incidence and prediction of periventricular-intraventricular hemorrhage in very preterm infants. J Perinat Med 1987;15:333–9.
56. Leviton A, Kuban KC, Pagano M, et al. Maternal toxemia and neonatal germinal matrix hemorrhage in intubated infants less than 1751g. Obstet Gynecol 1988;72:571–6.
57. Nelson KB, Grether JK. Can magnesium sulfate reduce the risk of cerebral palsy in very low birthweight infants? Pediatrics 1995;95:263–9.
58. Mittendorf R, Dambrosia J, Pryde PG, et al. Association between the use of antenatal magnesium sulfate in preterm labor and adverse health outcomes in infants. Am J Obstet Gynecol 2002;186:1111–8.
59. Magpie Trial Follow-up Study Collaborative Group. The Magpie Trial: a randomized trial comparing magnesium sulfate with placebo for pre-eclampsia. Outcome for children at 18 months. BJOG 2007;114:289–99.
60. Crowther CA, Hiller JE, Doyle LW, et al, Australian Collaborative Trial of Magnesium Sulfate (ACTOMgSO4) Collaborative Group. Effect of magnesium sulfate given for neuroprotection before preterm birth: a randomized control trial. JAMA 2003;290:2669–76.
61. Marret S, Marpeau L, Zupan-Simunek V, et al, PREMAG Trial Group. Magnesium sulphate given before very-preterm birth to protect infant brain: the randomized controlled PREMAG trial. BJOG 2007;114:310–8.
62. Rouse DJ, Hirtz DG, Thom E, et al, Eunice Kennedy Shriver National Institute of Child Health and Human Development Maternal-Fetal Medicine Units Network. A randomized, controlled trial of magnesium sulfate for the prevention of cerebral palsy. N Engl J Med 2008;359:895–905.

63. Dolye LW, Crowther CA, Middleton P, et al. Magnesium sulphate for women at risk of preterm birth for neuroprotection of the fetus. Cochrane Database Syst Rev 2009;(1):CD004661.

64. Rouse DJ, Gibbins KJ. Magnesium sulfate for cerebral palsy prevention. Semin Perinatol 2013;37(6):414–6.

65. Han S, Crowther CA, Moore V. Magnesium maintenance therapy for preventing preterm birth after threatened preterm labour. Cochrane Database Syst Rev 2010;(7):CD000940.

66. Papatsonis D, Flenady V, Cole S, et al. Oxytocin receptor antagonists for inhibiting preterm labour. Cochrane Database Syst Rev 2005;(3):CD004452.

67. King JF, Flenady V, Cole S, et al. Cyclo-oxygenase (COX) inhibitors for treating preterm labour. Cochrane Database Syst Rev 2005;(2):CD001992.

68. King JF, Flenady V, Papatsonis D, et al. Calcium channel blockers for inhibiting preterm labour. Cochrane Database Syst Rev 2003;(1):CD002255.

69. Anotayanonth S, Subhedar NV, Neilson JP, et al. Betamimetics for inhibiting preterm labour. Cochrane Database Syst Rev 2004;(4):CD004352.

70. Mackeen AD, Seibel-Seamon J, Grimes-Dennis J, et al. Tocolytics for preterm premature rupture of membranes. Cochrane Database Syst Rev 2011;(10):CD007062.

71. Van Vliet EO, Nijman TA, Schuit E, et al. Nifedipine versus atosiban for threatened preterm birth (APOSTEL III): a multicentre, randomised controlled trial. Lancet 2016;387(10033):2117–24.

72. Kashanian M, Bahasadri S, Zolali B. Comparison of the efficacy and adverse effects of nifedipine and indomethacin for the treatment of preterm labor. Int J Gynecol Obstetrics 2011;113:192–5.

Management of Extremely Low Birth Weight Infants in Delivery Room

Asma Nosherwan, MBBS[a,b], Po-Yin Cheung, MBBS, PhD[a,b],
Georg M. Schmölzer, MD, PhD[a,b],*

KEYWORDS

- Infants • Newborn • Neonatal resuscitation • Very low birth weight infants

KEY POINTS

- Establishing breathing and improving oxygenation after birth are vital for survival and long-term health of preterm infants.
- Approximately 50% of extremely low birth weight (ELBW) infants are hypothermic after admission to neonatal intensive care units (NICUs).
- Active measures to avoid hypothermia during stabilization in the delivery room (DR) should include the use of plastic wrapping; warming equipment, such as radiant warmers; warmed humidified resuscitation gases; and adequate temperature.
- Respiratory support at birth should aim to facilitate the early establishment of an effective functional residual capacity (FRC), initiate spontaneous breathing, facilitate gas exchange, and deliver an adequate tidal volume, without damaging the lung.
- Current neonatal resuscitation guidelines recommend the use of 21% to 30% oxygen during neonatal resuscitation at birth.

No reprints requested.

Conflict of Interest Statement: None.

Authors' Contributions: conception and design: A. Nosherwan, G.M. Schmölzer; drafting of the article: A. Nosherwan, G.M. Schmölzer; critical revision of the article for important intellectual content: A. Nosherwan, G.M. Schmölzer; and final approval of the article: A. Nosherwan, G.M. Schmölzer.

[a] Centre for the Studies of Asphyxia and Resuscitation, Royal Alexandra Hospital, 10240 Kingsway Avenue Northwest, Edmonton, Alberta T5H 3V9, Canada; [b] Department of Pediatrics, University of Alberta, 116 St & 85 Avenue, Edmonton, Alberta T6G 2R3, Canada

* Corresponding author. Neonatal Research Unit, Centre for the Studies of Asphyxia and Resuscitation, Royal Alexandra Hospital, 10240 Kingsway Avenue Northwest, Edmonton, Alberta T5H 3V9, Canada

E-mail address: georg.schmoelzer@me.com

INTRODUCTION

Establishing breathing and improving oxygenation after birth are vital for survival and long-term health of preterm infants. Very preterm infants often have difficulty in establishing effective breathing after birth because their lungs are structurally immature, surfactant deficient, and not supported by a stiff chest wall,[1] which render the lungs of very preterm infants uniquely susceptible to injury.[2,3] A majority of ELBW infants receive respiratory support in the DR. The DR is a stressful environment where decisions are made quickly and resuscitators need to be skilled in clinical assessment, decision making, and mask ventilation.[4] These tasks, however, are often more difficult than is widely appreciated, and it is possible that these infants are not optimally supported because of difficulties in ventilation and perfusion during initial resuscitation.[1,5,6]

CORD CLAMPING

For centuries a physiologic approach to clamping the cord was routinely used. In the middle of the twentieth century, this physiologic approach to cord clamping was changed to immediate cord clamping (ICC). One reason for this practice change was the thought that keeping the cord intact could contaminate the obstetric sterile field. The practice of ICC has recently been questioned as unphysiologic,[7] which is also reflected in the current neonatal resuscitation guidelines, which recommend delayed cord clamping (DCC) for at least 30 seconds.[4] Using DCC (defined by various definitions of time delays [eg, >30 seconds or until pulsation is no longer detected]) allows transfusion of blood to the newborn from the placenta; it can provide an infant with up to an additional 30% blood volume,[8] which may improve pulmonary blood flow and left ventricular preload.[9] In spontaneously breathing ELBW infants, DCC has short-term benefits on neonatal hemodynamic transition physiology.[10–12] A recent meta-analysis of preterm infants receiving DCC compared with ICC reported on 10 studies (199 infants).[13] Compared with ICC, DCC improves short-term outcomes of ELBW infants (mean difference 0.61; 95% CI, -2.52 to -1.92), including higher blood pressure and hemoglobin on admission and less frequent blood transfusions.[13] Although DCC has been shown to reduce overall intraventricular hemorrhage (IVH) (mainly lower grades 1 and 2) by 50%,[14,15] it has not been proved to reduce the incidence of severe (grade 3 or 4) IVH or death.[13] Furthermore, these short-term benefits have failed to translate into improved neurodevelopment outcomes at later age.[13,16]

Umbilical cord milking (UCM) is an alternate to DCC, is a faster technique of promoting placental transfusion, and takes approximately 5 seconds to 10 seconds.[12] The 2 interventions when compared showed no any difference in mean hemoglobin concentration at birth, number of blood transfusions in first 6 weeks of life,[17] or long-term neurodevelopmental follow-up.[17] Katheria and colleagues[12] showed UCM to be a more efficient technique than DCC to improve blood volume in premature infants when delivered by cesarean section. Alternative strategies include UCM[12] and initiation of resuscitation while the newborn remains attached to the cord.[18,19] Additional evidence is awaited, however, from ongoing clinical trials before this can be translated into clinical practice.

Practical Aspects

Currently, the evidence is equivocal; there is minimal advantage to DCC, which has, at minimum, hematologic benefits; it is suggested that ELBW infants not requiring immediate resuscitation should receive DCC for at least 30 seconds.[4] Infants could be either held above or below the level of the placenta.[20]

THERMOREGULATION

Maintenance of thermal homeostasis using a target range of 36.5°C to 37.5°C is one of the most critical supportive therapies during fetal to neonatal transition, in particular for preterm infants. Silverman and colleagues[21] first cited the association between survival and incubator temperature and hypothermia. On review of the data, only the ELBW infants had higher mortality in the cold (incubator temperature of 28.7°C) than the warm (31.7°C) groups. Both hypothermia and hyperthermia should be avoided during stabilization to prevent common morbidities.[22] Hypothermia remains problematic even when recommended routine thermal care guidelines are followed in the DR. ELBW infants are at a high risk of developing hypothermia due to an imbalance between heat loss by conduction (cold surface), radiation (cool walls), evaporation (thin epidermis with increased permeability), and convection (cool ambient room temperatures) to heat production (reduced quantities of subcutaneous brown fat and inadequate vasomotor responses).[18] There is a dose-related effect on mortality with an increased risk of approximately 30% for each degree below 36.5°C body temperature at admission. Therefore, the current neonatal resuscitation guidelines emphasize the importance of maintaining thermal homeostasis throughout neonatal stabilization. Strategies to minimize heat loss include (1) occlusive wrapping, (2) exothermic warming mattress, (3) warmed humidified resuscitation gases, (4) polyethylene caps, and (5) adequate DR temperature.[4]

A Cochrane review examined different barriers to prevent heat loss (eg, plastic wrap or bag, plastic cap, and stockinet cap).[23] Plastic wraps or bags were effective in reducing heat losses in infants less than 28 weeks' gestation (mean difference [95% CI] 0.68°C [0.45°C –0.91°C]). Plastic caps were effective in reducing heat losses in infants less than 29 weeks' gestation (mean difference [95% CI] 0.80°C [0.41°C –1.19°C]). The Cochrane review concluded that there was insufficient evidence to suggest that either plastic wraps or plastic caps reduce the risk of death during hospitalization,[23] and that stockinet caps were not effective in reducing heat loss.[23]

Using an external heat source (eg, skin-to-skin care [SSC] or a transwarmer mattress) can effectively reduce the risk of hypothermia compared with conventional incubator care for infants.[23] Using SSC or a transwarmer mattress reduces the incidence of hypothermia on admission to NICU in ELBW infants (relative risk [RR]: SSC 95% CI, 0.09 [0.01–0.64]; transwarmer mattress 95% CI, 0.30 [0.11–0.83]). Plastic wraps or bags, plastic caps, SSC, and transwarmer mattresses all keep preterm infants warmer, leading to higher temperatures on admission to neonatal units and less hypothermia. Furthermore, there is emerging evidence to use heated humidified gases for initial respiratory support during EBLW infant resuscitation, resulting in more infants with normothermia compared with cold dry gas (mean [SD] rectal temperature 35.9°C [0.6] vs 36.4°C [0.6] for cold and heated cohorts, respectively; $P = .0001$).[24]

It is recommended that DR temperature should be maintained at 23°C to 26°C.[4] Cold stress and incidence of hypothermia were reduced by increasing the DR temperature to that recommended by World Health Organization.[25] Duryea and colleagues[26] found that an increase in operating room temperature from 20°C to 23°C at the time of cesarean reduced the rate of neonatal and maternal hypothermia (without a measurable decrease in neonatal morbidity). Neonatal resuscitation guidelines (2015) recommend prewarming the DR to 26°C for infants with weight less than 1500 g.[4]

On the contrary, infants born to hyperthermic mothers seem to have increased neonatal mortality, seizures, and encephalopathy. Although there is an association between chorioamnionitis at the time of delivery with cerebral palsy, hyperthermia has many deleterious effects on the perinatal brain, including an increase in cellular metabolic rate and cerebral blood flow alteration; release of excitotoxic products, such as free radicals and glutamate; and hemostatic changes.[27] Therefore, hyperthermia (>38.0°C) should be avoided during stabilization of ELBW infants.[4]

The current evidence is limited by the small number of infants included in randomized trials. No long-term follow-up data are available to recommend any precise method for clinical practice.[23]

Practical Aspects

Active measures should be initiated and performed to avoid hypothermia in ELBW infants during stabilization in DR, including the use of plastic wrapping, warming equipment such as radiant warmer, warmed humidified resuscitation gases, and adequate DR temperature at 26°C. Especially for infants born to mothers with fever, however, vigilance in thermoregulation should be exercised to avoid hyperthermia.

Respiratory support in the delivery room

Although a majority of infants make the fetal-to-neonatal transition without help,[28] ELBW infants often need respiratory support at birth.[28] These infants often have difficulty establishing effective breathing after birth due to structurally immature surfactant-deficient lungs and not supported by a stiff chest wall,[1] which render the lungs of very preterm infants uniquely susceptible to injury. During the transition of spontaneously breathing ELBW infants, to facilitate the early establishment of an effective FRC, reduced atelectotrauma, and improved oxygenation, continuous positive airway pressure (CPAP) has been advocated at the initiation of respiratory support.[29–33] If an infant fails to initiate spontaneous breathing, current neonatal resuscitation guidelines recommend positive pressure ventilation (PPV) via a face mask[4] to establish FRC, facilitate gas exchange, deliver an adequate tidal volume (V_T), and initiate spontaneous breathing, without damaging the lung.[1] Further, using a sustained inflation (SI) may help lung liquid clearance, recruitment of FRC,[34] and positive end-expiratory pressure by preventing repeated collapse and opening of alveoli.[34]

CONTINUOUS POSITIVE AIRWAY PRESSURE

Observational studies in the era before the widespread use of antenatal steroids and the introduction of surfactant and the postsurfactant era have documented an association between lower rates of BPD and increased use of nasal CPAP in the DR.[31] Studies comparing centers predominantly using nasal CPAP in DR to centers using early mechanical ventilation (MV) and surfactant administration reported lower BPD rates in centers with a focus on nasal CPAP.[35–37] Van Marter and colleagues[37] reported higher rates of BPD in centers with more MV (75% vs 29%) and increased surfactant use (45% vs 10%) compared with centers with predominantly use of early nasal CPAP. These reports stimulated large randomized control trials comparing nasal CPAP or early endotracheal intubation at birth. A pooled analysis of a total of 2782 preterm infants less than 29 weeks' gestation (1296 infants in the nasal CPAP group and 1486 in the intubation group) showed a significant benefit for the combined outcome of death or BPD, or both, at 36 weeks' corrected gestation for babies treated with nasal CPAP (RR [95% CI] 0.91 [0.84–0.99]; risk difference −0.04, −0.07 to 0.00; number needed to treat 25). This suggests that 1 additional infant could survive to 36 weeks without BPD for every 25 babies treated with nasal CPAP in the DR rather than being intubated.[31]

SUSTAINED INFLATION

Animal studies have reported that SI (1) improves lung compliance without adverse circulatory effects,[38] (2) achieves lung aeration more uniformly,[39] (3) has an increased inspiratory volume and greater FRC compared with PPV alone,[34] and (4) does not cause overdistension of the lungs.[40]

Observational studies using SI during stabilization in the DR have reported a significant reduction in rates of intubation and MV, BPD, and use of oxygen,[41] which led to the design of several randomized controlled trials to compare SI with PPV alone. te Pas and colleagues[42] compared 2 different DR approaches —SI delivered via a T-piece and followed by early nasal CPAP compared with PPV with a self-inflating bag. They reported a significant reduction in intubation in the DR and BPD with SI and early nasal CPAP compared with traditional ventilator support in the DR. The studies comparing SI with nasal CPAP to CPAP alone did not find any difference in BPD in the 2 groups despite reduction in need of MV in first 72 hours.[43,44]

A recent meta-analysis of SI in DR reported a significant reduction in need for MV within the first 72 hours after birth in the SI group (RR [95% CI] 0.87 [0.77–0.97]; number needed to treat 10).[45] Neonatal mortality and BPD were similar, however, between the 2 groups. More concerning was the increase in patent ductus arteriosus treatment in infants receiving SI (RR [95% CI] 1.27 [1.05–1.54], number needed to harm 10).[45] The investigators speculated that early FRC establishment associated with reduction of pulmonary vascular resistance might induce rapid development of left-to-right shunting through the ductus.[45] A recent Cochrane review,[46] which was limited to infants who received a 15-second pressure-controlled SI versus standard inflations, reported no differences in mortality, intubation in the first 3 days of life, or BPD. In addition, there are several factors that may considerably influence the effectiveness of any SI intervention, including (1) skill of the clinical team, (2) interface by which an SI is delivered,[47] (3) an infant's intrinsic respiratory effort,[48] and (4) mask leak.[48] This suggests that an SI might not be the optimal approach in all apneic infants. These data suggest that more studies are needed before SI can be routinely used in the DR. Currently studies comparing SI to PPV alone are ongoing[49] and their results might help to inform the next cycle of the neonatal resuscitation guidelines in 2020. Until new results become available, SI should be limited to clinical trials.

OXYGEN USE IN THE DELIVERY ROOM

In 2010, neonatal resuscitation guidelines recommended use of blended air and oxygen to babies born at less than 32 weeks' gestation, and that FIO_2 should be guided by pulse oximetry.[50] These guidelines stated that resuscitation should be started with air in infants who were at least 32 weeks of gestation.[51] In 2015, the guidelines made a strong recommendation to initiate stabilization of preterm infants less than 35 weeks gestation with lower initial fraction of inspired oxygen (FIO_2) (0.21–0.3) and not higher FIO_2 (>0.65).[4] This approach is supported by a few small studies comparing different oxygen concentrations during neonatal resuscitation at birth. Wang and colleagues[52] reported that preterm infants ventilated in air required oxygen to achieve target oxygen saturation as measured by pulse oxymetry (SpO_2) and to overcome bradycardia. Although ELBW infants resuscitated with an initial FIO_2 of 0.3 compared with 0.9 had reduced oxidative stress and risk of BPD.[53] There was no difference in the overall risk of death or other common preterm morbidities when resuscitation is initiated at delivery with lower (≤ 0.30) or higher (≥ 0.6) FIO_2 in infants less than or equal to 28^{+6} weeks' gestation.[52–54] The opposing results for masked and unmasked trials may represent a type I error, emphasizing the need for larger, well-designed studies.[55]

A recent meta-analysis in 677 preterm infants less than or equal to 32 weeks' gestation showed no differences in morbidity, with a trend toward lower mortality in the lower (0.21–0.3 Fio_2) oxygen group compared with the higher (0.6–1.0 Fio_2) oxygen group.[56] These data support the current neonatal resuscitation recommendations to initiate stabilization of preterm infants less than 35 weeks' gestation with lower initial Fio_2 (0.21–0.3) and not higher Fio_2 (>0.65).[4]

There is recent evidence, however, from several studies that initiating stabilization of ELBW infants with lower initial Fio_2 (0.21–0.3) might increase morbidities and mortality in these infants. The Targeted Oxygenation in the Resuscitation of Premature Infants and Their Developmental Outcome (TO2RPIDO) trial compared Fio_2 of 1.0 versus 0.21 during DR resuscitation of preterm infants less than 32 weeks' gestation targeting for Spo_2 65% to 95% up to 5 minutes and 85% to 95% until admission. The study endpoints were mortality and neurodevelopmental outcome at 2 years of corrected age; however, the trail was closed prematurely due to slow enrollment. In 2015, Oei and colleagues reported that mortality was 16.2% versus 6% in the 0.21 versus the 1.0 Fio_2 group ($P = .013$), but only in a subgroup of babies less than 29 weeks' gestation.[57] In 2006 the Canadian Neonatal Resuscitation Program recommended use of either room air or an intermediate concentration of oxygen (eg, 0.3–0.4 Fio_2) in preterm infants and to adjust Fio_2 according to Spo_2 values. Rabi and colleagues[58] compared pre-epochs (use of 1.0 Fio_2) and post-epochs (titration of Fio_2) epochs on the effects on neonatal outcomes. The adjusted odds ratio (AOR) for the primary outcome of severe neurologic injury or death was higher in the lower oxygen group (AOR 1.36; 95% CI, 1.11–1.66) than those resuscitated in 100% oxygen (AOR 1.33; 95% CI, 1.04–1.69). These studies[57,58] (published after the current neonatal resuscitation guidelines) suggest that the current recommendations do not reflect the present state of uncertainty regarding best initial Fio_2 for ELBW infants and certainly not how to optimally titrate Fio_2.[55]

Practical Aspects

Since the 2010 resuscitation guidelines recommendations, there has been a change in practice in centers using 100% oxygen to initiate resuscitation. Overall, the number of units starting at 100% oxygen decreased from 56.3% (36/64) to 6.3% (4/64) and the rate of those using greater than 40% oxygen decreased from 76.6% (49/64) to 9.4% (6/64).[59] For the resuscitation and stabilization ELBW infants at birth, while waiting for the results from larger, well-designed studies on the comparison of low versus high oxygen concentrations, it seems appropriate to start with 21% to 30% oxygen.

MONITORING DURING NEONATAL TRANSITION

In the NICU, preterm infants are continuously monitored using an array of devices to assess arterial blood gases, heart rate (HR), oxygen saturation, end-tidal carbon dioxide, and respiratory functions to guide effectiveness of respiratory support. Although these methods are not commonly applied in the DR, there is an increasing interest in monitoring physiologic changes during neonatal transition.[60–64]

Heart Rate and Oxygen Saturation

The oxygen saturation and HR reflect adequate transition of newborn infants in the DR.[4] The pulse oximeter should be placed on the right hand or wrist of the infant to obtain both oxygen saturation and HR measurement.[4] Fetal life occurs in a hypoxic environment and it is well established that preterm preductal oxygen saturation reaches 80% to 90% between 5 minutes and 10 minutes of life.[65] Recently, oxygen percentiles have been established and are recommended to be used when ELBWs are supported in the DR.[65,66] The targeted oxygen saturation reference ranges for first 10 minutes of neonatal life are encouraged to be incorporated in neonatal resuscitation to titrate the inspired oxygen in the DR. During neonatal resuscitation, an increase in HR is an indicator for effective ventilation.[4,67] The neonatal HR dictates interventions in the DR and quick and reliable detection of HR improves the timeliness of critical interventions.[66] Traditional assessment techniques (eg, palpation of the umbilical cord or auscultation) have been demonstrated to be inaccurate.[68–71] Furthermore, newborn HR increases more slowly in (1) preterm vs term infants,[72] (2) after cesarean vs vaginal birth,[72] and (3) in newborns after maternal analgesia administration and DCC.[65,73] Recently there has been a trend to either use pulse oximetry or ECG to continuously display HR during resuscitation.[74,75] Potential limitations of ECG includes difficult ECG lead placement on the wet skin of ELBW infants, epidermal loss at the site of leads placement, and overestimation of HR in the setting of potential pulseless electric activity, thus delaying needed resuscitation efforts.

Respiratory Function Monitor

Effective mask PPV, however, can be compromised by mask leak, airway obstruction,[76,77] poor technique,[78,79] placing a hat, or drying the infant.[78] In addition, current neonatal resuscitation guidelines recommend a set peak inflation pressure with the assumption this delivers an adequate V_T; however, the V_T has rarely been measured.[80,81] Observational studies in the DR reported a delivered V_T between 0 mL/kg and 30 mL/kg when a set pressure was used.[80,81] This is concerning because animal studies have reported that only 6 inflations with a V_T of 35 mL/kg damage the lungs and alter the response to surfactant.[82]

Using a respiratory function monitor (RFM) can provide real-time assessment of airway pressures, gas flow, V_T, and leak[83] during neonatal training[84] and neonatal resuscitation.[48,83,85–88] Using an RFM in addition to clinical assessment compared with clinical assessment alone has the potential to lower the rate of excessive V_T delivery and reduce DR intubation.[85] Caregivers using an RFM during mask PPV, however, need to be familiar with their device and the waveforms displayed.[83] Further research is needed to determine whether the routine use of an RFM during neonatal training or neonatal resuscitation improves clinical outcomes.

Exhaled Carbon Dioxide

Spo_2 and HR in the DR guide oxygen delivery and respiratory support; these are further supplemented by using an RFM to measure gas flows and V_T. These parameters provide little information, however, on ventilation efficiency and the degree of gas exchange and provide limited feedback to guide clinical care when cardiorespiratory indicators fail to improve. CO_2 is produced in tissues as a byproduct of oxidative metabolism, enters the blood, and is eliminated from the body by diffusion across the alveolar epithelium before it is exhaled in the expired gas. Because CO_2 can only be present in expired gas if gas exchange has commenced, expired CO_2 (ECO_2) levels may indicate the degree and success of lung aeration and gas exchange.[89] Currently, colorimetric CO_2 detectors are commonly used in the DR to assess mask ventilation and to confirm correct endotracheal tube placement.[76,88,90–92] In addition, several observational studies have described the value of using ECO_2 to assess lung aeration and guide respiratory support in the DR.[64,93–95] Recent small trials using ECO_2 to guide respiratory support at birth reported no difference in admission blood gases[96] but a trend to lower rates of BPD.[45]

Near-infrared Spectroscopy

Near-infrared spectroscopy (NIRS) allows noninvasive continuous real-time measurement of the regional tissue oxygen saturation.[97] NIRS can also be used in conjunction with arterial pulse oximetry to calculate the fractional tissue oxygen extraction: the ratio of cerebral oxygen consumption to cerebral oxygen delivery. Pichler and colleagues[98] found spontaneously breathing premature infants (mean gestation 32 weeks) who received DCC had a lower initial (first 3 minutes of life) cerebral saturation whereas Baenziger and colleagues[99] found infants who received DCC had higher cerebral oxygenation levels at 4 hours and 24 hours of life compared with ICC. Similarly, infants who received UCM compared with DCC had a trend toward higher cerebral saturations between 3 hours and 24 hours after birth.[12] Low cerebral tissue oxygen saturation, as measured by NIRS in the first few days of life, has been shown associated with adverse neurologic outcome and IVH.[100] To prevent brain injury, the brain must have adequate tissue oxygen delivery.

Practical Aspects

Currently, Spo_2 monitoring should be used to titrate oxygen delivery during initial stabilization at birth.[4] Furthermore, ECG is the most accurate technique to assess HR at birth.[75] There is some evidence that during PPV an RFM can improve mask ventilation performance,[85] and ECO_2 can assess lung aeration.[89,93,96] In addition, using NIRS has the potential to monitor cerebral oxygen delivery.[101] Further evidence is needed before these techniques can be translated into routine care in the DR.

SURFACTANT DEFICIENCY

ELBW infants are born with structurally immature and surfactant-deficient lungs, which can be translated in difficult to maintain FRC and upper airway patency. Early administration of surfactant treatment, that is, within 2 hours after birth, has been shown to significantly decrease rates of death, air leak, and BPD, but comparing early surfactant in the DR against CPAP at birth, early surfactant does not show any benefit in the outcome with death or BPD.[30] The use of CPAP at birth can counteract the preterm RDS with reduced need of surfactant, ventilator dependence and BPD.[29,102]

Alternative surfactant administration methods (eg, intubation, surfactant, and extubation [INSURE] and minimal invasive surfactant therapy [MIST]) have been advocated to avoid MV after surfactant administration.[103–105] Verder and colleagues[106] first described INSURE in 1992 and reported that the need for subsequent MV after INSURE was significantly reduced to 43% compared with 85% in infants treated with CPAP alone (P = .003). A meta-analysis (n = 1551 preterm infant) comparing INSURE + CPAP vs CPAP alone, however, did not show any significant difference in either death or BPD. Side effects of INSURE include (1) CPAP failure rates of 10% to 50%, (2) sedation and analgesia, and (3) need for intubation and MV/PPV until extubation.

More recently, other strategies to administer surfactant by avoiding intubation and MV and/or analgesia/sedation have been described.[103–105] The Kribs technique[103] uses a thin feeding tube placed into the trachea using a Magill forceps during direct laryngoscopy. The procedure is performed without pharmacologic sedation and well tolerated.[103,107,108] Overall, the need for MV was reduced; however, no differences in BPD or death were observed.[103] The MIST technique uses a narrow-bore tracheal catheter during direct laryngoscopy without analgesia while receiving CPAP.[104,105] Observational studies using MIST reported a reduction for the need of MV in 25 weeks' to 28 weeks' gestation compared with controls (32% vs 68%; OR

[95% CI] 0.21, 0.083–0.55), with a similar trend at 29 weeks' gestation to 32 weeks' gestation (22% vs 45%; OR [95% CI] 0.34, 0.11–1.1).[104] Although MIST is feasible and potentially effective, further investigation in clinical trials are needed, particularly in the periviable period.

Practical Aspects

Currently, surfactant administration could be performed either after routine intubation or using the INSURE technique. MIST techniques are currently being investigated in multicenter randomized controlled trials and should only be used in the research environment.

EARLY USE OF CAFFEINE

Methylxanthines as treatment of apnea of prematurity have been demonstrated to reduce rates of BPD,[109] and caffeine improves survival without neurologic impairment or developmental delay at 18 months to 21 months of age.[110] Furthermore, early (prophylactic) use of caffeine is associated with less BPD and patent ductus arteriosus. Katheria and colleagues,[111] in a small feasibility study, randomized preterm infants to receive caffeine in the first 2 hours or 12 hours after birth. Administration of earlier caffeine administration was associated with improved blood pressure and superior vena cava flow without any differences in need for intubation or vasopressors. Currently, there is insufficient evidence to suggest routine caffeine administration in the DR, and larger studies are needed to determine the benefits of prophylactic caffeine.

Practical Aspects

Caffeine should be given to ELBW infants to reduce apnea of prematurity and BPD.[109] The timing of caffeine administration (DR or NICU), however, has not being determined.

SUMMARY

Extremely preterm infants face major challenges at birth due to their immature physiology leading to complicated transition. Multifactorial morbidities and lack of robust long-term neurodevelopmental outcome remain the main barriers in establishing clear well-defined guidelines for neonatal resuscitation for this vulnerable population.

ACKNOWLEDGMENTS

We would like to thank the public for donation of money to our funding agencies: G.M. Schmölzer is a recipient of the Heart and Stroke Foundation/University of Alberta Professorship of Neonatal Resuscitation, a National New Investigator of the Heart and Stroke Foundation Canada, and an Alberta New Investigator of the Heart and Stroke Foundation Alberta. The sponsors of the study had no role in study design, data collection, data analysis, data interpretation, or writing of the report.

REFERENCES

1. Schmölzer GM, te Pas AB, Davis PG, et al. Reducing lung injury during neonatal resuscitation of preterm infants. J Pediatr 2008;153:741–5.
2. Hooper SB, Siew ML, Kitchen M, et al. Establishing functional residual capacity in the non-breathing infant. Semin Fetal Neonatal Med 2013;18:336–43.

3. Hooper SB, te Pas AB, Kitchen M. Respiratory transition in the newborn: a three-phase process. Arch Dis Child Fetal Neonatal Ed 2016;101:F266–71.

4. Perlman J, Wyllie JP, Kattwinkel J, et al. Part 7: neonatal resuscitation: 2015 international consensus on cardiopulmonary resuscitation and emergency cardiovascular care science with treatment recommendations. Circulation 2015;132: S204–41.

5. Barton SK, Tolcos M, Miller SL, et al. Unraveling the links between the initiation of ventilation and brain injury in preterm infants. Front Pediatr 2015;3:280–9.

6. Barton SK, Tolcos M, Miller SL, et al. Ventilation-induced brain injury in preterm neonates: a review of potential therapies. Neonatology 2016;110:155–62.

7. Hooper SB, Polglase GR, te Pas AB. A physiological approach to the timing of umbilical cord clamping at birth. Arch Dis Child Fetal Neonatal Ed 2015;100: F355–60.

8. Yao AC, Moinian M, Lind J. Distribution of blood between infant and placenta after birth. Lancet 1969;2:871–3.

9. Bhatt S, Hooper SB, Pas te A, et al. Delaying cord clamping until ventilation onset improves cardiovascular function at birth in preterm lambs. J Physiol 2013;591:2113–26.

10. Hosono S, Mugishima H, Fujita H, et al. Umbilical cord milking reduces the need for red cell transfusions and improves neonatal adaptation in infants born at less than 29 weeks' gestation: a randomised controlled trial. Arch Dis Child Fetal Neonatal Ed 2008;93:F14–9.

11. Masaoka N, Yamamoto T. Blood pressure and urine output during the first 120 h of life in infants born at less than 29 weeks' gestation related to umbilical cord milking. Arch Dis Child Fetal Neonatal Ed 2009;94:F328–31.

12. Katheria AC, Leone TA, Woelkers D, et al. The effects of umbilical cord milking on hemodynamics and neonatal outcomes in premature neonates. J Pediatr 2014;164:1045–50.e1.

13. Ghavam S, Batra D, Mercer J, et al. Effects of placental transfusion in extremely low birthweight infants: meta-analysis of long- and short-term outcomes. Transfusion 2013;54:1192–8.

14. Rabe H. Cord clamping and neurodevelopmental outcome in very low birth weight infants. J Perinatol 2010;30:1.

15. Mercer JS. Delayed cord clamping in very preterm infants reduces the incidence of intraventricular hemorrhage and late-onset sepsis: a randomized, controlled trial. Pediatrics 2006;117:1235–42.

16. Mercer JS, Vohr BR, Erickson-Owens DA, et al. Seven-month developmental outcomes of very low birth weight infants enrolled in a randomized controlled trial of delayed versus immediate cord clamping. J Perinatol 2009;30:11–6.

17. Rabe H, Jewison A, Fernandez Alvarez R, et al. Milking compared with delayed cord clamping to increase placental transfusion in preterm neonates. Obstet Gynecol 2011;117:205–11.

18. Hutchon DJR. Ventilation before umbilical cord clamping improves physiological transition at birth or "umbilical cord clamping before ventilation is established destabilizes physiological transition at birth". Front Pediatr 2015;3:1–5.

19. Hutchon DJR. Evolution of neonatal resuscitation with intact placental circulation. Infant 2014;10(2):58–61.

20. Vain NE, Satragno DS, Gorenstein AN, et al. Effect of gravity on volume of placental transfusion: a multicentre, randomised, non-inferiority trial. Lancet 2014;384:235–40.

21. Silverman WA, Fertig JW, Berger AP. The influence of the thermal environment upon the survival of newly born premature infants. Pediatrics 1958;22:876–86.
22. Laptook AR, Salhab W, Bhaskar B, Neonatal Research Network. Admission temperature of low birth weight infants: predictors and associated morbidities. Pediatrics 2007;119:e643–9.
23. McCall EM, Alderdice F, Halliday HL, et al. Interventions to prevent hypothermia at birth in preterm and/or low birthweight infants. Cochrane Database Syst Rev 2010;(1):CD004210.
24. te Pas AB, Lopriore E, Dito I, et al. Humidified and heated air during stabilization at birth improves temperature in preterm infants. Pediatrics 2010;125:e1427–32.
25. World Health Organization. Born too soon: the global action report on preterm birth. 2012.
26. Duryea EL, Nelson DB, Wyckoff MH, et al. The impact of ambient operating room temperature on neonatal and maternal hypothermia and associated morbidities: a randomized controlled trial. Am J Obstet Gynecol 2016;214:505.e1–7.
27. Kasdorf E, Perlman J. Hyperthermia, inflammation, and perinatal brain injury. Pediatr Neurol 2013;49:8–14.
28. Aziz K, Chadwick M, Baker M, et al. Ante- and intra-partum factors that predict increased need for neonatal resuscitation. Resuscitation 2008;79:444–52.
29. Morley CJ, Davis PG, Doyle LW, et al. Nasal CPAP or intubation at birth for very preterm infants. N Engl J Med 2008;358:700–8.
30. SUPPORT Study Group of the Eunice Kennedy Shriver NICHD Neonatal Research Network, Finer N, Carlo WA, Walsh MC, et al. Early CPAP versus surfactant in extremely preterm infants. N Engl J Med 2010;362:1970–9.
31. Schmölzer GM, Kumar M, Pichler G, et al. Non-invasive versus invasive respiratory support in preterm infants at birth: systematic review and meta-analysis. BMJ 2013;347:f5980.
32. Dunn M, Kaempf J, de Klerk A, et al. Randomized trial comparing 3 approaches to the initial respiratory management of preterm neonates. Pediatrics 2011;128: e1069–76.
33. Sandri F, Ancora G, Plavka R, et al. Prophylactic or early selective surfactant combined with nCPAP in very preterm infants. Pediatrics 2010;125:e1402–9.
34. te Pas AB, Siew ML, Wallace MJ, et al. Establishing functional residual capacity at birth: the effect of sustained inflation and positive end-expiratory pressure in a preterm rabbit model. Pediatr Res 2009;65:537–41.
35. Avery ME, Tooley WH, Keller JB, et al. Is chronic lung disease in low birth weight infants preventable? A survey of eight centers. Pediatrics 1987;79:26–30.
36. Ammari A, Suri M, Milisavljevic V, et al. Variables associated with the early failure of nasal cpap in very low birth weight infants. J Pediatr 2005;147:341–7.
37. Van Marter LJ, Allred EN, Pagano M, et al. Do clinical markers of barotrauma and oxygen toxicity explain interhospital variation in rates of chronic lung disease? The Neonatology Committee for the Developmental Network. Pediatrics 2000;105(6):1194–201.
38. Sobotka KS, Hooper SB, Allison BJ, et al. An initial sustained inflation improves the respiratory and cardiovascular transition at birth in preterm lambs. Pediatr Res 2011;70:56–60.
39. te Pas AB, Siew ML, Wallace MJ, et al. Effect of sustained inflation length on establishing functional residual capacity at birth in ventilated premature rabbits. Pediatr Res 2009;66:295–300.
40. Hooper SB, Kitchen M, Siew ML, et al. Imaging lung aeration and lung liquid clearance at birth. FASEB J 2007;21:3329–37.

41. Lindner W, Pohlandt F, Vossbeck S, et al. Delivery room management of extremely low birth weight infants: spontaneous breathing or intubation? Pediatrics 1999;103:961–7.

42. te Pas AB, Walther FJ. A randomized, controlled trial of delivery-room respiratory management in very preterm infants. Pediatrics 2007;120:322–9.

43. Lista G, Boni L, Scopesi F, et al. Sustained lung inflation at birth for preterm infants: a randomized clinical trial. Pediatrics 2015;135:e457–64.

44. Lindner W, Högel J, Pohlandt F. Sustained pressure—controlled inflation or intermittent mandatory ventilation in preterm infants in the delivery room? A randomized, controlled trial on initial respiratory support via nasopharyngeal tube. Acta Paediatr 2005;94:303–9.

45. Schmölzer GM, Kumar M, Aziz K, et al. Sustained inflation versus positive pressure ventilation at birth: a systematic review and meta-analysis. Arch Dis Child Fetal Neonatal Ed 2014;100(4):F361–8.

46. O'Donnell CP, Bruschettini M, Davis PG. Sustained versus standard inflations during neonatal resuscitation to prevent mortality and improve respiratory outcomes. Cochrane Database Syst Rev 2015;(7):CD004953.

47. Keszler M. Sustained inflation during neonatal resuscitation. Curr Opin Pediatr 2015;27:145–51.

48. van Vonderen JJ, Hooper SB, Hummler HD, et al. Effects of a sustained inflation in preterm infants at birth. J Pediatr 2014;165:903–8.e1.

49. Foglia EE, Owen LS, Thio M, et al. Sustained aeration of infant lungs (SAIL) trial: study protocol for a randomized controlled trial. Trial 2015;16:189–97.

50. Kattwinkel J, Perlman J, Aziz K, et al. Part 15: neonatal resuscitation: 2010 American heart association guidelines for cardiopulmonary resuscitation and emergency cardiovascular care. Circulation 2010;122:S909–19.

51. Saugstad OD, Robertson NJ, Vento M. A critical review of the 2015 International Liaison Committee on Resuscitation treatment recommendations for resuscitating the newly born infant. Acta Paediatr 2016;105:442–4.

52. Wang CL, Finer N, Anderson CT, et al. Resuscitation of preterm neonates by using room air or 100% oxygen. Pediatrics 2008;121:1083–9.

53. Vento M, Escrig R, Arruza L, et al. Achievement of targeted saturation values in extremely low gestational age neonates resuscitated with low or high oxygen concentrations: a prospective, randomized trial. Pediatrics 2008;121:875–81.

54. Kapadia V, Chalak LF, Sparks JE, et al. Resuscitation of preterm neonates with limited versus high oxygen strategy. Pediatrics 2013;132:e1488–96.

55. Vento M, Schmölzer GM, Cheung P-Y, et al. What initial oxygen is best for preterm infants in the delivery room?-A response to the 2015 neonatal resuscitation guidelines. Resuscitation 2016;101:e7–8.

56. Saugstad OD, Aune D, Aguar M, et al. Systematic review and meta-analysis of optimal initial fraction of oxygen levels in the delivery room at ≤32 weeks. Acta Paediatr 2014;103(7):744–51.

57. Oei JL, Vento M, Rabi Y, et al. Higher or lower oxygen for delivery room resuscitation of preterm infants below 28 completed weeks gestation: a meta-analysis. Arch Dis Child Fetal Neonatal Ed 2017;102(1):F24–30.

58. Rabi Y, Lodha A, Soraisham A, et al. Outcomes of preterm infants following the introduction of room air resuscitation. Resuscitation 2015;96:252–9.

59. Trevisanuto D, Satariano I, Doglioni N, et al. Changes over time in delivery room management of extremely low birth weight infants in Italy. Resuscitation 2014;85:1072–6.

60. Pichler G, Binder-Heschl C, Avian A, et al. Reference ranges for regional cerebral tissue oxygen saturation and fractional oxygen extraction in neonates during immediate transition after birth. J Pediatr 2013;163:1558–63.
61. Baik N, Urlesberger B, Schwaberger B, et al. Reference ranges for cerebral tissue oxygen saturation index in term neonates during immediate neonatal transition after birth. Neonatology 2015;108:283–6.
62. Mian QN, Pichler G, Binder-Heschl C, et al. Tidal volumes in spontaneously breathing preterm infants supported with continuous positive airway pressure. J Pediatr 2014;165:702–6.e1.
63. Pichler G, Cheung P-Y, Binder-Heschl C, et al. Time course study of blood pressure in term and preterm infants immediately after birth. PLoS One 2014;9: e114504.
64. van Os S, Cheung P-Y, Pichler G, et al. Exhaled carbon dioxide can be used to guide respiratory support in the delivery room. Acta Paediatr 2014;103: 796–806.
65. Dawson JA, Kamlin COF, Vento M, et al. Defining the reference range for oxygen saturation for infants after birth. Pediatrics 2010;125:e1340–7.
66. Perlman J, Wyllie JP, Kattwinkel J, et al. Part 11: neonatal resuscitation: 2010 International consensus on cardiopulmonary resuscitation and emergency cardiovascular care science with treatment recommendations. Circulation 2010; 122(16 Suppl 2):S516–38.
67. Yam CH, Dawson JA, Schmölzer GM, et al. Heart rate changes during resuscitation of newly born infants. Arch Dis Child Fetal Neonatal Ed 2011;96:F102–7.
68. Kamlin COF, O'Donnell CP, Everest NJ, et al. Accuracy of clinical assessment of infant heart rate in the delivery room. Resuscitation 2006;71:319–21.
69. Wyllie JP, Voogdt KGJA, Morrison AC, et al. A randomised, simulated study assessing auscultation of heart rate at birth. Resuscitation 2010;81:1000–3.
70. Chitkara R, Rajani AK, Oehlert JW, et al. The accuracy of human senses in the detection of neonatal heart rate during standardized simulated resuscitation: implications for delivery of care, training and technology design. Resuscitation 2013;84:369–72.
71. Mizumoto H, Tomotaki S, Shibata H, et al. Electrocardiogram shows reliable heart rates much earlier than pulse oximetry during neonatal resuscitation. Pediatr Int 2011;54:205–7.
72. Dawson JA, Kamlin COF, Wong C, et al. Changes in heart rate in the first minutes after birth. Arch Dis Child Fetal Neonatal Ed 2010;95:F177–81.
73. Smit M, Dawson JA, Ganzeboom A, et al. Pulse oximetry in newborns with delayed cord clamping and immediate skin-to-skin contact. Arch Dis Child Fetal Neonatal Ed 2014;99:F309–14.
74. Kamlin COF, Dawson JA, O'Donnell CP, et al. Accuracy of pulse oximetry measurement of heart rate of newborn infants in the delivery room. J Pediatr 2008; 152:756–60.
75. Katheria AC, Rich W, Finer N. Electrocardiogram provides a continuous heart rate faster than oximetry during neonatal resuscitation. Pediatrics 2012;130: e1177–81.
76. Finer N, Rich W, Wang C, et al. Airway obstruction during mask ventilation of very low birth weight infants during neonatal resuscitation. Pediatrics 2009; 123:865–9.
77. Schmölzer GM, Dawson JA, Kamlin COF, et al. Airway obstruction and gas leak during mask ventilation of preterm infants in the delivery room. Arch Dis Child Fetal Neonatal Ed 2011;96:F254–7.

78. Chua C, Schmölzer GM, Davis PG. Airway manoeuvres to achieve upper airway patency during mask ventilation in newborn infants – an historical perspective. Resuscitation 2012;83:411–6.
79. Schilleman K, Siew ML, Lopriore E, et al. Auditing resuscitation of preterm infants at birth by recording video and physiological parameters. Resuscitation 2012;83:1135–9.
80. Poulton DA, Schmölzer GM, Morley CJ, et al. Assessment of chest rise during mask ventilation of preterm infants in the delivery room. Resuscitation 2011; 82:175–9.
81. Schmölzer GM, Kamlin COF, O'Donnell CP, et al. Assessment of tidal volume and gas leak during mask ventilation of preterm infants in the delivery room. Arch Dis Child Fetal Neonatal Ed 2010;95:F393–7.
82. Björklund LJ, Ingimarsson J, Curstedt T, et al. Manual ventilation with a few large Breaths at birth Compromises the Therapeutic effect of subsequent surfactant Replacement in immature lambs. Pediatr Res 1997;42:348–55.
83. Schmölzer GM, Kamlin COF, Dawson JA, et al. Respiratory monitoring of neonatal resuscitation. Arch Dis Child Fetal Neonatal Ed 2010;95:F295–303.
84. Schmölzer GM, Roehr C-C. Use of respiratory function monitors during simulated neonatal resuscitation. Klin Padiatr 2011;223:261–6.
85. Schmölzer GM, Morley CJ, Wong C, et al. Respiratory function monitor guidance of mask ventilation in the delivery room: a feasibility study. J Pediatr 2012;160: 377–81.e2.
86. Li ES-S, Cheung P-Y, Pichler G, et al. Respiratory function and near infrared spectroscopy recording during cardiopulmonary resuscitation in an extremely preterm newborn. Neonatology 2014;105:200–4.
87. van Vonderen JJ, van Zanten HA, Schilleman K, et al. Cardiorespiratory monitoring during neonatal resuscitation for direct feedback and audit. Front Pediatr 2016;4:336–7.
88. Finn D, Boylan GB, Ryan CA, et al. Enhanced monitoring of the preterm infant during stabilization in the delivery room. Front Pediatr 2016;4:249–311.
89. Hooper SB, Fouras A, Siew ML, et al. Expired CO_2 levels indicate degree of lung aeration at birth. PLoS One 2013;8:e70895.
90. Leone TA, Lange A, Rich W, et al. Disposable colorimetric carbon dioxide detector use as an indicator of a patent airway during noninvasive mask ventilation. Pediatrics 2006;118:e202–4.
91. Schmölzer GM, O'Reilly M, Davis PG, et al. Confirmation of correct tracheal tube placement in newborn infants. Resuscitation 2013;84:731–7.
92. Hawkes GA, Kelleher J, Ryan CA, et al. A review of carbon dioxide monitoring in preterm newborns in the delivery room. Resuscitation 2014;85(10):1315–9.
93. Kang LJ, Cheung P-Y, Pichler G, et al. Monitoring lung aeration during respiratory support in preterm infants at birth. PLoS One 2014;9:e102729.
94. Schmölzer GM, Hooper SB, Wong C, et al. Exhaled carbon dioxide in healthy term infants immediately after birth. J Pediatr 2015;166:844–9.e1–e3.
95. Mian QN, Cheung P-Y, O'Reilly M, et al. Spontaneously breathing preterm infants change in tidal volume to improve lung aeration immediately after birth. J Pediatr 2015;167(2):274–8.e1.
96. Kong JY, Rich W, Finer N, et al. Quantitative end-tidal carbon dioxide monitoring in the delivery room: a randomized controlled trial. J Pediatr 2013;163:104–8.e1.
97. Pichler G, Cheung P-Y, Aziz K, et al. How to monitor the brain during immediate neonatal transition and resuscitation? A systematic qualitative review of the literature. Neonatology 2014;105:205–10.

 98. Pichler G, Baik N, Urlesberger B, et al. Cord clamping time in spontaneously breathing preterm neonates in the first minutes after birth: impact on cerebral oxygenation - a prospective observational study. J Matern Fetal Neonatal Med 2016;29(10):1570–2.

 99. Baenziger O, Stolkin F, Keel M, et al. The influence of the timing of cord clamping on postnatal cerebral oxygenation in preterm neonates: a randomized, controlled trial. Pediatrics 2007;119:455–9.

100. Baik N, Urlesberger B, Schwaberger B, et al. Cerebral haemorrhage in preterm neonates: does cerebral regional oxygen saturation during the immediate transition matter? Arch Dis Child Fetal Neonatal Ed 2015;100(5):F422–7.

101. Pichler G, Urlesberger B, Baik N, et al. Cerebral oxygen saturation to guide oxygen delivery in preterm neonates for the immediate transition after birth: a 2-center randomized controlled pilot feasibility trial. J Pediatr 2016;170: 73–8.e1-e4.

102. Finer N, Carlo WA, Duara S, et al. Delivery room continuous positive airway pressure/positive end-expiratory pressure in extremely low birth weight infants: a feasibility trial. Pediatrics 2004;114:651–7.

103. Göpel W, Kribs A, Ziegler A, et al. Avoidance of mechanical ventilation by surfactant treatment of spontaneously breathing preterm infants (AMV): an open-label, randomised, controlled trial. Lancet 2011;378:1627–34.

104. Dargaville PA, Aiyappan A, De Paoli AG, et al. Minimally-invasive surfactant therapy in preterm infants on continuous positive airway pressure. Arch Dis Child Fetal Neonatal Ed 2013;98:F122–6.

105. Dargaville PA, Aiyappan A, Cornelius A, et al. Preliminary evaluation of a new technique of minimally invasive surfactant therapy. Arch Dis Child Fetal Neonatal Ed 2011;96:F243–8.

106. Verder H, Robertson B, Greisen G, et al. Surfactant therapy and nasal continuous positive airway pressure for newborns with respiratory distress syndrome. Danish-Swedish Multicenter Study Group. N Engl J Med 1994;331:1051–5.

107. Kribs A, Pillekamp F, Hünseler C, et al. Early administration of surfactant in spontaneous breathing with nCPAP: feasibility and outcome in extremely premature infants (postmenstrual age <27weeks). Paediatr Anaesth 2007;17:364–9.

108. Kribs A, Vierzig A, Hünseler C, et al. Early surfactant in spontaneously breathing with nCPAP in ELBW infants - a single centre four year experience. Acta Paediatr 2008;97:293–8.

109. Schmidt B, Roberts RS, Davis PG, et al. Caffeine therapy for apnea of prematurity. N Engl J Med 2006;354:2112–21.

110. Schmidt B, Roberts RS, Davis PG, et al. Long-term effects of caffeine therapy for apnea of prematurity. N Engl J Med 2007;357:1893–902.

111. Katheria AC, Sauberan J, Akotia D, et al. A pilot randomized controlled trial of early versus routine caffeine in extremely premature infants. Am J Perinatol 2015;32:879–86.

Hemodynamic Assessment and Monitoring of Premature Infants

Afif El-Khuffash, FRCPI, MD, DCh[a,b],
Patrick J. McNamara, MD, MSc[c,*]

KEYWORDS

- Hemodynamic assessment • Periviable • Preterm infant • Hypotension
- Echocardiography • NICOM • NIRS

KEY POINTS

- Management of the hemodynamic status of periviable premature infants is challenging owing to the multitude of etiologies and the unique characteristics of the circulatory system.
- There are difficulties in monitoring and identifying hemodynamic compromise and a lack of evidence supporting the current treatment approaches.
- A physiology-based approach to the diagnosis, monitoring and management of low blood flow sates in periviable infants is likely to produce the best outcomes.

INTRODUCTION

The cardiovascular care of critically ill preterm infants, particularly around the periviable period, remains a significant challenge in the neonatal intensive care unit for a multitude of reasons. First, the etiologic causes of hemodynamic compromise in this population are heterogeneous; second, the phenotypic presentation is oftentimes modified by the complex physiologic processes that occur during transition from fetal to neonatal life; third, the pharmacologic effects of therapeutic intervention are developmentally regulated; finally, thresholds to guide intervention, predominantly based on mean arterial pressure, lack scientific validation. Consequently, the approach to infants with low blood flow states needs to be individualized. The use of regimented protocols, which usually recommend the administration of fluids followed by stepwise incremental addition of specific cardiovascular agents, without consideration of their

Disclosure Statement: The authors have nothing to disclose.
[a] Department of Neonatology, The Rotunda Hospital, Parnell Square, Dublin 1, DO1 P5W9, Ireland; [b] Department of Paediatrics, School of Medicine, Royal College of Surgeons in Ireland, 123 St Stephen's Green, Dublin 2, Ireland; [c] Division of Neonatology, The Hospital for Sick Children, University of Toronto, 555 University Avenue, Toronto, Ontario MG5 1X8, Canada
* Corresponding author.
E-mail address: patrick.mcnamara@sickkids.ca

Clin Perinatol 44 (2017) 377–393
http://dx.doi.org/10.1016/j.clp.2017.02.001
0095-5108/17/© 2017 Elsevier Inc. All rights reserved.

biological appropriateness for the active pathophysiologic state, have failed to produce tangible improvements in short- and long-term outcomes. In fact, recent evidence points toward causing harm.[1] Another increasingly recognized challenge is the lack of feasible and robust measurements of systemic blood flow that facilitate the identification of hemodynamic compromise. The overreliance on blood pressure, which is a poor surrogate for systemic blood flow, may result in both overtreatment and undertreatment of infants in certain physiologic situations. Although methods for intermittent and/or continuous monitoring of cardiac output and systemic blood flow are becoming increasingly used, the unique physiologic environment of preterm infants (with the persistence of fetal shunts) add further challenges to using those methods. There remains a lack of reliable data on normal blood pressure and cardiac output values in the neonatal population during the early transitional period and beyond. Identification of thresholds or clinical scenarios where hemodynamic intervention may modify patient outcomes represents the most important challenge for neonatal intensivists. Relevant to the clinical decision making process are the active disease state, phase of physiologic transition, and competing interventions, yet these are often not considered.

TRANSITIONAL PHYSIOLOGY: CARDIOVASCULAR AND PHYSIOLOGIC CONCEPTS

The transition from fetal to neonatal life is accompanied by important physiologic changes in the circulatory system: There is a significant increase in systemic vascular resistance (SVR) resulting in an increase in left ventricular (LV) afterload. This increase is a consequence of the loss of low resistance placental circulation, and a surge in vasoconstrictor substances including vasopressin (through vasopressin receptors, which increase intracellular calcium release and upregulate adrenaline receptors) and thromboxane A_2 (a potent vasoconstrictor).[2] In addition, there is a decrease in pulmonary vascular resistance (PVR) as a consequence of pulmonary arterial vasodilatation. This decrease is facilitated by the increase in the partial pressure of oxygen accompanying lung aeration, and the increased production of potent pulmonary arterial vasodilators including prostaglandins, bradykinins, and histamine.[3] The increase in SVR and decrease in PVR redirects right ventricular output from shunting across the ductus arteriosus (and supplying the brain) toward the pulmonary vascular bed (to supply the lungs). This is a crucial step during the early transition, which ensures that LV preload (which was derived from the placental circulation during fetal life) is maintained by adequate pulmonary venous return. The maintenance of adequate LV preload is essential for sustaining an adequate LV output (LVO) in the face of a rising LV afterload. Consequently, right ventricular preload becomes dependent on systemic venous return, and right ventricular afterload remains low owing to decreasing PVR (**Figs. 1** and **2**).

The additional effects of the timing of cord clamping after birth need to be considered as an important part of the transitional process. The placenta is thought to hold 30% to 50% of the fetal circulating volume at any one time; therefore, early clamping of the cord may result in a significant reduction of LV preload and effective LVO. This is a consequence of the reduction in blood flow to the left atrium from the placental circulation, which is not restored effectively until pulmonary flow blow is established.[4] Deferring cord clamping until the infant begins to breath and establish pulmonary blood flow may result in fewer fluctuations in LVO by ensuring the maintenance of LV preload (from the placental circulation) until pulmonary venous return takes over.[5] Knowledge of the approach taken in a particular infant (early or deferred clamping of the umbilical cord) will help with the individualized approach to managing that particular infant if a low blood flow state is identified.

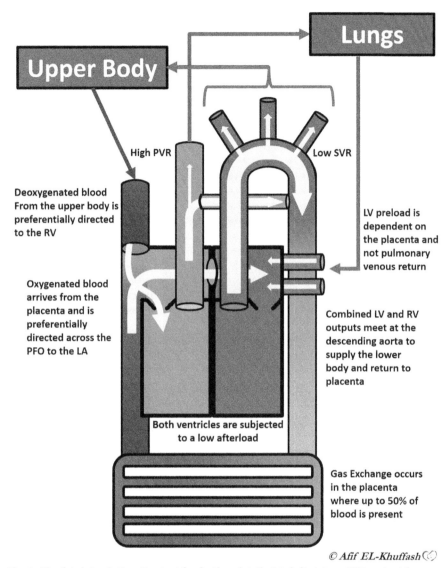

Fig. 1. The fetal circulation. See text for further details. LA, left atrium; PFO, patent foramen ovale; PVR, pulmonary vascular resistance; SVR, systemic vascular resistance.

The persistence of fetal shunts can add further complexity to the transitional circulation and may contribute to the evolution of hemodynamic compromise. During normal transition, the increasing left atrial pressure results in closure of foramen ovale flap with abolition of transatrial flow. In addition, owing to the increasing SVR and decreasing PVR, flow across the ductus arteriosus becomes exclusively left to right within the first 24 hours of life. The increase in oxygen tension, and decrease in prostaglandin levels postnatally, followed by local atherosclerotic-like processes within the ductal wall results in an arrest in flow across the ductus, usually within 48 hours.[5,6]

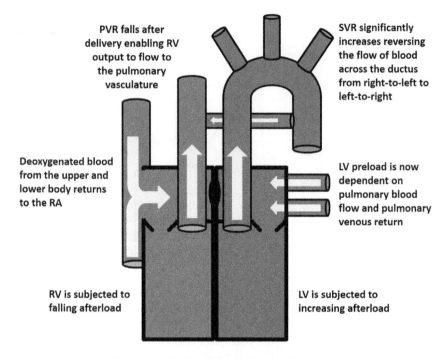

PVR falls after delivery enabling RV output to flow to the pulmonary vasculature

SVR significantly increases reversing the flow of blood across the ductus from right-to-left to left-to-right

Deoxygenated blood from the upper and lower body returns to the RA

LV preload is now dependent on pulmonary blood flow and pulmonary venous return

RV is subjected to falling afterload

LV is subjected to increasing afterload

Vascular Tone Regulation of Blood Vessels

NO acts cGMP on Calcium sensitive potassium channels & myosin phosphatases to cause vessel relaxation

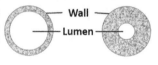

Wall — Lumen

Vasopressin increases tone via receptors that ↑ Ca^{++} release from sarcoplasmic reticulum, ↑ adrenaline receptors on smooth muscle walls and ↓NO synthesis

Prostaglandins are derived from cell membrane arachidonic acid by the actions of COX enzymes Prostaglandin E$_2$, a vasodilator, and Thromboxane A$_2$, a vasoconstrictor are both implicated in the early regulation of vascular tone

© Afif EL-Khuffash

Fig. 2. Circulation during early postnatal life. Ca^{++}, calcium ions; cGMP, cyclic guanine monophosphate; COX, cyclooxygenase; LV, left ventricle; NO, nitric oxide; PVR, pulmonary vascular resistance; RA, right atrium; SVR, systemic vascular resistance.

Important Considerations in Preterm Infants

The periviable preterm infant is faced with additional challenges that increase the risk of hemodynamic compromise, especially during the early transitional period. The myocardium of the preterm infant possesses an inefficient contractile mechanism (impaired systolic performance) and a preponderance of noncontractile, poorly compliant collagen, leading to impaired diastolic performance (**Fig. 3**).[7,8] In addition, owing to the relatively faster heart rate of preterm infants, the percentage of time spent in diastole (the time of LV filling) is considerably shorter.[9] As a result, it is poorly tolerant of increased afterload, and lacks the necessary reserve to cope with reduced preload, both of which are common occurrences during the transitional period as outlined. In addition to those challenges, preterm infants exhibit a high resting peripheral vascular

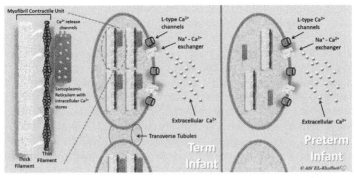

Fig. 3. Comparison between term and preterm infant myocytes. In term infants, extracellular calcium (*white circles*) enters the cell via L-type calcium channels. This in turn activates the release of large amounts intracellular calcium stored in the sarcoplasmic reticulum (SR) into the cytosol. This results in contraction of the myofilament. This whole process is facilitated by the proximity of the SR to the L-type Ca channels and by the presence of transverse tubules, which are invaginations of the myocyte cell wall into the cytosol. Relaxation is a result of active reuptake of cytosolic calcium into the SR. The small amount of calcium that entered the cell via L-type calcium channels is transported back to the extracellular compartment via the Na^+–Ca^{2+} exchanger. In preterm infants, the SR is physically separated from L-type Ca, the transverse tubules are absent, and the myocyte has a greater surface area to volume ratio. Consequently, contraction depends on extracellular calcium influx into the cells.

tone owing to the relatively higher concentration of vasoconstrictive (alpha) receptors at the expense of vasodilatory (beta receptors). The myocardium on the other hand lacks adequate adrenergic innervation limiting its ability to increase contractility (inotropy). Furthermore, preterm infants are unable to increase glucocorticoid production in response to stress owing to the underdeveloped hypothalamic–pituitary–adrenal axis.[10–12] In combination, these factors limit the ability of the preterm myocardium to respond to inotropes, which generally result in a predominant vasopressor effect in this population. Finally, left-to-right shunting across a patent ductus arteriosus (PDA) and a patent foramen ovale (PFO) may further compromise systemic blood flow and effective cardiac output by short circuiting blood to the lungs (pulmonary overcirculation) at the expense of the systemic circulation (systemic hypoperfusion).

Preterm infants around the periviable period may be particularly vulnerable to the effects of left-to-right shunting associated with a significant PDA. Left heart diastolic function may play a key role in handling the increased blood volume returning to the heart. In the setting of compromised diastolic function, the increased pulmonary venous return to the left atrium may result in increased left atrial pressure and eventual pulmonary venous congestion.[13] This process may explain the higher incidence of pulmonary hemorrhage in this population. Another important factor that compromises cardiac output is positive end-expiratory pressure. Infants born around the periviable period are more likely to have reduced respiratory drive at birth coupled with poor lung compliance and reduced thoracic wall muscle strength, resulting in a significant need for positive pressure support. Recent recommendations to maintain a relatively higher positive end-expiratory pressure may result in reduced cardiac output.[14] Increased airway pressure may lead to compression of the intraalveolar capillaries, increased PVR, and a reduction in effective pulmonary blood flow, pulmonary venous return, and LVO. This may occur with all modes of mechanical ventilation.[15]

Neonatal sepsis may also modulate hemodynamic change, particularly during the transitional period. Sepsis in term infants is associated with a decrease in both systolic and diastolic function, measured using the myocardial performance index and pulsed wave Doppler studies of the mitral inflow.[16] In addition, tissue Doppler–derived myocardial velocities reveal that both LV and right ventricular function are reduced in the presence of confirmed sepsis; nonsurvivors of neonatal sepsis have significantly higher troponin levels when compared with survivors.[17] Group B *Streptococcus* is a leading cause of early neonatal sepsis and induces myocardial injury through a cytotoxin (beta-hemolysin/cytolysin), which has deleterious effects on cardiomyocyte viability, contractility, and calcium exchange.[18] In addition to the direct myocardial effects, neonatal sepsis has a global effect on the cardiovascular system with the persistence of pulmonary arterial hypertension and an elevated SVR being the hallmarks of early disease (cold shock). Infants with *Escherichia coli* infection and other gram-negative organisms may present earlier with vasoactive shock (warm shock). The mortality in neonatal sepsis remains high.[19] A similar pattern is observed in necrotizing enterocolitis, which can also result in vasoactive shock owing to the release of cytokines and the alteration in endothelial function.

Importance of Low Blood Flow States on Neonatal Outcomes

The rationale to correct hypotension and low blood flow states stems from their association with adverse outcomes. Hypotension during the early transitional period (defined as the lower mean arterial pressure over the first 24 hours) is associated with adverse outcomes including severe intraventricular hemorrhage, chronic lung disease, and death.[20] However, several studies have also demonstrated that treatment of hypotension (irrespective of blood pressure) is also independently associated with death and significant neurodisability.[21,22] Similarly, a low LVO and superior vena cava flow (surrogate markers for systemic blood flow) are also associated with adverse short- and long-term outcomes, including severe intraventricular hemorrhage and neurodisability.[23–27] Correction of low blood flow states in an attempt to avoid those important outcomes has not been studied systematically.[28] The continued uncertainty regarding the association between hypotension (and its treatment) with adverse outcome highlights the need for reliable and valid methods for monitoring the hemodynamic status of periviable infants. This information will enable more robust trials on interventions to be implemented with the aim of reducing those adverse outcomes.

CURRENT METHODS OF HEMODYNAMIC ASSESSMENT

The complexity of the pathophysiologic processes that contribute to hemodynamic compromise highlights the fact that no one marker, in isolation, can be reliably used to characterize the degree of compromise. However, a holistic appraisal of all the clinical and laboratory measures of cardiovascular homeostasis, in addition to the use of imaging modalities (such as echocardiography), may provide a more complete and accurate picture of the cause of hemodynamic instability and offer a possible therapeutic approach. Commonly used markers include heart rate, blood pressure, and capillary refill time in addition to measures of end-organ functionality (urinary output, muscle tone, and the level of consciousness) and laboratory parameters such as arterial pH, lactate, urea, and creatinine.

Heart rate is an important determinant of cardiac output. However, stroke volume may play a more important role in maintaining cardiac output; recent data suggest that the increase in LVO seen soon after birth is a result of an increasing stroke volume rather than heart rate.[29] The value of elevated heart rate as a marker of hemodynamic instability, particularly in the setting of hypovolemia, needs to be considered in the context of confounders; specifically, these include pain, fever, caffeine use, anemia, and arrhythmias. Capillary refill time, as a sign of hemodynamic compromise, is also very unreliable, and does not indicate the adequacy of blood flow to internal organs. Although prolonged capillary refill time is associated with low blood flow, the correlation with echocardiography measurements of cardiac output is loose at best.[30,31] The assessment of renal perfusion in the early neonatal period is fraught with challenges. Urine output may indicate reduced renal perfusion in the absence of other pathologies (renal parenchymal disease and obstructive uropathies). Relative oliguria, may be normal in premature infants owing to renal tubular immaturity. Urine function tests may not reflect true neonatal renal function especially if taken within the first 24 hours of life. Anaerobic metabolism as a consequence of poor perfusion may lead elevated plasma lactate levels; however, its interpretation must be in combination with other markers of reduced perfusion. For example, an elevated lactate in isolation may be a consequence of increased glycogenolysis and inborn errors of metabolism. There may also be a delayed increase in serum lactate levels because poorly perfused areas will mot mobilize the produced lactate until after adequate blood flow is restored.[32] The relative time lag between the onset of shock and the change in those markers as outlined can make their clinical use less helpful.

A Focus on Blood Pressure

Mean blood pressure is most common bedside measure used by clinicians as a measure of the adequacy of perfusion in the neonates. The appeal stems from the relative simplicity of the measurement (both invasive and noninvasive) and its continuous nature. Theoretically, this enables care providers to monitor for hemodynamic compromise when it arises, and to monitor treatment response once therapy is instituted. However, there are several limitations to the current approach of the use of blood pressure to monitor and treat low blood flow states in preterm and term infants. Those limitations include a lack of robust normative dataset in both term and preterm populations, the dissociation between blood pressure and systemic blood flow when SVR is not taken into account, and the overreliance on mean blood pressure rather than the more important components of the measurement (systolic and diastolic blood pressures).

The definition of systemic hypotension is highly controversial, with several iterations currently in use. This lack of uniformity stems from the relative lack of a clear threshold below which autoregulation is impaired and organ perfusion (and cellular metabolism) are compromised. In fact, a single threshold may not even exist because it is likely to vary across different gestations, physiologic phases, and disease states. In practical terms, clinicians generally use 1 of 3 thresholds to define hypotension. The most widely used definition of hypotension is unfortunately the one with the least amount of supportive evidence: a mean blood pressure in mm Hg below the numerical gestational age of the infant in weeks. This arbitrary definition, although easy to remember, is not useful for identifying low blood flow states owing to the nonlinear and inverse relationship between these parameters.[33] Another threshold, used to define hypotension, is a mean blood pressure of less than 30 mm Hg. This cutoff is based on small studies that suggest there is a loss of cerebral autoregulation and cerebral white matter damage below this threshold.[34,35] There are, however, a lack of studies demonstrating any benefit to institution of treatment, using either inotropes and/or vasopressors, to correct blood pressure above those thresholds. A less commonly used approach to define hypotension that has recently been advocated is the use of normative centiles, derived from a large population set, of systolic and diastolic blood pressures.[36–38] This approach may be a more appropriate method of screening for potential hemodynamic compromise, especially when blood pressure falls below the third centiles for any given gestation; however, this approach is yet to be assessed systematically.

Appraisal of the relationship between blood pressure and cardiac output (systemic blood flow) must consider the SVR[39] because blood pressure is proportional to the product of cardiac output and SVR (blood pressure = cardiac output × SVR). A normal arterial pressure in the setting of a high SVR is usually accompanied by low cardiac output (such as infants with hypoxic ischemic encephalopathy). Conversely, a low blood pressure in the setting of low SVR may indicate normal or high cardiac output (such as infants with warm shock). As there are no ways to directly measure SVR in neonates, all assumptions are implied.

Considering blood pressure by its 2 distinct components, systolic and diastolic, may lead to a more physiologic basis for diagnosis and treatment of low blood flow states. Systolic blood pressure may reflect LV contractile force and effective cardiac output; therefore, a low value may indicate reduced stoke volume (which is influenced by preload, contractility, and afterload). Conversely, diastolic blood pressure may be more reflective of resting vascular tone (SVR) and intravascular blood volume (fluid status). Combined systolic and diastolic hypotension may be reflective of circulatory system failure, which may or may not have antecedent systolic or diastolic hypotension in isolation.[36] The physiologic impact of therapeutic intervention, based on these thresholds, and its relevance to neonatal outcomes needs prospective evaluation.

ENHANCED METHODS FOR ASSESSMENT OF THE HEMODYNAMIC STATUS

The limitations of clinical and laboratory indices support the need for a more comprehensive approach to the monitoring of hemodynamic status of sick neonates, identification of states of hemodynamic compromise, and evaluation of treatment response. Several new modalities have emerged over the last 15 to 20 years and are becoming increasingly used in daily clinical practice.

Neonatal Echocardiography

The use of echocardiography to evaluate cardiovascular well-being in neonates is common in many tertiary neonatal intensive care units.[40,41] When used in combination with clinical findings (to place the examination in context), neonatal echocardiography may be an invaluable tool for the identification of hemodynamic compromise, guiding therapeutic intervention, and monitoring treatment response. Over the last decade, there has been an increasing use of echocardiography performed by neonatologists around the world.[42] Neonatal echocardiography is most commonly used for the assessment of PDA significance, determining treatment benefit, and confirming PDA closure after treatment[43]; the prediction and management of hemodynamic instability after PDA ligation in preterm infants[44,45]; assessment of myocardial performance and monitoring treatment response in neonates with persistent pulmonary hypertension of the newborn and hypoxic ischemic encephalopathy[46–48]; and the assessment of central line positioning.[49,50] There are an increasing number of prospective studies that highlight the potential merits of neonatal echocardiography in identification of cardiovascular compromise and guiding neonatal cardiovascular care.[44,51–53] Regular use of echocardiography in the neonatal setting can lead to tangible improvement in the provision of care. Regular daily echocardiography once indomethacin treatment is instigated for PDA closure results in a reduction on the number of indomethacin doses given (and exposure to potential adverse effects) without increasing the number of treatment failures.[53] In addition, the use of echocardiography to provide targeted PDA treatment may result in a reduction of severe intraventricular hemorrhage and pulmonary haemorrhages.[51,52] For neonates undergoing PDA ligation, echocardiography is now used to identify potential infants at risk of hemodynamic compromise after the procedure and provide targeted therapy to avoid this compromise with significant success.[44,45] A detailed description of the use of echocardiography in various clinical scenarios in the preterm neonatal setting and its use to guide therapy has been described in detail by our group previously.[36,40] There is a clear need for the systematic evaluation of a targeted approach that guides an individualized treatment regimen of hypotension and low blood flow states and is physiologically based. This is of particular importance to the periviable infant population.

To ensure safe and effective use of this modality in the neonatal intensive care unit, there needs to be structured training programs designed to ensure competency and build clinical expertise in this field. There are currently 3 guidelines in existence with recommendations for training in basic and advanced echocardiography skills, building clinical expertise, maintenance of the acquired skills, and the infrastructure required for the implementation of a successful training program.[54–56] The only accredited training pathway for neonatal echocardiography currently in existence is the Neonatal Certificate in Clinician Performed Ultrasound, which is run by the Australian Society of Ultrasound Medicine (available from www.asum.com.au). The relative heterogeneity of these training programs (which is largely explained by the differing training needs across the various jurisdictions) highlights the need for the development of further accredited training bodies that hold the responsibility for training and ongoing maintenance of skills. The introduction of clinical programs should consider local expertise, patient populations, and proximity to pediatric echocardiography service; wherever possible, collaboration with pediatric echocardiography programs should be encouraged.

Noninvasive Techniques for Monitoring Cardiac Output

Although there are many advantages to imaging-guided care, the techniques required considerable skill and can only provide discrete intermittent measurements. The ability to provide continuous monitoring of cardiac output and possibly SVR in the neonatal population would be a welcome addition. In older children, and in adults, this can be achieved using thermodilution with a pulmonary artery catheter, an arterial catheter for pulse contour analysis, an intratracheal tube for partial CO_2 rebreathing, or an intraoesophageal probe for continuous Doppler velocity flow assessment. Thermodilution is regarded as the gold standard for continuous hemodynamic monitoring; however, this method is not feasible in the neonates owing to the invasive nature of the technique and the size constrains of the population of interest. Two relatively new noninvasive approaches for continuous monitoring of cardiac output based on the expanded theory of bioimpedance have recently emerged, namely, transthoracic bioreactance (TBR) and electrical velocimetry (EV).

TBR derives an estimate of stroke volume of the blood ejected from the aorta by measuring the degree of phase shift of an electrical current as it traverses the thorax (rather than measuring the attenuation of amplitude—bioimpedance). The system contains an algorithm that uses the degree of phase shift to derive stroke volume. Cardiac output can be derived by multiplying stroke volume by the heart rate. Interestingly, TBR can also be used to derive the SVR when invasive blood pressure readings are known, adding the potential advantage of knowing the 3 components that determine flow. This method has been validated extensively in the adult population against thermodilution with good agreement demonstrated.[57] TBR also possesses high sensitivity and specificity for predicting significant hemodynamic changes in critically ill adults, with good precision and responsiveness, in a wide range of intensive care circulatory situations when compared with thermodilution.[58] Validation studies in neonates have focused on comparing this technique with echocardiography. There is a strong correlation between TBR-derived LVO and both stroke volume and echocardiography derived parameters; however, there seems to be a systematic underestimation in TBR-derived values on the order of 30%.[59] TBR may also detect important hemodynamic changes occurring after PDA ligation in preterm infants.[60] Validation in small animal models with stroke volumes comparable to those in neonates (1–3 mL) demonstrated good agreement between TBR and invasive measurement of aortic blood flow.[61] The effect of significant intracardiac (PFO) and extracardiac (PDA) shunts on this technique has not been investigated to date in sick neonates. Current research using TBR is directed at delineating the hemodynamic profile on infants with hypoxic ischemic encephalopathy and persistent pulmonary hypertension of the newborn, with an assessment of the impact of therapeutic interventions on those parameters.

EV is based on the theory that the conductivity of blood in the aorta is higher during systole when all red blood cells are aligned in the direction of flow and lower in diastole when the red blood cells are randomly oriented. The mean rate of change in conductivity may be used to derive aortic stroke volume. There is evidence that EV-derived estimates of cardiac output are comparable with those obtained using echocardiography, with a mean difference of 4 mL/min. This method, however, demonstrates relatively wide limits of agreement ranging between −234 and 242 mL/min, with an adjusted percentage bias of 31.6%.[62] In addition, EV estimates of cardiac output are significantly influenced by a PDA and PFO. The presence of a high-volume shunt across the PDA increased the bias between the 2 methods from −6 to −36 mL/min in 1 study.[63] In another study, a PDA and PFO had a cumulative effect on EV measurements leading to an overestimation of EV-derived values when compared with echocardiography.[64] Further studies are required for both modalities to further demonstrate their potential benefit in the management of the hemodynamic status of neonates before widespread clinical use.

Near Infrared Spectroscopy

Near infrared spectroscopy (NIRS) offers the ability to assess target organ blood flow. It offers additional information regarding organ perfusion, which supplements data provided by echocardiography and other modalities.[65] The use of NIRS to assess cerebral perfusion is also subject to scientific adjudication. Early studies from adults demonstrated the benefit of NIRS in measuring cerebral perfusion during therapeutic hypothermia after cardiac arrest and during cardiac surgery.[66,67] Cerebral NIRS may also possess important prognostic abilities after cardiac arrest in adults.[68,69] Some of the first studies of NIRS in neonates also examined its use after cardiac surgery.[70,71]

In preterm infants, NIRS-derived fractional tissue oxygen extraction and regional cerebral oxygen saturation reference values, particularly over the first 72 hours of life, are emerging.[72] NIRS may provide novel insights into the effect of various disease states on end-organ flow. Recently, the use of NIRS was studied in infants with a hemodynamically significant PDA and demonstrated a decrease in regional cerebral oxygen saturation when a PDA persisted.[73] NIRS can also be used to assess regional saturations and fractional tissue oxygen extraction in the splanchnic vasculature with evidence, suggesting that this technique may be able to distinguish between complicated and uncomplicated necrotizing enterocolitis.[74] However, one of the most exciting uses of NIRS is its use in guiding the treatment of potential hemodynamic compromise and cerebral hypoxia in the preterm population. In a multicenter, randomized, controlled trial, infants monitored with NIRS and treated for evolving cerebral hypoxia had a lower cerebral hypoxic burden when compared with infants who were not treated based on NIRS findings.[75,76] The long-term benefit of this approach has yet to be elucidated. The role of NIRS as an ancillary monitoring device to support cardiovascular decision making in the neonatal intensive care unit is yet to be elucidated and should remain an investigative tool.

Cardiac MRI

Cardiovascular MRI, using balanced steady-state free precession, has been used recently in preterm infants to provide a more accurate delineation of myocardial volume, function, dimension, and flow across important shunts, such as a PDA. It has been validated recently in the neonatal population.[77,78] Its use in the preterm population remains in the research area at present, but this technique may provide novel insights.

A PATHOPHYSIOLOGY-BASED APPROACH TO THE MANAGEMENT OF LOW BLOOD FLOW STATES

Advances in neonatal intensive care, coupled with our enhanced understanding of preterm infant transitional physiology and the introduction of the enhanced methods of assessment as outlined, can pave the way for a more holistic approach to the management of low blood flow states and hypotension. Periviable preterm infants, with their inherent challenges, are the population most likely to benefit from this approach. The principles of this approach include a more objective assessment of the cardiovascular system as a whole, including a focus of target organ flow. This objective assessment needs to be performed on a continuous basis during the critical transitional period. This monitoring will enable a targeted and tailored approach to each physiologic situation (**Fig. 4**).

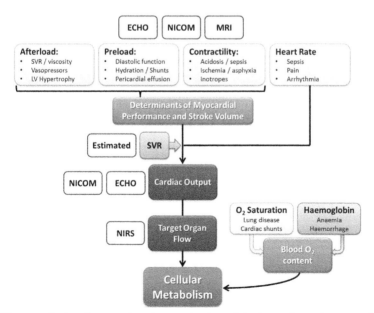

Fig. 4. The complexity of comprehensive monitoring of the hemodynamic status of periviable infants. ECHO, echocardiography; LV, left ventricular; NICOM, noninvasive cardiac output monitoring; NIRS, near infrared spectroscopy; SVR, systemic vascular resistance.

Treatment of low blood pressure in isolation may not necessarily translate into an improvement in systemic blood flow, because many cardiotropic agents (eg, dopamine) act by increasing SVR but at the expense of cardiac output. This approach does not take into account the maturity of the infant, the underlying cause, the presumed physiology, or other potential iatrogenic influences on systemic blood flow, including other medications, mechanical ventilation, or the presence of a PDA. There is limited evidence supporting the use of current therapeutic agents. Rather, the ultimate goal of treatment should be to maintain adequate oxygen delivery and tissue oxygenation to ensure normal cellular metabolism and not "normalizing" the blood pressure. Other factors influencing the adequacy of cellular oxygen delivery include hemoglobin and oxygen saturation, as well as factors influencing myocardial performance. Oxygen consumption should also be minimized by ensuring adequate sedation if necessary, pain control, and normothermia. A suggested approach to management is summarized in **Fig. 5**.

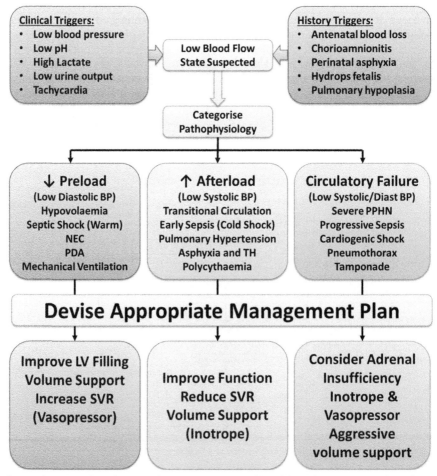

Fig. 5. Physiology-based approach to management of low blood flow states. BP, blood pressure; NEC, necrotizing enterocolitis; PDA, patent ductus arteriosus; PPHN, persistent pulmonary hypertension of the newborn; SVR, systemic vascular resistance.

SUMMARY

Preterm infants, particularly infants around the periviable period, provide a considerable challenge in the management of hemodynamic compromise. The pathophysiology and etiology is varied and depends on a variety of antenatal factors, transitional events, and postnatal stressors. This variation has precluded the benefit of a standardized approach to management. Individualized care is likely to be the most appropriate pathway to ensure optimal outcomes. To achieve this care and devise an initialized approach, reliable, precise and valid methods are needed to offer optimal and continuous monitoring.

REFERENCES

1. Kuint J, Barak M, Morag I, et al. Early treated hypotension and outcome in very low birth weight infants. Neonatology 2009;95(4):311–6.
2. Liedel JL, Meadow W, Nachman J, et al. Use of vasopressin in refractory hypotension in children with vasodilatory shock: five cases and a review of the literature. Pediatr Crit Care Med 2002;3(1):15–8.
3. Lang JA, Pearson JT, te Pas AB, et al. Ventilation/perfusion mismatch during lung aeration at birth. J Appl Physiol (1985) 2014;117(5):535–43.
4. van Vonderen JJ, Roest AA, Siew ML, et al. Measuring physiological changes during the transition to life after birth. Neonatology 2014;105(3):230–42.
5. Hooper SB, Polglase GR, te Pas AB. A physiological approach to the timing of umbilical cord clamping at birth. Arch Dis Child Fetal Neonatal Ed 2014;100(4): F355–60.
6. Hermes-DeSantis ER, Clyman RI. Patent ductus arteriosus: pathophysiology and management. J Perinatol 2006;26(Suppl 1):S14–8.
7. Rowland DG, Gutgesell HP. Noninvasive assessment of myocardial contractility, preload, and afterload in healthy newborn infants. Am J Cardiol 1995;75(12): 818–21.
8. Noori S, Seri I. Pathophysiology of newborn hypotension outside the transitional period. Early Hum Dev 2005;81(5):399–404.
9. Ali I, Ryan CA. Transient renal failure in twins with maternal Cox-1/Cox-2 use in pregnancy. Ir Med J 2005;98(10):249–50.
10. Ng PC, Lee CH, Lam CW, et al. Transient adrenocortical insufficiency of prematurity and systemic hypotension in very low birthweight infants. Arch Dis Child Fetal Neonatal Ed 2004;89(2):F119–26.
11. Ng PC, Lam CW, Fok TF, et al. Refractory hypotension in preterm infants with adrenocortical insufficiency. Arch Dis Child Fetal Neonatal Ed 2001;84(2):F122–4.
12. Noori S, Friedlich P, Wong P, et al. Hemodynamic changes after low-dosage hydrocortisone administration in vasopressor-treated preterm and term neonates. Pediatrics 2006;118(4):1456–66.
13. Dokainish H. Left ventricular diastolic function and dysfunction: central role of echocardiography. Glob Cardiol Sci Pract 2015;2015:3.
14. Fajardo MF, Claure N, Swaminathan S, et al. Effect of positive end-expiratory pressure on ductal shunting and systemic blood flow in preterm infants with patent ductus arteriosus. Neonatology 2014;105(1):9–13.
15. Polglase GR, Miller SL, Barton SK, et al. Respiratory support for premature neonates in the delivery room: effects on cardiovascular function and the development of brain injury. Pediatr Res 2014;75(6):682–8.
16. Tomerak RH, El-Badawy AA, Hussein G, et al. Echocardiogram done early in neonatal sepsis: what does it add? J Investig Med 2012;60(4):680–4.

17. Abdel-Hady HE, Matter MK, El-Arman MM. Myocardial dysfunction in neonatal sepsis: a tissue Doppler imaging study. Pediatr Crit Care Med 2012;13(3): 318–23.
18. Hensler ME, Miyamoto S, Nizet V. Group B streptococcal beta-hemolysin/ cytolysin directly impairs cardiomyocyte viability and function. PLoS One 2008; 3(6):e2446.
19. Barrington KJ. Common hemodynamic problems in the neonate. Neonatology 2013;103(4):335–40.
20. Faust K, Hartel C, Preuss M, et al. Short-term outcome of very-low-birthweight infants with arterial hypotension in the first 24 h of life. Arch Dis Child Fetal Neonatal Ed 2015;100(5):F388–92.
21. Batton B, Li L, Newman NS, et al. Early blood pressure, antihypotensive therapy and outcomes at 18-22 months' corrected age in extremely preterm infants. Arch Dis Child Fetal Neonatal Ed 2016;101(3):F201–6.
22. Szpecht D, Szymankiewicz M, Nowak I, et al. Intraventricular hemorrhage in neonates born before 32 weeks of gestation-retrospective analysis of risk factors. Childs Nerv Syst 2016;32(8):1399–404.
23. Kluckow M, Evans N. Low superior vena cava flow and intraventricular haemorrhage in preterm infants. Arch Dis Child Fetal Neonatal Ed 2000;82(3):F188–94.
24. Osborn DA, Evans N, Kluckow M. Hemodynamic and antecedent risk factors of early and late periventricular/intraventricular hemorrhage in premature infants. Pediatrics 2003;112(1 Pt 1):33–9.
25. Hunt RW, Evans N, Rieger I, et al. Low superior vena cava flow and neurodevelopment at 3 years in very preterm infants. J Pediatr 2004;145(5):588–92.
26. Noori S, McCoy M, Anderson MP, et al. Changes in cardiac function and cerebral blood flow in relation to peri/intraventricular hemorrhage in extremely preterm infants. J Pediatr 2014;164(2):264–70.
27. James AT, Corcoran JD, Franklin O, et al. Clinical utility of right ventricular fractional area change in preterm infants. Early Hum Dev 2016;92:19–23.
28. Paradisis M, Evans N, Kluckow M, et al. Pilot study of milrinone for low systemic blood flow in very preterm infants. J Pediatr 2006;148(3):306–13.
29. van Vonderen JJ, Roest AA, Siew ML, et al. Noninvasive measurements of hemodynamic transition directly after birth. Pediatr Res 2014;75(3):448–52.
30. Osborn D, Evans N, Kluckow M. Randomized trial of dobutamine versus dopamine in preterm infants with low systemic blood flow. J Pediatr 2002;140(2): 183–91.
31. Gale C. Question 2. Is capillary refill time a useful marker of haemodynamic status in neonates? Arch Dis Child 2010;95(5):395–7.
32. de Boode WP. Clinical monitoring of systemic hemodynamics in critically ill newborns. Early Hum Dev 2010;86(3):137–41.
33. Stranak Z, Semberova J, Barrington K, et al. International survey on diagnosis and management of hypotension in extremely preterm babies. Eur J Pediatr 2014;173(6):793–8.
34. Munro MJ, Walker AM, Barfield CP. Hypotensive extremely low birth weight infants have reduced cerebral blood flow. Pediatrics 2004;114(6):1591–6.
35. Borch K, Lou HC, Greisen G. Cerebral white matter blood flow and arterial blood pressure in preterm infants. Acta Paediatr 2010;99(10):1489–92.
36. Giesinger RE, McNamara PJ. Hemodynamic instability in the critically ill neonate: an approach to cardiovascular support based on disease pathophysiology. Semin Perinatol 2016;40(3):174–88.

37. Hegyi T, Anwar M, Carbone MT, et al. Blood pressure ranges in premature infants: II. The first week of life. Pediatrics 1996;97(3):336–42.
38. Hegyi T, Carbone MT, Anwar M, et al. Blood pressure ranges in premature infants. I. The first hours of life. J Pediatr 1994;124(4):627–33.
39. Kluckow M, Evans N. Relationship between blood pressure and cardiac output in preterm infants requiring mechanical ventilation. J Pediatr 1996;129(4):506–12.
40. El-Khuffash AF, McNamara PJ. Neonatologist-performed functional echocardiography in the neonatal intensive care unit. Semin Fetal Neonatal Med 2011;16(1): 50–60.
41. Weisz DE, Poon WB, James A, et al. Low cardiac output secondary to a malpositioned umbilical venous catheter: value of targeted neonatal echocardiography. AJP Rep 2014;4(1):23–8.
42. Evans N, Gournay V, Cabanas F, et al. Point-of-care ultrasound in the neonatal intensive care unit: international perspectives. Semin Fetal Neonatal Med 2011; 16(1):61–8.
43. El-Khuffash A, Weisz DE, McNamara PJ. Reflections of the changes in patent ductus arteriosus management during the last 10 years. Arch Dis Child Fetal Neonatal Ed 2016;101(5):F474–8.
44. Jain A, Sahni M, El-Khuffash A, et al. Use of targeted neonatal echocardiography to prevent postoperative cardiorespiratory instability after patent ductus arteriosus ligation. J Pediatr 2012;160(4):584–9.
45. El-Khuffash AF, Jain A, Weisz D, et al. Assessment and treatment of post patent ductus arteriosus ligation syndrome. J Pediatr 2014;165(1):46–52.
46. James AT, Corcoran JD, McNamara PJ, et al. The effect of milrinone on right and left ventricular function when used as a rescue therapy for term infants with pulmonary hypertension. Cardiol Young 2016;26(1):90–9.
47. Sehgal A, Wong F, Menahem S. Speckle tracking derived strain in infants with severe perinatal asphyxia: a comparative case control study. Cardiovasc Ultrasound 2013;11:34.
48. McNamara PJ, Shivananda SP, Sahni M, et al. Pharmacology of milrinone in neonates with persistent pulmonary hypertension of the newborn and suboptimal response to inhaled nitric oxide. Pediatr Crit Care Med 2013;14(1):74–84.
49. Jain A, McNamara PJ, Ng E, et al. The use of targeted neonatal echocardiography to confirm placement of peripherally inserted central catheters in neonates. Am J Perinatol 2012;29(2):101–6.
50. El-Khuffash A, Herbozo C, Jain A, et al. Targeted neonatal echocardiography (TnECHO) service in a Canadian neonatal intensive care unit: a 4-year experience. J Perinatol 2013;33(9):687–90.
51. O'Rourke DJ, El-Khuffash A, Moody C, et al. Patent ductus arteriosus evaluation by serial echocardiography in preterm infants. Acta Paediatr 2008;97(5):574–8.
52. Kluckow M, Jeffery M, Gill A, et al. A randomised placebo-controlled trial of early treatment of the patent ductus arteriosus. Arch Dis Child Fetal Neonatal Ed 2014; 99(2):F99–104.
53. Carmo KB, Evans N, Paradisis M. Duration of indomethacin treatment of the preterm patent ductus arteriosus as directed by echocardiography. J Pediatr 2009; 155(6):819–22.
54. Singh Y, Gupta S, Groves AM, et al. Expert consensus statement 'Neonatologist-performed echocardiography (NoPE)'-training and accreditation in UK. Eur J Pediatr 2016;175(2):281–7.
55. Mertens L, Seri I, Marek J, et al. Targeted neonatal echocardiography in the neonatal intensive care unit: practice guidelines and recommendations for

training writing group of the American Society of Echocardiography (ASE) in collaboration with the European Association of Echocardiography (EAE) and the Association for European Pediatric Cardiologists (AEPC). J Am Soc Echocardiogr 2011;24(10):1057–78.

56. de Boode WP, Singh Y, Gupta S, et al. Recommendations for neonatologist performed echocardiography in Europe: consensus statement endorsed by European Society for Paediatric Research (ESPR) and European Society for Neonatology (ESN). Pediatr Res 2016;80(4):465–71.

57. Squara P, Denjean D, Estagnasie P, et al. Noninvasive cardiac output monitoring (NICOM): a clinical validation. Intensive Care Med 2007;33(7):1191–4.

58. Marque S, Cariou A, Chiche JD, et al. Comparison between Flotrac-Vigileo and Bioreactance, a totally noninvasive method for cardiac output monitoring. Crit Care 2009;13(3):R73.

59. Weisz DE, Jain A, McNamara PJ, et al. Non-invasive cardiac output monitoring in neonates using bioreactance: a comparison with echocardiography. Neonatology 2012;102(1):61–7.

60. Weisz DE, Jain A, Ting J, et al. Non-invasive cardiac output monitoring in preterm infants undergoing patent ductus arteriosus ligation: a comparison with echocardiography. Neonatology 2014;106(4):330–6.

61. Heerdt PM, Wagner CL, Demais M, et al. Noninvasive cardiac output monitoring with bioreactance as an alternative to invasive instrumentation for preclinical drug evaluation in beagles. J Pharmacol Toxicol Methods 2011;64(2):111–8.

62. Noori S, Drabu B, Soleymani S, et al. Continuous non-invasive cardiac output measurements in the neonate by electrical velocimetry: a comparison with echocardiography. Arch Dis Child Fetal Neonatal Ed 2012;97(5):F340–3.

63. Torigoe T, Sato S, Nagayama Y, et al. Influence of patent ductus arteriosus and ventilators on electrical velocimetry for measuring cardiac output in very-low/low birth weight infants. J Perinatol 2015;35(7):485–9.

64. Blohm ME, Hartwich J, Obrecht D, et al. Effect of patent ductus arteriosus and patent foramen ovale on left ventricular stroke volume measurement by electrical velocimetry in comparison to transthoracic echocardiography in neonates. J Clin Monit Comput 2016. [Epub ahead of print].

65. Murkin JM, Arango M. Near-infrared spectroscopy as an index of brain and tissue oxygenation. Br J Anaesth 2009;103(Suppl 1):i3–13.

66. Suffoletto B, Kristan J, Rittenberger JC, et al. Near-infrared spectroscopy in post-cardiac arrest patients undergoing therapeutic hypothermia. Resuscitation 2012; 83(8):986–90.

67. Senanayake E, Komber M, Nassef A, et al. Effective cerebral protection using near-infrared spectroscopy monitoring with antegrade cerebral perfusion during aortic surgery. J Cardiovasc Surg 2012;27(2):211–6.

68. Shin'oka T, Nollert G, Shum-Tim D, et al. Utility of near-infrared spectroscopic measurements during deep hypothermic circulatory arrest. Ann Thorac Surg 2000;69(2):578–83.

69. Abdul-Khaliq H, Schubert S, Troitzsch D, et al. Dynamic changes in cerebral oxygenation related to deep hypothermia and circulatory arrest evaluated by near-infrared spectroscopy. Acta Anaesthesiol Scand 2001;45(6):696–701.

70. Abdul-Khaliq H, Troitzsch D, Schubert S, et al. Cerebral oxygen monitoring during neonatal cardiopulmonary bypass and deep hypothermic circulatory arrest. Thorac Cardiovasc Surg 2002;50(2):77–81.

71. Toet MC, Flinterman A, Laar I, et al. Cerebral oxygen saturation and electrical brain activity before, during, and up to 36 hours after arterial switch procedure

in neonates without pre-existing brain damage: its relationship to neurodevelopmental outcome. Exp Brain Res 2005;165(3):343–50.

72. Alderliesten T, Dix L, Baerts W, et al. Reference values of regional cerebral oxygen saturation during the first 3 days of life in preterm neonates. Pediatr Res 2016;79(1–1):55–64.

73. Dix L, Molenschot M, Breur J, et al. Cerebral oxygenation and echocardiographic parameters in preterm neonates with a patent ductus arteriosus: an observational study. Arch Dis Child Fetal Neonatal Ed 2016. [Epub ahead of print].

74. Schat TE, Schurink M, van der Laan ME, et al. Near-infrared spectroscopy to Predict the Course of Necrotizing enterocolitis. PLoS One 2016;11(5):e0154710.

75. Pellicer A, Greisen G, Benders M, et al. The SafeBoosC phase II randomised clinical trial: a treatment guideline for targeted near-infrared-derived cerebral tissue oxygenation versus standard treatment in extremely preterm infants. Neonatology 2013;104(3):171–8.

76. Plomgaard AM, van Oeveren W, Petersen TH, et al. The SafeBoosC II randomized trial: treatment guided by near-infrared spectroscopy reduces cerebral hypoxia without changing early biomarkers of brain injury. Pediatr Res 2016;79(4):528–35.

77. Broadhouse KM, Price AN, Durighel G, et al. Assessment of PDA shunt and systemic blood flow in newborns using cardiac MRI. NMR Biomed 2013;26(9): 1135–41.

78. Price AN, Malik SJ, Broadhouse KM, et al. Neonatal cardiac MRI using prolonged balanced SSFP imaging at 3T with active frequency stabilization. Magn Reson Med 2013;70(3):776–84.

Nutrition for the Extremely Preterm Infant

Kera McNelis, MD, Ting Ting Fu, MD, Brenda Poindexter, MD, MS*

KEYWORDS

- Extremely preterm • Infant • Neonate • Nutrition • Growth faltering
- Necrotizing enterocolitis • Breast milk

KEY POINTS

- Complete parenteral nutrition, including intravenous lipid emulsions, should be delivered to extremely preterm infants on the day of birth.
- A standardized feeding protocol and the preferential use of human milk are important steps in the prevention of necrotizing enterocolitis.
- Early breast milk fortification should be used to meet the needs of extremely preterm infants, and implementation of a strategy for fortification of donor breast milk is necessary to avoid growth faltering.

INTRODUCTION

With advancements in the care of preterm infants, the goals in nutritional care have expanded from survival and mimicking fetal growth to optimizing neurodevelopmental outcomes.[1] Among infants born at the limits of viability, the challenges of providing optimal nutritional support are magnified and the consequences of failing to do so are greatest. The management challenges these infants present relate to not having appropriate tools to monitor growth, availability of nutritional products (both parenteral and enteral) designed to support the most immature, and a myriad of morbidities that complicate the ability to deliver optimal nutrition.

NORMAL POSTNATAL GROWTH OF EXTREMELY PRETERM INFANTS

Healthy fetal growth rates must first be established as the basis for reference to assess neonatal growth.[2] Despite the availability of more intrauterine growth curves, constructed and validated from a large, racially diverse US population that may now be used as a more representative tool for neonatal growth assessment,[3] these curves

Disclosure Statement: The authors have nothing to disclose.
Perinatal Institute, Cincinnati Children's Hospital Medical Center, 3333 Burnet Avenue, Cincinnati, OH 45229-3026, USA
* Corresponding author.
E-mail address: Brenda.Poindexter@cchmc.org

are still hindered by the fact that they reflect cross-sectional data of infants born prematurely. Indeed, this was recognized by Dr Lubchenco and colleagues[4] in the 1960s when she acknowledged the limitation of her landmark estimate of intrauterine growth as follows: "The sample has an undeterminable bias because premature birth itself is probably related to non-physiological states of variable duration in either mother or fetus." In addition to this inherent limitation, the number of 22- to 24-week gestational age infants included in cohorts from which these curves were constructed is extremely small (1175 and 5510 infants, respectively; **Table 1**), which further limits their use in this population. There are observational studies suggesting that customized fetal growth charts, incorporating gestational age, fetal sex, parity, ethnicity, maternal age, height, and weight, may better predict constitutional versus pathologic growth restriction, but there is a paucity of high-quality evidence for the use of these growth charts.[5–7] Comparing neonatal growth in the first weeks of life to predicted fetal growth does not account for the contraction of body water compartments or initial catabolic state, although postnatal weight loss may be absent in the extremely preterm infants.[8,9] Early nutritional care to support an adequate initial postnatal growth rate (18–20 g/kg/d) is correlated to improved neurodevelopmental outcomes in comparison with late catch-up growth.[10,11] The Fenton Preterm Growth Charts were recently revised to account for the new World Health Organization Growth Standard Preterm Multicentre Growth study and the fetal-infant growth reference.[12,13] The International Fetal and Newborn Growth Consortium (INTERGROWTH-21st) project used serial ultrasound measurements and anthropometric measurements to assess fetal growth in a multiethnic population, but given that the study targeted healthy pregnancies without any evidence of fetal growth restriction, very few infants born at less than 33 weeks' estimated gestational age met eligibility criteria for inclusion in the study.[14–16] As a result, even this large population-based study does not offer additional help to clinicians to assess growth of the most immature infants. For the most preterm infants, there currently is no method to differentiate small-for-gestational-age infants (constitutionally small) versus those infants who suffered intrauterine growth restriction (pathologically small). This characterization could potentially stratify the risk of necrotizing enterocolitis (NEC) and postnatal growth faltering.

GROWTH FALTERING OF EXTREMELY PRETERM INFANTS

The incidence of growth faltering is inversely related to gestational age and is associated with higher morbidity and adverse long-term outcomes.[8,17,18] Independent risk factors for growth include length of ventilatory support, length of hospitalization,

Table 1
Number of infants from 22 to 24 weeks' gestational age included in reference growth curves

Gestational Age (wk)	Olsen et al,[3] 2010 (Total N = 257,855)	Fenton & Kim,[12] 2013 (Total N = 3,986,456)	Lubchenco et al,[4] 1963; Villar et al,[16] 2016 (Total N = 5636)
22	—	816	—
23	286	1682	—
24	889	3012	24
Total n (% of cohort)	1175 (0.46%)	5510[a] (0.14%)	24 (0.43%)

[a] The revised Fenton curves include infants in Olsen curves.
Data from Refs.[3,4,12,16]

bronchopulmonary dysplasia, and NEC.[18–20] Inadequate nutritional support may be a risk factor for major complications of prematurity; conversely, higher disease burden is a risk for growth restriction. The birth of an extremely preterm infant represents a nutritional emergency, and early provision of protein is correlated with improved growth.[21,22] Frequently, actual delivery of energy and macronutrients falls short of intended intake.[23] Early energy and macronutrient deficits can be difficult to overcome with later nutritional practices.[24] Adoption of early high parenteral nutritional support and early standardized feeding practices leads to lower incidence of growth faltering in this population.[25–29]

GROWTH BEYOND MEASURE: ADVANCED TECHNIQUES IN BODY COMPOSITION

Anthropometric measurements are ubiquitous in neonatal nutritional care, as these measurements are well studied, affordable, and noninvasive. Length more accurately reflects lean body mass growth and is an important biomarker to predict long-term developmental outcomes, but is a less reliable measurement.[9,30] Obtaining accurate linear growth can be challenging when measurements are deferred, while the extremely preterm infant is clinically unstable or with concerns for inadvertent extubation. A more complete measurement of neonatal growth includes proportionality indices. Body mass index z-score is emerging as an additional indicator of growth in term infants, but this is poorly studied in preterm infants at the limits of viability.[31] Likewise, measuring midarm circumference is an affordable technique to estimate adiposity that could be readily incorporated into standard intensive care practice, but past studies have focused on preterm infants that are not at the earliest gestational age.[32] Body composition measurements through air displacement plethysmography, dual-energy X-ray absorptiometry, or MRI are well studied, but this technology is cost prohibitive for many neonatal intensive care units.[33–35] Body composition measurements through air displacement plethysmography may only be done for infants in room air, and preterm infants delivered at the limits of viability frequently have a lengthy duration of supplemental oxygen requirements.[36]

EARLY SUPPORT THROUGH PARENTERAL NUTRITION

The birth of an extremely preterm infant represents a nutritional emergency, because the high rate of fetal accretion of nutrient supply through placental flow must be replaced. Parenteral nutrition supports energy and nutrient needs during early postnatal life of the extremely preterm infant until enteral feeding is established.

Amino Acids

Early amino acid intake in very low-birth-weight infants results in an anabolic state and is positively correlated with neurodevelopmental outcomes.[37,38] Variation in policies and practices between neonatal intensive care units is a barrier to meeting recommendations of early amino acid administration despite supportive evidence.[39] The amino acid composition of parenteral nutrition was designed to mimic the plasma amino acid profile of healthy, term, breast-fed infants.[40] Conversely, the amino acid profile of a healthy fetus at the equivalent postmenstrual age of the extremely preterm infant is unknown. The normal fetal amino acid profile represents an opportunity for new study. Currently used amino acid solutions are not specifically designed for the extremely preterm infant, as the particular needs of essential and conditionally essential amino acids are not well studied. The need for essential and conditionally essential amino acids represents an opportunity for improvement in our practice because extremely preterm infants may not have the equivalent synthetic capacity as other populations.

Carbohydrate

Glucose is the main energy source in fetal life, and in early postnatal life, extremely preterm infants are at risk of altered glucose homeostasis.[41] Early continuous glucose infusion is required to provide a continuous energy source to the brain and vital organs.[42] Early provision of amino acid has been the focus of neonatal nutrition research, but the early provision of sufficient glucose and energy is equally important. Hyperglycemia is a common challenge in early postnatal life of extremely preterm infants, and it can be precipitated by iatrogenic glucose delivery and stressors, such as NEC, infection, and surgery.[43] Hyperglycemia in very low-birth-weight infants is associated with increased length of hospital stay and morbidity.[44–46]

Lipids

Intravenous lipid emulsions provide a main energy source for preterm neonates and essential fatty acids. Provision of lipid emulsion must be sufficient to prevent essential fatty acid deficiency and match metabolic demands. Although the current recommendation is to begin intravenous lipid emulsion at 2 g/kg/d on the day of birth, this practice is not ubiquitous.[47] There is evidence that early lipid emulsion delivery is associated with later neurologic development in very preterm infants.[48] Currently, only soy-oil product is approved for use in the United States, although other products are available in Europe and may be available for compassionate use or research protocols.[49] There is emerging evidence that fish-oil lipid emulsion (Omegaven), which is high in omega-3 fatty acids, may prevent parenteral nutrition-associated liver disease.[50] A lipid emulsion containing medium-chain triglycerides, olive, and fish oils (SMOFlipid) is associated with a lower risk of retinopathy of prematurity and an improved fatty acid profile.[51–54] There is a weak association of use of non-soy-oil lipid emulsions with a lower risk of sepsis.[55] Large randomized controlled trials are needed to guide optimal dose, timing, and product choice of lipid emulsions for extremely preterm infants. Although use of soy-oil lipid emulsion was implemented before prospective clinical trials, the introduction of alternative lipid emulsion product for neonates should be preceded by a sufficiently large study to insure safety.

Special Concerns Regarding Other Components of Parenteral Nutrition

Within the United States, there is a constantly changing supply of parenteral nutrition components.[56] Extremely preterm infants are a particularly vulnerable population, as enteral substitutes are not always an option.[57] For zinc and phosphorus in particular, there are case reports of deleterious effects of dose restriction of parenteral nutrient components in preterm infants subjected to national shortages.[58,59] In times of shortages, strategies to prioritize the most preterm infants should be enacted. The American Society for Parenteral and Enteral Nutrition Web site maintains up-to-date parenteral nutrition component shortage management strategies for clinicians (www.nutritioncare.org).[60,61]

Unfortunately, parenteral nutrition is a source of aluminum toxicity, which is associated with anemia, osteopenia, neurologic defects, and parenteral nutrition–associated liver disease. Prolonged use of parenteral nutrition leads to excessive manganese deposition in the brain. These diseases are already a risk for the extremely preterm infant.[62,63] The use and solubility of calcium chloride and sodium phosphate rather than calcium gluconate and potassium phosphate have been studied to decrease aluminum concentration in parenteral nutrition.[64] Development of new compositions for parenteral nutrition solutions that deliver appropriate nutrient concentrations within the constraints of osmolarity is an opportunity for improvement.

ENTERAL NUTRITION FOR THE EXTREMELY PRETERM INFANT
What to Feed: Beginning with Maternal Breast Milk and Fortifying

Maternal breast milk is the preferred choice for feeding extremely preterm infants, because it confers a decreased risk of NEC, late-onset sepsis, and death.[65–67] The protection conferred by human milk is dose dependent.[68] Although breast milk is the optimal choice for feeding, it has insufficient nutrients, including calcium, phosphorus, and protein, to meet the needs of the extremely preterm infant, so human milk fortifier must be used to improve nutrient delivery and enhance growth.[69–71] Past concerns about the osmolarity and delayed gastric emptying leading to feeding intolerance and NEC have been negated with recent research.[72,73] There is emerging evidence that early fortification of feeds may be well tolerated and improve growth.[74,75]

However, fortification is complicated and challenging in this population. Fortification products vary in nutritional content based on the manufacturer alone, and liquid fortifiers, which are now the most commonly used products, carry the disadvantage of displacing maternal milk. Furthermore, major manufacturers assume the protein content of human preterm milk to be 1.4 to 1.6 g/dL (Abbott Nutrition, Mead Johnson Nutrition), but in reality, the macronutrient composition of human milk at baseline is highly variable and depends on individual mothers, gestational age, stage of lactation, duration of lactation, and method of expression.[66] Thus, standard fortifiers may not consistently provide adequate protein and calorie intake, but newer bovine milk protein–based fortification products with higher protein content result in improved growth.[76]

Other approaches to alleviate this problem include adjustable and targeted fortification strategies in which providers fortify based on blood urea nitrogen levels of patients or point-of-care macronutrient analysis of human milk, respectively. However, targeted fortification is very labor intensive and may have limited clinical availability.[77,78]

Another concern regarding the fortification of human milk revolves around the risk for developing NEC associated with bovine protein–based preterm formula.[79] The most frequently used fortifiers contain bovine protein, which may be antigenic; thus, some practitioners choose to use ProLactPlus fortifiers (Prolacta Bioscience), a human milk–based human milk fortifier. Although there are no randomized controlled trials comparing an exclusive human milk–based diet and the use of human milk fortified with bovine milk–based fortifiers, there are small studies with limited evidence that a complete human milk diet can improve feeding tolerance and decrease incidence of NEC. The limited available evidence is a result of studies funded by the manufacturers of the human milk fortifiers.[80–83] Although the human milk–based fortifier provides lower protein than bovine-based fortifiers, growth and neurodevelopment outcomes of extremely low-birth-weight infants can still be supported on an exclusive human milk–based diet.[84]

Donor Breast Milk Supplementation

Although maternal breast milk is the preferred enteral nutrition substrate, only 30% of mothers of extremely preterm infants produce enough milk to supply the entirety of their child's feeds.[85] Pasteurized donor breast milk (DBM) is often used as an alternative to formula, either for supplementation or for primary diet, but concerns regarding its nutritional content still remain as the vast majority of donors are mothers of term babies in later stages of lactation. Compared with preterm milk, term milk contains less protein, lipid, and total calories, and these concentrations decrease as lactation progresses over time.[67] Studies analyzing the composition of DBM reported average concentrations of 0.9 to 1.0 g/dL protein and 14.6 to 19.8 kcal/oz.[86,87] Protein in particular is necessary for growth and optimal neurodevelopment.[79] For extremely premature infants, enteral protein and caloric intakes should be targeted around 4.0 to 4.5 g/kg/d and 110 to 135 kcal/kg/d, respectively, to counter losses and facilitate accretion, and this may be more difficult to achieve using DBM.[88,89]

Another concern regarding DBM is the effect of pasteurization on the bioactive components of breast milk. Secretory immunoglobulin A (sIgA) and lactoferrin are the most abundant immune components found in breast milk, and Holder pasteurization has been shown to retain 67% to 100% of sIgA activity but only 27% to 43% of lactoferrin activity.[90] It is unclear the extent of immunoprotection the remaining bioactivity offers. Furthermore, lipoprotein lipase and bile salt–activated lipase, which aid in digestion of triglycerides, are completely inactivated by pasteurization.[90]

When and How: Feeding Protocol Choices

Beliefs regarding minimizing the risk of NEC lead to delayed introduction or advancement of enteral feeding; yet enteral feeding is essential to promote gastrointestinal development, and the poor use of the gastrointestinal tract blunts intestinal mucosal growth.[91] There is little evidence that delaying enteral feedings decreases the risk of NEC.[92] Use of a standardized feeding protocol to minimize clinical practice variability allows preterm infants to achieve full enteral feeds faster, decreases the rates of NEC, and promotes improved neurodevelopment.[93–95] Still, there is great variability between intensive care units' feeding regimens.[96,97] Some units practice a slow feeding advancement protocol based on observational studies demonstrating a reduced incidence of NEC.[98,99] However, a systemic review demonstrated that slow feeding advancement does not reduce the incidence of NEC and prolongs the time to achieve full enteral feeding.[100]

NUTRITION AFTER ACUTE ILLNESS

After surgical NEC, maternal breast milk remains the gold standard when enteral feedings are reintroduced. Hydrolyzed or elemental formulas are frequently used when maternal breast milk is insufficient because of an unfounded concern for immune response to bovine milk protein.[101,102] Although these formulas are frequently used, these products were not designed to meet the extraordinary needs of the extremely preterm infant.

Postdischarge nutrition requires careful consideration by the care team. Prescriptive preterm formulas or fortifications are expensive and not readily available to the general public. Newborn intensive care units may have variable resources, and extremely preterm infants may not be able to be followed by a skilled nutritionist following discharge or provided with a supply of special formula. The discharging care team should carefully consider the home-going feeding plan based on the resources at hand so that catch-up growth can continue to be supported.[103]

SUMMARY

With advancements in the care of preterm infants, the goals in nutritional care have expanded from survival and mimicking fetal growth to optimizing neurodevelopmental outcomes. Inadequate nutritional support may be a risk factor for major complications of prematurity; conversely, higher disease burden is a risk for growth restriction. Early complete parenteral nutrition support, including intravenous lipid emulsion, should be adopted, and the next challenge that should be addressed is parenteral nutrition customized to fit the specific needs and metabolism of the extremely preterm infant.

Standardized feeding protocols should be adopted, which include early introduction to enteral feeding, preferential use of human milk, early fortification, and targeted fortification of DBM.

REFERENCES

1. Ehrenkranz RA, Dusick AM, Vohr BR, et al. Growth in the neonatal intensive care unit influences neurodevelopmental and growth outcomes of extremely low birth weight infants. Pediatrics 2006;117(4):1253–61.
2. Clark RH, Olsen IE, Spitzer AR. Assessment of neonatal growth in prematurely born infants. Clin Perinatol 2014;41(2):295–307.
3. Olsen IE, Groveman SA, Lawson ML, et al. New intrauterine growth curves based on United States data. Pediatrics 2010;125(2):e214–24.
4. Lubchenco LO, Hansman C, Dressler M, et al. Intrauterine growth as estimated from liveborn birth-weight data at 24 to 42 weeks of gestation. Pediatrics 1963; 32:793–800.
5. Carberry AE, Gordon A, Bond DM, et al. Customised versus population-based growth charts as a screening tool for detecting small for gestational age infants in low-risk pregnant women. Cochrane Database Syst Rev 2011;(12):CD008549.
6. Chauhan SP, Gupta LM, Hendrix NW, et al. Intrauterine growth restriction: comparison of American College of Obstetricians and Gynecologists practice bulletin with other national guidelines. Am J Obstet Gynecol 2009;200(4): 409.e1-6.
7. Gardosi J. Customised assessment of fetal growth potential: implications for perinatal care. Arch Dis Child Fetal Neonatal Ed 2012;97(5):F314–7.
8. Cole TJ, Statnikov Y, Santhakumaran S, et al. Birth weight and longitudinal growth in infants born below 32 weeks' gestation: a UK population study. Arch Dis Child Fetal Neonatal Ed 2014;99(1):F34–40.
9. Moyer-Mileur LJ. Anthropometric and laboratory assessment of very low birth weight infants: the most helpful measurements and why. Semin Perinatol 2007;31(2):96–103.
10. Fanaro S. Which is the ideal target for preterm growth? Minerva Pediatr 2010; 62(3 Suppl 1):77–82.
11. Franz AR, Pohlandt F, Bode H, et al. Intrauterine, early neonatal, and postdischarge growth and neurodevelopmental outcome at 5.4 years in extremely preterm infants after intensive neonatal nutritional support. Pediatrics 2009;123(1): e101–9.
12. Fenton TR, Kim JH. A systematic review and meta-analysis to revise the Fenton growth chart for preterm infants. BMC Pediatr 2013;13:59.
13. Fenton TR, Nasser R, Eliasziw M, et al. Validating the weight gain of preterm infants between the reference growth curve of the fetus and the term infant. BMC Pediatr 2013;13:92.
14. Giuliani F, Cheikh Ismail L, Bertino E, et al. Monitoring postnatal growth of preterm infants: present and future. Am J Clin Nutr 2016;103(2):635S–47S.
15. Villar J, Altman DG, Purwar M, et al. The objectives, design and implementation of the INTERGROWTH-21st Project. BJOG 2013;120(Suppl 2):9–26, v.
16. Villar J, Giuliani F, Fenton TR, et al. INTERGROWTH-21st very preterm size at birth reference charts. Lancet 2016;387(10021):844–5.
17. Ruth VA. Extrauterine growth restriction: a review of the literature. Neonatal Netw 2008;27(3):177–84.

18. Ehrenkranz RA, Younes N, Lemons JA, et al. Longitudinal growth of hospitalized very low birth weight infants. Pediatrics 1999;104(2 Pt 1):280–9.

19. Shan HM, Cai W, Cao Y, et al. Extrauterine growth retardation in premature infants in Shanghai: a multicenter retrospective review. Eur J Pediatr 2009; 168(9):1055–9.

20. Theile AR, Radmacher PG, Anschutz TW, et al. Nutritional strategies and growth in extremely low birth weight infants with bronchopulmonary dysplasia over the past 10 years. J Perinatol 2012;32(2):117–22.

21. Poindexter BB, Langer JC, Dusick AM, et al. Early provision of parenteral amino acids in extremely low birth weight infants: relation to growth and neurodevelopmental outcome. J Pediatr 2006;148(3):300–5.

22. Su BH. Optimizing nutrition in preterm infants. Pediatr Neonatol 2014;55(1): 5–13.

23. Olsen IE, Richardson DK, Schmid CH, et al. Intersite differences in weight growth velocity of extremely premature infants. Pediatrics 2002;110(6):1125–32.

24. Embleton NE, Pang N, Cooke RJ. Postnatal malnutrition and growth retardation: an inevitable consequence of current recommendations in preterm infants? Pediatrics 2001;107(2):270–3.

25. Ehrenkranz RA. Extrauterine growth restriction: is it preventable? J Pediatr (Rio J) 2014;90(1):1–3.

26. Prince A, Groh-Wargo S. Nutrition management for the promotion of growth in very low birth weight premature infants. Nutr Clin Pract 2013;28(6):659–68.

27. Bloom BT, Mulligan J, Arnold C, et al. Improving growth of very low birth weight infants in the first 28 days. Pediatrics 2003;112(1 Pt 1):8–14.

28. Cormack BE, Bloomfield FH. Increased protein intake decreases postnatal growth faltering in ELBW babies. Arch Dis Child Fetal Neonatal Ed 2013; 98(5):F399–404.

29. Dinerstein A, Nieto RM, Solana CL, et al. Early and aggressive nutritional strategy (parenteral and enteral) decreases postnatal growth failure in very low birth weight infants. J Perinatol 2006;26(7):436–42.

30. Ramel SE, Demerath EW, Gray HL, et al. The relationship of poor linear growth velocity with neonatal illness and two-year neurodevelopment in preterm infants. Neonatology 2012;102(1):19–24.

31. De Cunto A, Paviotti G, Ronfani L, et al. Can body mass index accurately predict adiposity in newborns? Arch Dis Child Fetal Neonatal Ed 2014;99(3):F238–9.

32. Daly-Wolfe KM, Jordan KC, Slater H, et al. Mid-arm circumference is a reliable method to estimate adiposity in preterm and term infants. Pediatr Res 2015; 78(3):336–41.

33. Rigo J, Nyamugabo K, Picaud JC, et al. Reference values of body composition obtained by dual energy X-ray absorptiometry in preterm and term neonates. J Pediatr Gastroenterol Nutr 1998;27(2):184–90.

34. Olhager E, Thuomas KA, Wigstrom L, et al. Description and evaluation of a method based on magnetic resonance imaging to estimate adipose tissue volume and total body fat in infants. Pediatr Res 1998;44(4):572–7.

35. Johnson MJ, Wootton SA, Leaf AA, et al. Preterm birth and body composition at term equivalent age: a systematic review and meta-analysis. Pediatrics 2012; 130(3):e640–9.

36. Pryhuber GS, Maitre NL, Ballard RA, et al. Prematurity and respiratory outcomes program (PROP): study protocol of a prospective multicenter study of respiratory outcomes of preterm infants in the United States. BMC Pediatr 2015;15:37.

37. Yang J, Chang SS, Poon WB. Relationship between amino acid and energy intake and long-term growth and neurodevelopmental outcomes in very low birth weight infants. JPEN J Parenter Enteral Nutr 2016;40(6):820–6.

38. Vlaardingerbroek H, Roelants JA, Rook D, et al. Adaptive regulation of amino acid metabolism on early parenteral lipid and high-dose amino acid administration in VLBW infants—a randomized, controlled trial. Clin Nutr 2014;33(6): 982–90.

39. Ehrenkranz RA. Early, aggressive nutritional management for very low birth weight infants: what is the evidence? Semin Perinatol 2007;31(2):48–55.

40. Heird WC, Dell RB, Helms RA, et al. Amino acid mixture designed to maintain normal plasma amino acid patterns in infants and children requiring parenteral nutrition. Pediatrics 1987;80(3):401–8.

41. Mitanchez D. Glucose regulation in preterm newborn infants. Horm Res 2007; 68(6):265–71.

42. Farrag HM, Cowett RM. Glucose homeostasis in the micropremie. Clin Perinatol 2000;27(1):1–22, v.

43. Decaro MH, Vain NE. Hyperglycaemia in preterm neonates: what to know, what to do. Early Hum Dev 2011;87(Suppl 1):S19–22.

44. Alaedeen DI, Walsh MC, Chwals WJ. Total parenteral nutrition-associated hyperglycemia correlates with prolonged mechanical ventilation and hospital stay in septic infants. J Pediatr Surg 2006;41(1):239–44 [discussion: 239–44].

45. Kao LS, Morris BH, Lally KP, et al. Hyperglycemia and morbidity and mortality in extremely low birth weight infants. J Perinatol 2006;26(12):730–6.

46. Heimann K, Peschgens T, Kwiecien R, et al. Are recurrent hyperglycemic episodes and median blood glucose level a prognostic factor for increased morbidity and mortality in premature infants </=1500 g? J Perinat Med 2007; 35(3):245–8.

47. Lapillonne A. Enteral and parenteral lipid requirements of preterm infants. In: Koletzko B, Poindexter B, Uauy R, editors. Nutritional care of preterm infants scientific basis and practical guidelines. Munich (Germany): Karger; 2014. p. 82–98.

48. dit Trolli SE, Kermorvant-Duchemin E, Huon C, et al. Early lipid supply and neurological development at one year in very low birth weight (VLBW) preterm infants. Early Hum Dev 2012;88(Suppl 1):S25–9.

49. Abrams SA. Impact of new-generation parenteral lipid emulsions in pediatric nutrition. Adv Nutr 2013;4(5):518–20.

50. Nandivada P, Carlson SJ, Cowan E, et al. Role of parenteral lipid emulsions in the preterm infant. Early Hum Dev 2013;89(Suppl 2):S45–9.

51. Rayyan M, Devlieger H, Jochum F, et al. Short-term use of parenteral nutrition with a lipid emulsion containing a mixture of soybean oil, olive oil, medium-chain triglycerides, and fish oil: a randomized double-blind study in preterm infants. JPEN J Parenter Enteral Nutr 2012;36(1 Suppl):81S–94S.

52. Beken S, Dilli D, Fettah ND, et al. The influence of fish-oil lipid emulsions on retinopathy of prematurity in very low birth weight infants: a randomized controlled trial. Early Hum Dev 2014;90(1):27–31.

53. D'Ascenzo R, D'Egidio S, Angelini L, et al. Parenteral nutrition of preterm infants with a lipid emulsion containing 10% fish oil: effect on plasma lipids and long-chain polyunsaturated fatty acids. J Pediatr 2011;159(1):33–38 e31.

54. Tomsits E, Pataki M, Tolgyesi A, et al. Safety and efficacy of a lipid emulsion containing a mixture of soybean oil, medium-chain triglycerides, olive oil, and fish

oil: a randomised, double-blind clinical trial in premature infants requiring parenteral nutrition. J Pediatr Gastroenterol Nutr 2010;51(4):514–21.

55. Vlaardingerbroek H, Veldhorst MA, Spronk S, et al. Parenteral lipid administration to very-low-birth-weight infants—early introduction of lipids and use of new lipid emulsions: a systematic review and meta-analysis. Am J Clin Nutr 2012;96(2):255–68.

56. Holcombe B. Parenteral nutrition product shortages: impact on safety. JPEN J Parenter Enteral Nutr 2012;36(2 Suppl):44S–7S.

57. Hanson C, Thoene M, Wagner J, et al. Parenteral nutrition additive shortages: the short-term, long-term and potential epigenetic implications in premature and hospitalized infants. Nutrients 2012;4(12):1977–88.

58. Ruktanonchai D, Lowe M, Norton SA, et al. Zinc deficiency-associated dermatitis in infants during a nationwide shortage of injectable zinc—Washington, DC, and Houston, Texas, 2012-2013. MMWR Morb Mortal Wkly Rep 2014; 63(2):35–7.

59. McNelis K, Viswanathan S. Effects of parenteral phosphorus dose restriction in preterm infants. J Neonatal Perinatal Med 2016;9(2):153–8.

60. Guenter P, Holcombe B, Mirtallo JM, et al. Parenteral nutrition utilization: response to drug shortages. JPEN J Parenter Enteral Nutr 2014;38(1):11–2.

61. Vanek VW, Borum P, Buchman A, et al. A.S.P.E.N. position paper: recommendations for changes in commercially available parenteral multivitamin and multi-trace element products. Nutr Clin Pract 2012;27(4):440–91.

62. Hall AR, Arnold CJ, Miller GG, et al. Infant parenteral nutrition remains a significant source for aluminum toxicity. JPEN J Parenter Enteral Nutr 2016. [Epub ahead of print].

63. Aschner JL, Anderson A, Slaughter JC, et al. Neuroimaging identifies increased manganese deposition in infants receiving parenteral nutrition. Am J Clin Nutr 2015;102(6):1482–9.

64. Migaki EA, Melhart BJ, Dewar CJ, et al. Calcium chloride and sodium phosphate in neonatal parenteral nutrition containing trophamine: precipitation studies and aluminum content. JPEN J Parenter Enteral Nutr 2012;36(4):470–5.

65. Meinzen-Derr J, Poindexter B, Wrage L, et al. Role of human milk in extremely low birth weight infants' risk of necrotizing enterocolitis or death. J Perinatol 2009;29(1):57–62.

66. Tudehope DI. Human milk and the nutritional needs of preterm infants. J Pediatr 2013;162(3 Suppl):S17–25.

67. Underwood MA. Human milk for the premature infant. Pediatr Clin North Am 2013;60(1):189–207.

68. Patel AL, Johnson TJ, Engstrom JL, et al. Impact of early human milk on sepsis and health-care costs in very low birth weight infants. J Perinatol 2013;33(7): 514–9.

69. Groh-Wargo S, Sapsford A. Enteral nutrition support of the preterm infant in the neonatal intensive care unit. Nutr Clin Pract 2009;24(3):363–76.

70. Kuschel CA, Harding JE. Multicomponent fortified human milk for promoting growth in preterm infants. Cochrane Database Syst Rev 2004;(1):CD000343.

71. Arslanoglu S, Moro GE, Ziegler EE, The WAPM Working Group on Nutrition. Optimization of human milk fortification for preterm infants: new concepts and recommendations. J Perinat Med 2010;38(3):233–8.

72. Pearson F, Johnson MJ, Leaf AA. Milk osmolality: does it matter? Arch Dis Child Fetal Neonatal Ed 2013;98(2):F166–9.

73. Yigit S, Akgoz A, Memisoglu A, et al. Breast milk fortification: effect on gastric emptying. J Matern Fetal Neonatal Med 2008;21(11):843–6.
74. Tillman S, Brandon DH, Silva SG. Evaluation of human milk fortification from the time of the first feeding: effects on infants of less than 31 weeks gestational age. J Perinatol 2012;32(7):525–31.
75. Senterre T, Rigo J. Optimizing early nutritional support based on recent recommendations in VLBW infants and postnatal growth restriction. J Pediatr Gastroenterol Nutr 2011;53(5):536–42.
76. Moya F, Sisk PM, Walsh KR, et al. A new liquid human milk fortifier and linear growth in preterm infants. Pediatrics 2012;130(4):e928–35.
77. Arslanoglu S, Moro GE, Ziegler EE. Preterm infants fed fortified human milk receive less protein than they need. J Perinatol 2009;29(7):489–92.
78. Fusch G, Rochow N, Choi A, et al. Rapid measurement of macronutrients in breast milk: how reliable are infrared milk analyzers? Clin Nutr 2015;34(3): 465–76.
79. Adamkin DH, Radmacher PG. Fortification of human milk in very low birth weight infants (VLBW <1500 g birth weight). Clin Perinatol 2014;41(2):405–21.
80. Assad M, Elliott MJ, Abraham JH. Decreased cost and improved feeding tolerance in VLBW infants fed an exclusive human milk diet. J Perinatol 2016;36(3): 216–20.
81. Herrmann K, Carroll K. An exclusively human milk diet reduces necrotizing enterocolitis. Breastfeed Med 2014;9(4):184–90.
82. Sullivan S, Schanler RJ, Kim JH, et al. An exclusively human milk-based diet is associated with a lower rate of necrotizing enterocolitis than a diet of human milk and bovine milk-based products. J Pediatr 2010;156(4):562–7.e1.
83. Abrams SA, Schanler RJ, Lee ML, et al. Greater mortality and morbidity in extremely preterm infants fed a diet containing cow milk protein products. Breastfeed Med 2014;9(6):281–5.
84. Colacci M, Murthy K, DeRegnier RO, et al. Growth and development in extremely low birth weight infants after the introduction of exclusive human milk feedings. Am J Perinatol 2017;34(2):130–7.
85. Schanler RJ, Lau C, Hurst NM, et al. Randomized trial of donor human milk versus preterm formula as substitutes for mothers' own milk in the feeding of extremely premature infants. Pediatrics 2005;116(2):400–6.
86. Cooper AR, Barnett D, Gentles E, et al. Macronutrient content of donor human breast milk. Arch Dis Child Fetal Neonatal Ed 2013;98(6):F539–41.
87. Radmacher PG, Lewis SL, Adamkin DH. Individualizing fortification of human milk using real time human milk analysis. J Neonatal Perinatal Med 2013;6(4): 319–23.
88. Ziegler EE. Meeting the nutritional needs of the low-birth-weight infant. Ann Nutr Metab 2011;58(Suppl 1):8–18.
89. Koletzko B, Poindexter B, Uauy R. Recommended nutrient intake levels for stable, fully enterally fed very low birth weight infants. World Rev Nutr Diet 2014; 110:297–9.
90. Tully DB, Jones F, Tully MR. Donor milk: what's in it and what's not. J Hum Lact 2001;17(2):152–5.
91. Neu J. Gastrointestinal development and meeting the nutritional needs of premature infants. Am J Clin Nutr 2007;85(2):629S–34S.
92. Morgan J, Bombell S, McGuire W. Early trophic feeding versus enteral fasting for very preterm or very low birth weight infants. Cochrane Database Syst Rev 2013;(3):CD000504.

93. Isaacs EB, Gadian DG, Sabatini S, et al. The effect of early human diet on caudate volumes and IQ. Pediatr Res 2008;63(3):308–14.

94. Jadcherla SR, Dail J, Malkar MB, et al. Impact of process optimization and quality improvement measures on neonatal feeding outcomes at an all-referral neonatal intensive care unit. JPEN J Parenter Enteral Nutr 2016;40(5):646–55.

95. Gephart SM, Hanson CK. Preventing necrotizing enterocolitis with standardized feeding protocols: not only possible, but imperative. Adv Neonatal Care 2013; 13(1):48–54.

96. Hans DM, Pylipow M, Long JD, et al. Nutritional practices in the neonatal intensive care unit: analysis of a 2006 neonatal nutrition survey. Pediatrics 2009; 123(1):51–7.

97. Klingenberg C, Embleton ND, Jacobs SE, et al. Enteral feeding practices in very preterm infants: an international survey. Arch Dis Child Fetal Neonatal Ed 2012; 97(1):F56–61.

98. Viswanathan S, McNelis K, Super D, et al. Standardized slow enteral feeding protocol and the incidence of necrotizing enterocolitis in extremely low birth weight infants. JPEN J Parenter Enteral Nutr 2015;39(6):644–54.

99. Henderson G, Craig S, Brocklehurst P, et al. Enteral feeding regimens and necrotising enterocolitis in preterm infants: a multicentre case-control study. Arch Dis Child Fetal Neonatal Ed 2009;94(2):F120–3.

100. Morgan J, Young L, McGuire W. Slow advancement of enteral feed volumes to prevent necrotising enterocolitis in very low birth weight infants. Cochrane Database Syst Rev 2015;(10):CD001241.

101. Jones KD, Howarth LJ. Intestinal failure following necrotizing enterocolitis: a clinical approach. Early Hum Dev 2016;97:29–32.

102. Lapillonne A, Matar M, Adleff A, et al. Use of extensively hydrolysed formula for refeeding neonates postnecrotising enterocolitis: a nationwide survey-based, cross-sectional study. BMJ Open 2016;6(7):e008613.

103. Kim JH, Chan CS, Vaucher YE, et al. Challenges in the practice of human milk nutrition in the neonatal intensive care unit. Early Hum Dev 2013;89(Suppl 2): S35–8.

The Microbiota of the Extremely Preterm Infant

Mark A. Underwood, MD, MAS*, Kristin Sohn, MD

KEYWORDS

- Microbiota • Dysbiosis • Intestinal tract • Skin • Oral cavity
- Necrotizing enterocolitis • Late-onset sepsis

KEY POINTS

- The intestinal microbiota of the extremely preterm infant differs dramatically from that of term infants, children, and adults with decreased diversity and high numbers of γ-proteobacteria and Firmicutes and low numbers of common commensal microbes.
- Alterations in the intestinal microbiota of the preterm infant precede the onset of necrotizing enterocolitis and sepsis.
- Altering the intestinal microbiota with diet, antibiotics, and prebiotic and probiotic supplements may be less effective in extremely preterm infants, prompting the need for novel approaches to dysbiosis in this population.

INTRODUCTION

Colonization of the fetal skin and intestinal tract begins in utero and is influenced by maternal microbial communities (particularly those that inhabit the distal intestinal tract, the mouth, the vagina, and the skin), timing of rupture of membranes, maternal genetic factors, medications and supplements. Colonization is further influenced by mode of delivery and postpartum environmental exposures and medical procedures, infant genetic factors, medications and supplements, enteral feeding, and maturity of the infant innate and adaptive immune systems. Breakthroughs in recent decades in the analysis of complex communities of bacteria and viruses and studies in germ-free and gnotobiotic animals have vastly expanded our understanding of the importance of interactions between host and microbe. The composition of the microbial community of the intestinal tract and skin impacts inflammatory pathways and is thus important in the pathogenesis of a wide variety of disease processes (**Box 1**).

Disclosure of Funding Sources and Conflicts of Interest: The authors have no conflicts of interest to disclose. Dr M.A. Underwood has received funding from the National Institutes of Health (R01 HD059127).
Department of Pediatrics, University of California Davis, 2516 Stockton Boulevard, Sacramento, CA 95817, USA
* Corresponding author.
E-mail address: munderwood@ucdavis.edu

Box 1
Diseases and conditions in which the microbiota plays a role in pathogenesis

Antibiotic-associated diarrhea	Traveler's diarrhea
Necrotizing enterocolitis	Infectious diarrheas
Preterm birth	Sepsis
Infant colic	*Clostridium difficile* colitis
Inflammatory bowel disease	Food and environmental allergies
Irritable bowel syndrome	Celiac disease
Obesity	Diabetes mellitus (types 1 and 2)
Atherosclerosis	Cancer
Atopic eczema	Psoriasis
Seborrhea	Rheumatoid arthritis
Alzheimer and other neurodegenerative diseases	Mood disorders, schizophrenia, and autism

Novel mechanisms by which the microbiota influences host immunity and inflammation have recently been described.[1–3]

The importance of the intestinal microbiota in extremely preterm infants is most clearly evident in considering the risks of developing necrotizing enterocolitis (NEC) and sepsis. The roles of the skin microbiota in sepsis risk and the oral microbiota in pneumonia risk are less clear. Perhaps most compelling is the role of colonizing microbes in shaping and influencing the developing innate and adaptive immune responses in extremely preterm infants and the long-term impact of these host-microbe interactions. An additional layer of complexity is emerging with the realization that nutrients (eg, human milk, infant formulas and fortifiers, vitamins and minerals) are consumed by both host and bacterial cells, often with keen competition and overlapping effects. Host-microbe-nutrient interactions are likely to be particularly important in such processes as growth, brain development, immune development, and disease risk for the most preterm infants. In this article, we use the terms microbiota to refer to the composition of bacteria in a given anatomic niche and dysbiosis to mean an alteration in the microbiota associated with disease. There is evidence of significant colonization of the extremely preterm infant with yeasts, bacteriophages, and other viruses,[4] but discussion of these microbes is beyond the scope of this article.

DEVELOPMENT OF THE INFANT MICROBIOTA
In Utero

The development of tools to characterize the microbiota based on identification of bacterial DNA rather than relying on cultures has expanded understanding of the initial colonization of the neonate tremendously. **Table 1** summarizes the primary bacterial taxa that colonize the preterm infant. It has long been believed that the fetus grows in a sterile environment and that colonization begins at the time of rupture of the fetal membranes. More recent careful studies have shown that the amniotic fluid is not sterile, suggesting that colonization of the fetal skin and gut begins in utero.[5] The role of microbes in triggering preterm labor is perhaps the most clinically relevant observation related to this observation. Chorioamnionitis has long been recognized as a trigger of preterm labor and neonatal infection (particularly in preterm infants). The preponderance of evidence suggests a causal relationship between maternal periodontal disease and preterm labor.[6] For instance, the presence of specific bacteria (eg, *Peptostreptococcus micros* or *Campylobacter rectus*) in maternal gingival plaque was associated with increased risk of preterm delivery.[7] Treatment of periodontal

Table 1
Key bacterial taxa in the preterm infant

Phylum	Class	Order	Family	Genus
Firmicutes	Bacilli	Bacillales	Staphylococcaceae	*Staphylococcus*
		Lactobacillales	Streptococcaceae	*Streptococcus*
			Enterococcaceae	*Enterococcus*
			Lactobacillaceae	*Lactobacillus*
	Clostridia	Clostridiales	Clostridiaceae	*Clostridium*
	Negativicutes	Selenomonadales	Veillonellaceae	*Veillonella*
	Mollicutes	Mycoplasmatales	Mycoplasmataceae	*Ureaplasma*
Proteobacteria	γ-Proteobacteria	Enterobacteriales	Enterobacteriaceae	*Klebsiella*
				Escherichia
				Proteus
				Serratia
				Enterobacter
				Cronobacter
		Pseudomonadales	Pseudomonadaceae	*Pseudomonas*
			Moraxellaceae	*Acinetobacter*
Bacteroidetes	Bacteroidetes	Bacteroidales	Bacteroidaceae	*Bacteroides*
Actinobacteria	Actinobacteria	Bifidobacteriales	Bifidobacteriaceae	*Bifidobacterium*
		Propionibacteriales	Propionibacteriaceae	*Propionibacterium*

disease during pregnancy is associated with decreased risk of preterm labor.[8] The demonstration of the same microbes in the amniotic fluid and periodontal plaques in women delivering preterm,[9] the observation that the most common bacterium identified in amniotic fluid from women delivering preterm is *Fusobacterium nucleatum* (a common oral microbe in adults),[10] and the observation that dental infection with *Porphyromonas gingivalis* (a common bacterium in periodontal disease) causes preterm birth, low birth weight, and colonization of the placenta in mice[11] suggests actual colonization of the placenta and fetus.

Detailed studies of the microbiota of the placenta have shed some light on early colonization of the fetus. The placenta has a low bacterial load and is easily contaminated during vaginal delivery. Analysis of placentas obtained at term cesarean delivery without rupture of the fetal membranes showed similarities among the microbiota of the placenta, the amniotic fluid, and meconium, suggesting in utero gut colonization with changes in the infant fecal samples in the first 3 to 4 days after birth reflecting the acquisition of microbes in colostrum.[12] Colonization of the placenta with *Ureaplasma* species increases the risks of preterm labor and intraventricular hemorrhage in extremely preterm infants[13] and of chorioamnionitis in moderate and late preterm infants.[14]

Shortly after birth, the neonatal microbiota in the *term* infant is heavily influenced by mode of delivery with vaginally delivered infants colonized with organisms from the maternal vagina and infants delivered by cesarean colonized with organisms from the maternal skin and no real differences in neonatal microbial communities among the mouth, nasopharynx, skin, and meconium.[15] In *preterm* infants, the microbiota of the skin diverges from that of the stool and saliva by day 8 of life, and the microbiota of the saliva and stool diverge by day 15.[16] In a study of the microbiota of meconium in preterm infants, *Staphylococcus* was the dominant genus and *Staphylococcus epidermidis* the most common species. Among those infants with gestational age less than 28 weeks, *S epidermidis* was present in meconium of 3 of the 4 infants delivered by cesarean and 1 of the 3 delivered vaginally.[17]

Fecal Microbiota

Changes in the fecal microbiota of the extremely preterm infant over the first weeks of life have been characterized.[4,17–22] The following patterns are consistent across multiple studies: (1) bacterial diversity is low in meconium and increases over time; (2) an early dominance of Firmicutes (predominantly staphylococci, enterococci, and in some studies streptococci) changes to a dominance of Proteobacteria (predominantly Enterobacteriaceae); (3) *Clostridium* and *Veillonella* species appear late compared with term infants, with *Veillonella* least common in infants born at <27 weeks; (4) diet and antibiotic exposure have a lesser impact on the fecal microbiota in extremely preterm infants than is seen in term infants (eg, the human milk oligosaccharide [HMO]-consuming organisms, bifidobacteria and *Bacteroides*, are uncommon even in exclusively human milk–fed preterm infants); and (5) postmenstrual age significantly influences the fecal microbiota. These observations suggest that environmental factors and maturation of the host immune response are the primary shapers of the developing gut microbiota in preterm infants. It is worth noting how strikingly the fecal microbiota of the preterm infant differs from that of the healthy term infant with the former often containing 1 to 2 orders of magnitude higher levels of γ-Proteobacteria and the latter commonly dominated by bifidobacteria and *Bacteroides*.

Gastric Microbiota

Gastric aspirates have recently been studied using bacterial DNA techniques. Analysis of 22 neonates with an average gestational age of 27.7 weeks (± 2.8) demonstrated a relative paucity of species in the stomach, with *Bacteroides* spp predominant in the first 4 weeks of life and *Bifidobacterium* colonization significantly higher in infants receiving human milk. These results differ dramatically from studies of the fecal microbiota and raise the possibility that, although rare in the feces of preterm infants, the 2 genera of bacteria capable of consuming HMOs may be present in their small bowel.[23] In this study, *Helicobacter pylori* and *Ureaplasma* were not identified; however, a different study of 12 neonates with an average gestational age of 27 weeks (± 0.5) found the predominant species in the first week of life to be *Ureaplasma*, with a predominance of *S epidermidis* in subsequent weeks. By the fourth week, Proteobacteria and Firmicutes each accounted for 50% of the total gastric organisms.[24] The reasons for this disparity are unclear, but may represent differences in technique (denaturing gradient gel electrophoresis in the first study and direct sequencing of polymerase chain reaction [PCR]-amplified clones in the second), differences in population (both studies were performed in the United States, but diversity in maternal colonization with *Ureaplasma* may have played a role), or the relatively small numbers of infants analyzed.

Oral Microbiota

Investigations of the development of the oral microbiota in extremely preterm infants are limited. The largest study to date included 110 preterm infants with birth weight less than 1000 g with weekly oral swabs for the first 6 weeks of life, but used culture techniques rather than bacterial DNA-based approaches. At birth the oral swabs did not show significant growth of culturable bacteria, but by week one, 21 infants were colonized with methicillin-resistant *Staphylococcus aureus* (MRSA), 6 infants had other pathogenic bacteria (*S aureus,* Enterobacteriaceae, *Escherichia coli*), 56 infants were colonized with "nonpathogenic bacteria" (*S epidermidis* was most common followed by *Corynebacterium, Lactobacillus,* and *Streptococcus*), and 22 infants still showed no significant growth of culturable bacteria. By 6 weeks, 60 of the infants were colonized with MRSA. It is noteworthy that MRSA sepsis cases were less common in those infants with early oral colonization with the "nonpathogenic" microbes.[25] Smaller studies of preterm infants using culture-only technology have shown colonization of the mouth in the first 10 days of life with coagulase-negative staphylococci, enterococci, Enterobacteriaceae, *Pseudomonas*, and *Candida*.[26] A study using bacterial DNA-based technology included 1 infant with gestational age 24 weeks; the saliva microbiota differed from the other 4 preterm infants analyzed (gestational age 30–31 weeks) in that there were Enterobacteriaceae at days 8 and 10 and *Pseudomonas* and *Mycoplasma* at days 15, 18, and 21 that were not seen in the older preterm infants.[16] We analyzed the oral microbiota of 7 preterm infants (gestational age 25–27 weeks) with bacterial DNA techniques at 3 time points in the first 5 days of life and found a predominance of Mycoplasmataceae and Moraxellaceae in the first 36 hours of life and Staphylococcaceae and Planococcaceae by day of life 5.[27]

Skin Microbiota

The skin of the extremely preterm infant changes dramatically in the first weeks of life. The stratum corneum, which functions as the epidermal barrier, is nearly absent at 23 weeks' gestation, has a few cornified layers at 26 weeks, and is not fully mature until approximately 34 weeks' gestation.[28] When infants are born preterm, the epidermis matures fairly rapidly, and even the most immature neonate has functionally and histologically mature epidermis by approximately 2 weeks postnatal age.[29] Studies of the skin microbiota of the extremely preterm infant are limited. Several studies have demonstrated that pathogens commonly colonize the skin of preterm infants (mostly staphylococci, enterococci, Enterobacteriaceae, Pseudomonadales, and *Candida*) and that MRSA colonization is more common in the preterm infant; however, these studies were not designed to analyze the broader skin microbiota.[30–32] The previously noted study comparing changes over time in the saliva, skin, and feces included 1 infant with gestational age 24 weeks. The skin of this infant was dominated by staphylococci during the time of testing (day 8 to day 21) and did not differ from the older preterm infants.[16] Environmental factors that influence the skin microbiota include parental skin, feeding type, environmental surfaces and caregiving equipment, health care provider skin, and antibiotic use.[33]

THE MICROBIOTA AND DISEASE RISK IN EXTREMELY PRETERM INFANTS
The Fecal Microbiota and Necrotizing Enterocolitis and Sepsis

The incidences of NEC and sepsis are highest in the most preterm infants, likely due to immaturity of intestinal and skin barriers and immaturity of immune responses. Cases and outbreaks of NEC have been associated with a striking variety of organisms (**Table 2**), suggesting that there is not a single organism responsible. The evidence that the early or colonizing microbiota of the intestine influences the risk for subsequent development of NEC and/or sepsis has become quite compelling. The observation that NEC is most common in infants born at less than 28 weeks gestation and most commonly occurs at 30 to 32 weeks corrected gestational age[34] suggests that maturation of the host immune response and/or maturation of the intestinal microbiota are important in NEC pathogenesis. The Paneth cells of the small intestine produce large quantities of antimicrobial peptides that shape the intestinal microbiota.[35] It is not likely coincidental that Paneth cells increase in numbers and become immunecompetent at 29 weeks corrected gestational age.[36,37] Lower fecal bacterial diversity and/or richness is common in extremely preterm infants and has been demonstrated

Table 2
Microbes associated with cases or outbreaks of necrotizing enterocolitis

Gram-Positive Bacteria	Gram-Negative Bacteria	Fungi	Viruses
Enterococcus faecalis	Klebsiella pneumoniae	Candida albicans	Coronavirus
Clostridium perfringens	Escherichia coli	Candida parapsilosis	Coxsackie B2 virus
Clostridium butyricum	Pseudomonas aeruginosa	Candida glabrata	Rotavirus
Clostridium neonatale	Enterobacter cloacae	Aspergillus	Adenovirus
Clostridium difficile	Cronobacter sakazakii	Mucoraceae	Torovirus
Staphylococcus aureus	Cronobacter muytjensii		Astrovirus
Staphylococcus	Shigella		Echovirus 22
epidermidis	Salmonella		Norovirus
			Cytomegalovirus

in some studies of infants with NEC compared with matched controls,[22,38–40] although this is not universal.[41,42] Studies investigating the fecal microbiota before the onset of NEC compared with matched controls are summarized in **Table 3**.[40,41,43–54] These studies demonstrate the following: (1) colonization patterns differ between preterm infants who subsequently develop NEC and those who do not; (2) these differences are heavily influenced by maturation, NICU location, antibiotic exposure, and perhaps feeding type; (3) it remains unclear whether NEC risk is associated with the absence of potentially protective microbes (eg, Propionibacterium, Bifidobacterium, Bacteroides, or Veillonella species) or the dominance of potentially pathogenic microbes (eg, Enterobacteriaceae or Clostridium species); and (4) it remains unclear whether dysbiosis is the cause of NEC or a marker of alterations in host genetics or immune development. Two observations support the hypothesis that Enterobacteriaceae are important in the pathogenesis of NEC: (1) recognition of lipopolysaccharide in the cell wall of Gram-negative Enterobacteriaceae by Toll-like receptor 4 triggers a proinflammatory response and an influx of lymphocytes that in animal models is essential to the development of NEC,[55] and (2) Enterobacteriaceae have unique metabolic pathways by which they both trigger inflammation and use the products of the host inflammatory response as an energy source allowing them to outcompete other gut microbes.[56]

Many of the organisms responsible for late-onset sepsis (LOS), including staphylococci, in extremely preterm infants originate in the intestinal tract.[57] Several studies have demonstrated organisms in the feces before or concurrent with the onset of LOS caused by the identical organism in extremely preterm infants.[58–60] Decreased bacterial diversity and a predominance of staphylococci in early fecal specimens were associated with later sepsis in one small study of infants with gestational age 24 to 27 weeks.[61]

The Skin Microbiota and Sepsis

Efforts to decrease LOS with emphasis on the skin microbiota (eg, hand washing, protocols for line placement and care, early removal of central lines) have been partially successful, suggesting that a portion of these infections originate in the skin. Studies correlating skin colonization with LOS have relied on culture-based approaches and therefore likely give a limited view of the microbiota.[62]

The Oral and Gastric Microbiota and Pneumonia

In critically ill adults and children, attention to oral care has been shown to decrease the risk of ventilator-associated pneumonia, suggesting that aspirated oral microbes may play a role in pathogenesis. No studies to date have demonstrated similar decreases in ventilated preterm infants. Tracheal pepsin has been proposed as a marker of aspiration of gastric contents and appears to be common in preterm infants.[63] Bacterial DNA techniques have demonstrated an association between the gastric microbiota and chronic lung disease, with *Ureaplasma* the most common genus.[64]

The Tracheal Microbiota and Chronic Lung Disease

The lower airway is not sterile in the preterm infant. Tracheal aspirates from very preterm intubated infants have predominantly been studied with culture-based techniques.[65] A study of 25 preterm infants using bacterial DNA techniques demonstrated a predominance of Actinobacteria, which decreased over time in infants who subsequently developed chronic lung disease (gestational age 26.2 ± 1.9 weeks) but remained stable over time in the infants who did not (gestational age 28.9 ± 1.4 weeks). In the former group, *Staphylococcus* increased over time and bacterial diversity was lower.[66] A study of 10 infants with birth weight 500 to 1250 g who were intubated for more than 21 days demonstrated a predominance of *Staphylococcus, Ureaplasma, Pseudomonas, Enterococcus,* and *Escherichia.*[67] In both culture-based and DNA-based studies there appear to be differences in the tracheal microbiota between infants who subsequently develop chronic lung disease and those who do not; however, distinguishing between colonization of the airway and infection remains challenging.

Environmental Microbes and Disease Risk

The impact of the NICU environment on colonization, immune responses, and risk for nosocomial infection in the extremely preterm infant has not been fully characterized. The composition of the surface and airborne microbiota is influenced by building design and utilization with hospital surfaces more likely to contain human pathogens than other office settings.[68] Two studies of NICU surfaces using bacterial DNA techniques, found significant diversity between NICUs and demonstrated common neonatal pathogens (eg, *Enterobacter, Pseudomonas, Streptococcus, Staphylococcus, Escherichia, Enterococcus, Acinetobacter,* and *Candida albicans*) on NICU surfaces.[69,70] Intensive cleaning has been shown to significantly reduce the total microbial load and reshape the diversity toward nonpathogenic organisms. Interestingly, many of the common NICU enteric genera (*Enterococcus, Klebsiella, Escherichia,* and *Pseudomonas*) were not significantly altered by an intensive cleaning regimen, and routine cleaning of environmental surfaces with antibacterial wipes may be just as effective to reduce potentially pathogenic bacteria.[70]

Examples of environmental studies of NICU infectious outbreaks are abundant. In one NICU, during high-risk respiratory syncytial virus season, 4% of clothing swabs, and 9% of environmental "high-touch" surface swabs (beds, side tables, countertops, chairs, tables, and computers) tested positive for the virus by PCR.[71] Using DNA sequencing, a sink drain was shown to be the source of a *Pseudomonas aeruginosa* outbreak and replacing the sink and plumbing appeared to eradicate the outbreak.[72] A *Burkholderia cepacia* outbreak, in which 12 neonates developed clinical and/or laboratory evidence of sepsis was traced to contaminated intravenous solution and water for humidification of ventilator circuits.[73] A cluster of *Bacillus cereus* colitis cases,[74] an extended-spectrum beta-lactamase *E coli* outbreak,[75] and case reports of Group B *Streptococcus* septicemia in preterm infants[76] have all been attributed to contaminated breast milk. *Cronobacter* species have been identified as a contaminant of powdered milk formulas, with sporadic outbreaks linked to NEC, bacteremia, and

Table 3
Studies of the fecal microbiota before the onset of NEC (only studies that included infants with gestational age <28 weeks are included)

	Gestational Age at Birth[a]	NEC	Controls	Meconium	Early Stools	Just Before NEC Onset
De la Cochetiere et al,[43] 2004	24–29	3	9		*Clostridium perfringens* ↑	
Mai et al,[41] 2011	23–29	9	9		Firmicutes ↑ Actinobacteria ↓ Bacteroidetes ↓	Proteobacteria ↑
Stewart et al,[44] 2012	24–28	7	21		Coagulase-negative staphylococci ↑ Enterococci ↓	
Smith et al,[45] 2012	23–30	15	128	No differences at 3 time points: 0–5 d, day 10, and day 30		
Morrow et al,[40] 2013	25.5 (1.8)	11	21	*Propionibacterium* ↓	Staphylococci ↑ Enterococci ↑ Enterobacteriaceae ↑	
Normann et al,[46] 2013	22–25	10	16		Trends: Enterobacteriaceae ↑ Bacillales ↑ Enterococci ↓	
Torrazza et al,[47] 2013	27.4 (2.6)	18	35	*Klebsiella*-like sp ↑	Proteobacteria ↑ Actinobacteria ↑ Bifidobacteria ↓ Bacteroidetes ↓	
Jenke et al,[48] 2013	24–27	12	56		Lactobacilli ↑ *Escherichia coli* ↓	*E coli* ↑
McMurtry et al,[49] 2015	27.2 (2.8)	21	74			Actinobacteria ↓ Clostridia ↓ *Veillonella* ↓ Streptococci ↓

Study	Gestational age[a]	n	n		
Sim et al,[50] 2015	25–28	12	36	Klebsiella ↑	Klebsiella ↑ Clostridia ↑
Zhou et al,[39] 2015	24–31	12	26		Clostridia ↑ Staphylococci ↓
Heida et al,[51] 2016	24–29	11	22	C perfringens ↑ Bacteroides dorei ↑	C perfringens ↑ Staphylococci ↓
Warner et al,[22] 2016[b]	26.0 (24.7–27.9)	46	120		γ-Proteobacteria ↑ Negativicutes ↓ Clostridia ↓
Ward et al,[52] 2016	26 (23–28)	7	37	No differences in samples from days 3–16. Days 17–22: Uropathogenic E coli ↑ Veillonella ↓	
Twin studies					
Stewart et al, 2013[53]	26–30	5	5		Escherichia ↑
Claud et al,[54] 2013		1	1		Proteobacteria ↑ Veillonella ↓

Arrows represent significant differences in NEC compared with control specimens.

Abbreviation: NEC, necrotizing enterocolitis.

[a] Range or mean (SD) or median (interquartile range).

[b] The associations were most strong for infants with gestational age at birth <27 weeks with strong time-by-NEC interactions.

meningitis.[77,78] Bacteria also can colonize unlikely sources. *B cepacia* and *Enterobacter cloacae* have the ability to hydrolyze, render inactive, and proliferate in parabens, which are esters of para-hydroxybenzoic acid that are usually antimicrobial and used as preservatives in ultrasound gel (implicated in a *B cepacia* outbreak in a NICU).[79,80] *Serratia marcescens* outbreaks in NICUs have been linked to stored water and incubator surfaces,[81] the exit port of a high-frequency oscillatory ventilator,[82] contaminated parenteral nutrition,[83] soap dispensers,[84] and baby shampoo.[85]

MANIPULATING THE MICROBIOTA OF THE EXTREMELY PRETERM INFANT
Diet

Breast-fed *term* infants generally become colonized in the first weeks after birth with gut microbes that are able to consume HMOs and other human milk glycans (bifidobacteria and *Bacteroides*), whereas formula-fed infants tend to become colonized with a more diverse mixture of microbes. As noted previously, in the extremely preterm infant, the provision of human milk does not have a marked influence on the fecal microbiota with "human milk–consuming" microbes consistently either absent or present in low abundance across multiple studies. In a small study, neither the addition of a mixture rich in HMOs to preterm infant formula nor the "all-human diet" (human milk fortified with a fortifier made from donor human milk) led to a significant change in the fecal microbiota.[86] Nevertheless, careful analysis of the composition of HMOs in ingested milk and undigested HMOs in feces in preterm infants showed that different HMO structures are differentially consumed in the preterm gut with increased fucosylated HMOs in milk associated with a decrease in Proteobacteria in the infant feces.[87]

Probiotics

To date, a total of 41 randomized placebo-controlled trials of probiotics in preterm infants have been published in English; 37 of these trials included NEC, sepsis, and/or death as an outcome. In spite of differences in probiotic choice and dose administered, several meta-analyses have reached the same conclusion: probiotics decrease the risk of NEC, death, and sepsis in preterm infants and decrease the time to full enteral feeding in preterm infants receiving human milk.[88–90] In addition, there have been 11 cohort studies published in English comparing periods of no probiotic to periods of universal probiotic administration in preterm infants with a meta-analysis of these studies demonstrating a decrease in NEC and mortality with probiotic administration.[91] **Table 4** summarizes the nonweighted results of the randomized controlled trials and the cohort studies.[92–96] In spite of this astounding level of evidence and the relative lack of risk, routine probiotic administration is not recommended in the United States due to concerns from the Food and Drug Administration and other experts regarding the lack of commercial probiotic products that meet high standards of purity and viability. Whether these recommendations are justifiable given the incidence, cost, and severity of NEC and the relative paucity of evidence of harm associated with probiotic administration is hotly debated. In addition, it has been widely reported that although probiotic products appear to be beneficial for preterm infants with birth weight greater than 1000 g, data supporting a benefit for extremely low birth weight infants are lacking.[21] **Tables 5** and **6** summarize the data available from the randomized controlled trials and the cohort studies for the smallest preterm infants, including unweighted totals and percentages.[96–114] Although the level of support is not as compelling as that for larger preterm infants, these data suggest potential benefit and certainly no convincing evidence of harm for this population.

Table 4
Unweighted summary of probiotic studies in preterm infants

Number Enrolled		NEC Cases Stage 2 or 3		Culture-Positive Sepsis		Deaths	
Probiotic	Control	Probiotic	Control	Probiotic	Control	Probiotic	Control
7 randomized placebo-controlled trials with 200 or more preterm infants in each arm							
2520	2554	98	151	236	244	129	169
% of those reporting the outcome	3.9	5.9		10	11	5.1	6.6
7 cohort studies with 200 or more preterm infants in each group							
6779	5099	201	299	648	530	498	434
% of those reporting the outcome	3.0	5.9		11	13	7.3	8.5
37 randomized placebo-controlled trials (includes the infants in the 7 larger trials above)							
4710	4675	153	283	475	548	224	315
% of those reporting the outcome	3.3	6.2		12	14	5.1	7.2
11 cohort studies (includes the infants in the 7 larger studies above)							
7742	7592	224	408	737	667	556	493
% of those reporting the outcome	2.9	5.3		12	14	7.7	9.0

Details of 33 of the randomized controlled trials and 10 of the cohort studies are presented in **Tables 1** and **2** of Ref.[90] with the additional studies in Refs.[91–94,108]

Antibiotics

Five clinical trials of oral administration of antibiotics that are unlikely to be absorbed systemically (gentamicin, kanamycin, or vancomycin) demonstrated a decrease in the incidence of NEC.[115] Although this approach has been adopted in some NICUs, the concerns of emergence of resistant organisms have precluded widespread adoption. A recent report of the emergence of colistin-resistant extended-spectrum beta-lactamase–producing Enterobacteriaceae following oral administration to preterm infants for NEC prophylaxis underscores the validity of these concerns.[116]

Buccal Colostrum

Administration of colostrum directly into the buccal pouch has been proposed as oral hygiene to decrease the risk of ventilator-associated pneumonia in intubated neonates. To date, studies have shown an impact on the oropharyngeal lymphatic tissues[117] and the oral microbiota,[27] a decrease in clinical sepsis,[117] but no clear decrease in pneumonia. A multicenter trial of this intervention is under way.[118]

Cleaning Agents

Early studies of the value of environmental disinfection as a strategy to decrease hospital-acquired infections were limited and disappointing.[119] More recent studies suggest that novel interventions may be helpful in interrupting and preventing infectious hospital outbreaks.[120] Demonstrations that chlorhexidine bathing is associated with decreased risk of hospital-acquired infections compared with soap and water[121] have prompted widespread adoption of this practice for children and adults. For similar reasons, frequent use of hand-sanitizing gels and foams among health care providers has become widespread. Unfortunately, we have no data about the

Table 5
Randomized controlled trials evaluating probiotics published in English and specifically evaluating infants <1 kg

Author	Country	Probiotic Species	n <1 kg		NEC Cases ≥ stage 2		Culture + Sepsis		Deaths	
			Pro	Pla	Pro	Pla	Pro	Pla	Pro	Pla
Costeloe et al,[98] 2016	UK	Bifidobacterium breve	317	327	50	53	63	61	46	53
Kanic et al,[93] 2015[a]	Slovenia	Lactobacillus acidophilus + Enterococcus faecium + Bifidobacterium infantum	13	17	0	5	8	6	3	3
Van Niekirk et al,[99] 2015[a]	South Africa	Bifidobacterium infantis + Lactobacillus rhamnosus	43	49	0	4	–	–	5	5
Sangtawesin et al,[97] 2014[a]	Thailand	L acidophilus + Bifidobacterium bifida	3	4	1	1	2	1	0	0
Tewari et al,[100] 2015[a]	India	Bacillus clausii	23	22	0	0	6	8	8	9
Oncel et al,[101] 2014	Turkey	Lactobacillus reuteri	93	103	5	9	6	19	11	17
Patole et al,[102] 2014[a]	Australia	B breve	28	29	–	–	11	6	0	0
Totsu et al,[103] 2014[a,b]	Japan	Bifidobacterium bifidum	76	66	0	0	5	10	2	0
Jacobs et al,[104] 2013[c]	Australia + NZ	B infantis + Streptococcus thermophilus + Bifidobacterium lactis	235	239	10	14	53	58	–	–
Al-Hosni et al,[105] 2012	US	B infantis + L rhamnosus	50	51	2	2	13	16	3	4
Mihatsch et al,[106] 2010[d]	Germany	B lactis	91	89	2	4	28	29	2	1
Rouge et al,[107] 2009	France	Bifidobacterium longum + L rhamnosus	16	22	–	–	12	14	–	–
Underwood et al,[96] 2009	US	L rhamnosus OR combination (L acidophilus + B infantis + B longum + B bifidum)	9	7	0	1	4	0	0	0
Lin et al,[108] 2008[e]	Taiwan	L acidophilus + B bifidum	102	79	4	7	28	14	0	6
Wang et al,[109] 2007[a]	Japan	B breve	11	11	0	0	–	–	–	–
Bin-Nun et al,[110] 2005[a]	Israel	B infantis + S thermophilus + B lactis	25	17	2	6	4	10	6	9
Total			1140	1137	77	106	248	254	86	107
Percentage of those reporting the outcome			–	–	6.8	9.5	23	24	9.8	12

Abbreviations: NEC, necrotizing enterocolitis; Pla, placebo; Pro, probiotic.
[a] Personal communication from the author.
[b] Culture-positive sepsis at greater than 7 days of life.
[c] In regression model, reduction of NEC significant in subgroup analysis of less than 1 kg infants (RR [relative risk] 0.73).
[d] These infants were less than 29 weeks (birth weight <1.16 kg).
[e] Death and NEC were significantly lower in the probiotic group for infants 500 to 750 g (P = .02).

Table 6
Cohort studies evaluating probiotics published in English and specifically evaluating infants <1 kg

Author	Country	Probiotic Species	n <1 kg		NEC Cases ≥ Stage 2		Culture + Sepsis		Deaths	
			Pro	Con	Pro	Con	Pro	Con	Pro	Con
Guthman et al,[111] 2016	Switzerland	*Lactobacillus acidophilus* + *Bifidobacterium infantis*	238	250	6	16	–	–	16	26
Janvier et al,[112] 2014	Canada	*Bifidobacterium bifidum* + *Bifidobacterium breve* + *B infantis* + *B longum* + *Lactobacillus rhamnosus*	98	109	10	18	30	38	14	27
Hunter et al,[113] 2012	US	*Lactobacillus reuteri*	79	232	2	35	18	72	–	–
Luoto et al,[114] 2010	Finland	*L rhamnosus*	218	879	17	45	–	–	–	–
Total			633	1470	35	114	48	110	30	53
% of those reporting the outcome			–	–	5.5	7.8	27	32	8.9	15

Abbreviations: Con, control; NEC, necrotizing enterocolitis; Pro, probiotic.

long-term impact of these interventions on the skin microbiota or systemic absorption of these products for either the health care provider or the patient (particularly for highly vulnerable patients like the extremely preterm infant).

Emollients

Topical application of ointments, oils, or other emollients to the skin of the preterm infant has not demonstrated any significant decrease in rates of invasive infection or death.[122] Studies of the impact of this approach on the skin microbiota are limited to culture studies, with 1 study showing no differences[123] and 2 studies showing nonspecific changes.[30,124]

Functionalized Surfaces

Creation of novel surfaces that are resistant to colonization with potentially pathogenic microbes is a promising approach. Although this field is still in its infancy, the most promising result may be decreased surface contamination with viruses.[125] Isolettes with pathogen-resistant surfaces and medical devices coated with commensal or probiotic organisms may someday be commonplace.

SUMMARY

The study of microbes that colonize extremely preterm infants and the devices and surfaces with which they come in contact holds great promise for decreasing the high morbidity and mortality in this evolutionarily new population. Understanding and preventing dysbiosis may be crucial to the prevention of common and devastating processes such as NEC, chronic lung disease, and sepsis, but also may impact growth, development, immune function, and risk for a broad variety of chronic diseases and conditions.

Best Practices

What is the current practice?

- The American Academy of Pediatrics recommends mother's own milk for preterm infants and pasteurized donor human milk if the mother is unable to provide sufficient milk

- In many countries, prophylactic probiotic supplements are routine for preterm infants

What changes in current practice are likely to improve outcomes?

- Increased utilization of probiotics that reach high standards of purity and viability will decrease NEC in infants with birth weight greater than 1000 g (Centre for Evidence-Based Medicine, Oxford, 1a)

- Increased utilization of probiotics may decrease NEC and sepsis in smaller preterm infants (Centre for Evidence-Based Medicine, Oxford, 1b) and may decrease risk of childhood and adult onset diseases (Centre for Evidence-Based Medicine, Oxford, 5)

- Development of targeted approaches to decrease dysbiosis of the mouth, stomach, intestines, skin, and trachea may decrease diseases of extremely preterm infants associated with acute or chronic inflammation (Centre for Evidence-Based Medicine, Oxford, 5)

Data from Oxford Centre for Evidence-based Medicine – Levels of Evidence (March 2009). Centre for Evidence Based Medicine. Available at: http://www.cebm.net/oxford-centre-evidence-based-medicine-levels-evidence-march-2009/. Accessed March 6, 2017.

REFERENCES

1. Vatanen T, Kostic AD, d'Hennezel E, et al. Variation in microbiome LPS immunogenicity contributes to autoimmunity in humans. Cell 2016;165(4):842–53.
2. Taira R, Yamaguchi S, Shimizu K, et al. Bacterial cell wall components regulate adipokine secretion from visceral adipocytes. J Clin Biochem Nutr 2015;56(2):149–54.
3. Cani PD, Plovier H, Van Hul M, et al. Endocannabinoids–at the crossroads between the gut microbiota and host metabolism. Nature reviews. Endocrinology 2016;12(3):133–43.
4. LaTuga MS, Ellis JC, Cotton CM, et al. Beyond bacteria: a study of the enteric microbial consortium in extremely low birth weight infants. PLoS One 2011;6(12):e27858.
5. Wassenaar TM, Panigrahi P. Is a foetus developing in a sterile environment? Lett Appl Microbiol 2014;59(6):572–9.
6. Boggess KA, Society for Maternal-Fetal Medicine Publications Committee. Maternal oral health in pregnancy. Obstet Gynecol 2008;111(4):976–86.
7. Buduneli N, Baylas H, Buduneli E, et al. Periodontal infections and pre-term low birth weight: a case-control study. J Clin Periodontol 2005;32(2):174–81.
8. Lopez NJ, Smith PC, Gutierrez J. Periodontal therapy may reduce the risk of preterm low birth weight in women with periodontal disease: a randomized controlled trial. J Periodontol 2002;73(8):911–24.
9. Ercan E, Eratalay K, Deren O, et al. Evaluation of periodontal pathogens in amniotic fluid and the role of periodontal disease in pre-term birth and low birth weight. Acta Odontol Scand 2013;71(3–4):553–9.

10. Han YW, Shen T, Chung P, et al. Uncultivated bacteria as etiologic agents of intra-amniotic inflammation leading to preterm birth. J Clin Microbiol 2009; 47(1):38–47.

11. Ao M, Miyauchi M, Furusho H, et al. Dental infection of *Porphyromonas gingivalis* induces preterm birth in mice. PLoS One 2015;10(8):e0137249.

12. Collado MC, Rautava S, Aakko J, et al. Human gut colonisation may be initiated in utero by distinct microbial communities in the placenta and amniotic fluid. Sci Rep 2016;6:23129.

13. Olomu IN, Hecht JL, Onderdonk AO, et al, Extremely low gestational age newborn study I. Perinatal correlates of *Ureaplasma urealyticum* in placenta parenchyma of singleton pregnancies that end before 28 weeks of gestation. Pediatrics 2009;123(5):1329–36.

14. Sweeney EL, Kallapur SG, Gisslen T, et al. Placental infection with *Ureaplasma* species is associated with histologic chorioamnionitis and adverse outcomes in moderately preterm and late-preterm infants. J Infect Dis 2016;213(8):1340–7.

15. Dominguez-Bello MG, Costello EK, Contreras M, et al. Delivery mode shapes the acquisition and structure of the initial microbiota across multiple body habitats in newborns. Proc Natl Acad Sci U S A 2010;107(26):11971–5.

16. Costello EK, Carlisle EM, Bik EM, et al. Microbiome assembly across multiple body sites in low-birthweight infants. MBio 2013;4(6):e00782-13.

17. Moles L, Gomez M, Heilig H, et al. Bacterial diversity in meconium of preterm neonates and evolution of their fecal microbiota during the first month of life. PLoS One 2013;8(6):e66986.

18. Schwiertz A, Gruhl B, Lobnitz M, et al. Development of the intestinal bacterial composition in hospitalized preterm infants in comparison with breast-fed, full-term infants. Pediatr Res 2003;54(3):393–9.

19. La Rosa PS, Warner BB, Zhou Y, et al. Patterned progression of bacterial populations in the premature infant gut. Proc Natl Acad Sci U S A 2014;111(34): 12522–7.

20. Ferraris L, Butel MJ, Campeotto F, et al. Clostridia in premature neonates' gut: incidence, antibiotic susceptibility, and perinatal determinants influencing colonization. PLoS One 2012;7(1):e30594.

21. Warner BB, Tarr PI. Necrotizing enterocolitis and preterm infant gut bacteria. Semin Fetal Neonatal Med 2016;21(6):394–9.

22. Warner BB, Deych E, Zhou Y, et al. Gut bacteria dysbiosis and necrotising enterocolitis in very low birthweight infants: a prospective case-control study. Lancet 2016;387(10031):1928–36.

23. Patel K, Konduru K, Patra AK, et al. Trends and determinants of gastric bacterial colonization of preterm neonates in a NICU setting. PLoS One 2015;10(7): e0114664.

24. Milisavljevic V, Garg M, Vuletic I, et al. Prospective assessment of the gastroesophageal microbiome in VLBW neonates. BMC Pediatr 2013;13:49.

25. Shimizu A, Shimizu K, Nakamura T. Non-pathogenic bacterial flora may inhibit colonization by methicillin-resistant *Staphylococcus aureus* in extremely low birth weight infants. Neonatology 2008;93(3):158–61.

26. Makhoul IR, Sujov P, Ardekian L, et al. Factors influencing oral colonization in premature infants. Isr Med Assoc J 2002;4(2):98–102.

27. Sohn K, Kalanetra KM, Mills DA, et al. Buccal administration of human colostrum: impact on the oral microbiota of premature infants. J Perinatol 2016; 36(2):106–11.

28. Visscher MO, Adam R, Brink S, et al. Newborn infant skin: physiology, development, and care. Clin Dermatol 2015;33(3):271–80.

29. Evans NJ, Rutter N. Development of the epidermis in the newborn. Biol Neonate 1986;49(2):74–80.

30. Erdemir A, Kahramaner Z, Yuksel Y, et al. The effect of topical ointment on neonatal sepsis in preterm infants. J Matern Fetal Neonatal Med 2015;28(1): 33–6.

31. Choi Y, Saha SK, Ahmed AS, et al. Routine skin cultures in predicting sepsis pathogens among hospitalized preterm neonates in Bangladesh. Neonatology 2008;94(2):123–31.

32. Huang YC, Chou YH, Su LH, et al. Methicillin-resistant Staphylococcus aureus colonization and its association with infection among infants hospitalized in neonatal intensive care units. Pediatrics 2006;118(2):469–74.

33. Hartz LE, Bradshaw W, Brandon DH. Potential NICU environmental influences on the neonate's microbiome: a systematic review. Adv Neonatal Care 2015; 15(5):324–35.

34. Yee WH, Soraisham AS, Shah VS, et al. Incidence and timing of presentation of necrotizing enterocolitis in preterm infants. Pediatrics 2012;129(2):e298–304.

35. Salzman NH, Bevins CL. Dysbiosis–a consequence of Paneth cell dysfunction. Semin Immunol 2013;25(5):334–41.

36. Heida FH, Beyduz G, Bulthuis ML, et al. Paneth cells in the developing gut: when do they arise and when are they immune competent? Pediatr Res 2016; 80(2):306–10.

37. McElroy SJ, Underwood MA, Sherman MP. Paneth cells and necrotizing enterocolitis: a novel hypothesis for disease pathogenesis. Neonatology 2013;103(1): 10–20.

38. Wang Y, Hoenig JD, Malin KJ, et al. 16S rRNA gene-based analysis of fecal microbiota from preterm infants with and without necrotizing enterocolitis. ISME J 2009;3(8):944–54.

39. Zhou Y, Shan G, Sodergren E, et al. Longitudinal analysis of the premature infant intestinal microbiome prior to necrotizing enterocolitis: a case-control study. PLoS One 2015;10(3):e0118632.

40. Morrow AL, Lagomarcino AJ, Schibler KR, et al. Early microbial and metabolomic signatures predict later onset of necrotizing enterocolitis in preterm infants. Microbiome 2013;1(1):13.

41. Mai V, Young CM, Ukhanova M, et al. Fecal microbiota in premature infants prior to necrotizing enterocolitis. PLoS One 2011;6(6):e20647.

42. Mshvildadze M, Neu J, Shuster J, et al. Intestinal microbial ecology in premature infants assessed with non-culture-based techniques. J Pediatr 2010;156(1): 20–5.

43. de la Cochetiere MF, Piloquet H, des Robert C, et al. Early intestinal bacterial colonization and necrotizing enterocolitis in premature infants: the putative role of Clostridium. Pediatr Res 2004;56(3):366–70.

44. Stewart CJ, Marrs EC, Magorrian S, et al. The preterm gut microbiota: changes associated with necrotizing enterocolitis and infection. Acta Paediatr 2012; 101(11):1121–7.

45. Smith B, Bode S, Skov TH, et al. Investigation of the early intestinal microflora in premature infants with/without necrotizing enterocolitis using two different methods. Pediatr Res 2012;71(1):115–20.

46. Normann E, Fahlen A, Engstrand L, et al. Intestinal microbial profiles in extremely preterm infants with and without necrotizing enterocolitis. Acta Paediatr 2013;102(2):129–36.
47. Torrazza RM, Ukhanova M, Wang X, et al. Intestinal microbial ecology and environmental factors affecting necrotizing enterocolitis. PLoS One 2013;8(12): e83304.
48. Jenke AC, Postberg J, Mariel B, et al. S100A12 and hBD2 correlate with the composition of the fecal microflora in ELBW infants and expansion of *E. coli* is associated with NEC. Biomed Res Int 2013;2013:150372.
49. McMurtry VE, Gupta RW, Tran L, et al. Bacterial diversity and *Clostridia* abundance decrease with increasing severity of necrotizing enterocolitis. Microbiome 2015;3:11.
50. Sim K, Shaw AG, Randell P, et al. Dysbiosis anticipating necrotizing enterocolitis in very premature infants. Clin Infect Dis 2015;60(3):389–97.
51. Heida FH, van Zoonen AG, Hulscher JB, et al. A necrotizing enterocolitis-associated gut microbiota is present in the meconium: results of a prospective study. Clin Infect Dis 2016;62(7):863–70.
52. Ward DV, Scholz M, Zolfo M, et al. Metagenomic sequencing with strain-level resolution implicates uropathogenic *E. coli* in necrotizing enterocolitis and mortality in preterm infants. Cell Rep 2016;14(12):2912–24.
53. Stewart CJ, Marrs EC, Nelson A, et al. Development of the preterm gut microbiome in twins at risk of necrotising enterocolitis and sepsis. PLoS One 2013; 8(8):e73465.
54. Claud EC, Keegan KP, Brulc JM, et al. Bacterial community structure and functional contributions to emergence of health or necrotizing enterocolitis in preterm infants. Microbiome 2013;1(1):20.
55. Egan CE, Sodhi CP, Good M, et al. Toll-like receptor 4-mediated lymphocyte influx induces neonatal necrotizing enterocolitis. J Clin Invest 2016;126(2): 495–508.
56. Winter SE, Baumler AJ. Dysbiosis in the inflamed intestine: chance favors the prepared microbe. Gut Microbes 2014;5(1):71–3.
57. Tarr PI, Warner BB. Gut bacteria and late-onset neonatal bloodstream infections in preterm infants. Semin Fetal Neonatal Med 2016;21(6):388–93.
58. Shaw AG, Sim K, Randell P, et al. Late-onset bloodstream infection and perturbed maturation of the gastrointestinal microbiota in premature infants. PLoS One 2015;10(7):e0132923.
59. Taft DH, Ambalavanan N, Schibler KR, et al. Center variation in intestinal microbiota prior to late-onset sepsis in preterm infants. PLoS One 2015;10(6): e0130604.
60. Carl MA, Ndao IM, Springman AC, et al. Sepsis from the gut: the enteric habitat of bacteria that cause late-onset neonatal bloodstream infections. Clin Infect Dis 2014;58(9):1211–8.
61. Madan JC, Salari RC, Saxena D, et al. Gut microbial colonisation in premature neonates predicts neonatal sepsis. Arch Dis Child 2012;97(6):F456–62.
62. Ponnusamy V, Perperoglou A, Venkatesh V, et al. Skin colonisation at the catheter exit site is strongly associated with catheter colonisation and catheter-related sepsis. Acta Paediatr 2014;103(12):1233–8.
63. Garland JS, Alex CP, Johnston N, et al. Association between tracheal pepsin, a reliable marker of gastric aspiration, and head of bed elevation among ventilated neonates. J Neonatal Perinatal Med 2014;7(3):185–92.

64. Oue S, Hiroi M, Ogawa S, et al. Association of gastric fluid microbes at birth with severe bronchopulmonary dysplasia. Arch Dis Child 2009;94(1):F17–22.
65. Young KC, Del Moral T, Claure N, et al. The association between early tracheal colonization and bronchopulmonary dysplasia. J Perinatol 2005;25(6):403–7.
66. Lohmann P, Luna RA, Hollister EB, et al. The airway microbiome of intubated premature infants: characteristics and changes that predict the development of bronchopulmonary dysplasia. Pediatr Res 2014;76(3):294–301.
67. Mourani PM, Harris JK, Sontag MK, et al. Molecular identification of bacteria in tracheal aspirate fluid from mechanically ventilated preterm infants. PLoS One 2011;6(10):e25959.
68. Kembel SW, Jones E, Kline J, et al. Architectural design influences the diversity and structure of the built environment microbiome. ISME J 2012;6(8):1469–79.
69. Hewitt KM, Mannino FL, Gonzalez A, et al. Bacterial diversity in two neonatal intensive care units (NICUs). PLoS One 2013;8(1):e54703.
70. Bokulich NA, Mills DA, Underwood MA. Surface microbes in the neonatal intensive care unit: changes with routine cleaning and over time. J Clin Microbiol 2013;51(8):2617–24.
71. Homaira N, Sheils J, Stelzer-Braid S, et al. Respiratory syncytial virus is present in the neonatal intensive care unit. J Med Virol 2016;88(2):196–201.
72. Davis RJ, Jensen SO, Van Hal S, et al. Whole genome sequencing in real-time investigation and management of a Pseudomonas aeruginosa outbreak on a neonatal intensive care unit. Infect Control Hosp Epidemiol 2015;36(9):1058–64.
73. Paul LM, Hegde A, Pai T, et al. An outbreak of Burkholderia cepacia bacteremia in a neonatal intensive care unit. Indian J Pediatr 2016;83(4):285–8.
74. Decousser JW, Ramarao N, Duport C, et al. Bacillus cereus and severe intestinal infections in preterm neonates: putative role of pooled breast milk. Am J Infect Control 2013;41(10):918–21.
75. Nakamura K, Kaneko M, Abe Y, et al. Outbreak of extended-spectrum beta-lactamase-producing Escherichia coli transmitted through breast milk sharing in a neonatal intensive care unit. J Hosp Infect 2016;92(1):42–6.
76. Salamat S, Fischer D, van der Linden M, et al. Neonatal group B streptococcal septicemia transmitted by contaminated breast milk, proven by pulsed field gel electrophoresis in 2 cases. Pediatr Infect Dis J 2014;33(4):428.
77. Xu F, Li P, Ming X, et al. Detection of Cronobacter species in powdered infant formula by probe-magnetic separation PCR. J Dairy Sci 2014;97(10):6067–75.
78. van Acker J, de Smet F, Muyldermans G, et al. Outbreak of necrotizing enterocolitis associated with Enterobacter sakazakii in powdered milk formula. J Clin Microbiol 2001;39(1):293–7.
79. Hutchinson J, Runge W, Mulvey M, et al. Burkholderia cepacia infections associated with intrinsically contaminated ultrasound gel: the role of microbial degradation of parabens. Infect Control Hosp Epidemiol 2004;25(4):291–6.
80. Nannini EC, Ponessa A, Muratori R, et al. Polyclonal outbreak of bacteremia caused by Burkholderia cepacia complex and the presumptive role of ultrasound gel. Braz J Infect Dis 2015;19(5):543–5.
81. Morillo A, Gonzalez V, Aguayo J, et al. A six-month Serratia marcescens outbreak in a neonatal intensive care unit. Enferm Infecc Microbiol Clin 2016;34(10):645–51.
82. Macdonald TM, Langley JM, Mailman T, et al. Serratia marcescens outbreak in a neonatal intensive care unit related to the exit port of an oscillator. Pediatr Crit Care Med 2011;12(6):e282–6.

83. Arslan U, Erayman I, Kirdar S, et al. *Serratia marcescens* sepsis outbreak in a neonatal intensive care unit. Pediatr Int 2010;52(2):208–12.

84. Buffet-Bataillon S, Rabier V, Betremieux P, et al. Outbreak of *Serratia marcescens* in a neonatal intensive care unit: contaminated unmedicated liquid soap and risk factors. J Hosp Infect 2009;72(1):17–22.

85. Madani TA, Alsaedi S, James L, et al. *Serratia marcescens*-contaminated baby shampoo causing an outbreak among newborns at King Abdulaziz University Hospital, Jeddah, Saudi Arabia. J Hosp Infect 2011;78(1):16–9.

86. Underwood MA, Kalanetra KM, Bokulich NA, et al. Prebiotic oligosaccharides in premature infants. J Pediatr Gastroenterol Nutr 2014;58(3):352–60.

87. Underwood MA, Gaerlan S, De Leoz ML, et al. Human milk oligosaccharides in premature infants: absorption, excretion, and influence on the intestinal microbiota. Pediatr Res 2015;78(6):670–7.

88. Aceti A, Gori D, Barone G, et al. Probiotics and time to achieve full enteral feeding in human milk-fed and formula-fed preterm infants: systematic review and meta-analysis. Nutrients 2016;8(8):471.

89. Rao SC, Athalye-Jape GK, Deshpande GC, et al. Probiotic supplementation and late-onset sepsis in preterm infants: a meta-analysis. Pediatrics 2016;137(3): e20153684.

90. Alfaleh K, Anabrees J. Probiotics for prevention of necrotizing enterocolitis in preterm infants. Cochrane Database Syst Rev 2014;(4):CD005496.

91. Olsen R, Greisen G, Schroder M, et al. Prophylactic probiotics for preterm infants: a systematic review and meta-analysis of observational studies. Neonatology 2016;109(2):105–12.

92. Vongbhavit K, Underwood MA. Prevention of necrotizing enterocolitis through manipulation of the intestinal microbiota of the premature infant. Clin Ther 2016;38(4):716–32.

93. Kanic Z, Micetic Turk D, Burja S, et al. Influence of a combination of probiotics on bacterial infections in very low birthweight newborns. Wien Klin Wochenschr 2015;127(Suppl 5):S210–5.

94. Xu L, Wang Y, Wang Y, et al. A double-blinded randomized trial on growth and feeding tolerance with *Saccharomyces boulardii* CNCM I-745 in formula-fed preterm infants. J Pediatr (Rio J) 2016;92(3):296–301.

95. Manzoni P, Meyer M, Stolfi I, et al. Bovine lactoferrin supplementation for prevention of necrotizing enterocolitis in very-low-birth-weight neonates: a randomized clinical trial. Early Hum Dev 2014;90(Suppl 1):S60–5.

96. Underwood MA, Salzman NH, Bennett SH, et al. A randomized placebo-controlled comparison of 2 prebiotic/probiotic combinations in preterm infants: impact on weight gain, intestinal microbiota, and fecal short-chain fatty acids. J Pediatr Gastroenterol Nutr 2009;48(2):216–25.

97. Saengtawesin V, Tangpolkaiwalsak R, Kanjanapattankul W. Effect of oral probiotics supplementation in the prevention of necrotizing enterocolitis among very low birth weight preterm infants. J Med Assoc Thai 2014;97(Suppl 6):S20–5.

98. Costeloe K, Hardy P, Juszczak E, et al, Probiotics in Preterm Infants Study Collaborative Group. Bifidobacterium breve BBG-001 in very preterm infants: a randomised controlled phase 3 trial. Lancet 2016;387(10019):649–60.

99. Van Niekerk E, Nel DG, Blaauw R, et al. Probiotics reduce necrotizing enterocolitis severity in HIV-exposed premature infants. J Trop Pediatr 2015;61(3): 155–64.

100. Tewari VV, Dubey SK, Gupta G. *Bacillus clausii* for prevention of late-onset sepsis in preterm infants: a randomized controlled trial. J Trop Pediatr 2015; 61(5):377–85.
101. Oncel MY, Sari FN, Arayici S, et al. *Lactobacillus reuteri* for the prevention of necrotising enterocolitis in very low birthweight infants: a randomised controlled trial. Arch Dis Child 2014;99(2):F110–5.
102. Patole S, Keil AD, Chang A, et al. Effect of *Bifidobacterium breve* M-16V supplementation on fecal bifidobacteria in preterm neonates–a randomised double blind placebo controlled trial. PLoS One 2014;9(3):e89511.
103. Totsu S, Yamasaki C, Terahara M, et al, Probiotics Study Group in Japan. Bifidobacterium and enteral feeding in preterm infants: cluster-randomized trial. Pediatr Int 2014;56(5):714–9.
104. Jacobs SE, Tobin JM, Opie GF, et al. Probiotic effects on late-onset sepsis in very preterm infants: a randomized controlled trial. Pediatrics 2013;132(6): 1055–62.
105. Al-Hosni M, Duenas M, Hawk M, et al. Probiotics-supplemented feeding in extremely low-birth-weight infants. J Perinatol 2012;32(4):253–9.
106. Mihatsch WA, Vossbeck S, Eikmanns B, et al. Effect of *Bifidobacterium lactis* on the incidence of nosocomial infections in very-low-birth-weight infants: a randomized controlled trial. Neonatology 2010;98(2):156–63.
107. Rouge C, Piloquet H, Butel MJ, et al. Oral supplementation with probiotics in very-low-birth-weight preterm infants: a randomized, double-blind, placebo-controlled trial. Am J Clin Nutr 2009;89(6):1828–35.
108. Lin HC, Hsu CH, Chen HL, et al. Oral probiotics prevent necrotizing enterocolitis in very low birth weight preterm infants: a multicenter, randomized, controlled trial. Pediatrics 2008;122(4):693–700.
109. Wang C, Shoji H, Sato H, et al. Effects of oral administration of *Bifidobacterium breve* on fecal lactic acid and short-chain fatty acids in low birth weight infants. J Pediatr Gastroenterol Nutr 2007;44(2):252–7.
110. Bin-Nun A, Bromiker R, Wilschanski M, et al. Oral probiotics prevent necrotizing enterocolitis in very low birth weight neonates. J Pediatr 2005;147(2):192–6.
111. Guthmann F, Arlettaz Mieth RP, Bucher HU, et al. Short courses of dual-strain probiotics appear to be effective in reducing necrotising enterocolitis. Acta Paediatr 2016;105(3):255–9.
112. Janvier A, Malo J, Barrington KJ. Cohort study of probiotics in a North American neonatal intensive care unit. J Pediatr 2014;164(5):980–5.
113. Hunter C, Dimaguila MA, Gal P, et al. Effect of routine probiotic, *Lactobacillus reuteri* DSM 17938, use on rates of necrotizing enterocolitis in neonates with birthweight < 1000 grams: a sequential analysis. BMC Pediatr 2012;12:142.
114. Luoto R, Matomaki J, Isolauri E, et al. Incidence of necrotizing enterocolitis in very-low-birth-weight infants related to the use of Lactobacillus GG. Acta Paediatr 2010;99(8):1135–8.
115. Bury RG, Tudehope D. Enteral antibiotics for preventing necrotizing enterocolitis in low birthweight or preterm infants. Cochrane Database Syst Rev 2001;(1):CD000405.
116. Strenger V, Gschliesser T, Grisold A, et al. Orally administered colistin leads to colistin-resistant intestinal flora and fails to prevent faecal colonisation with extended-spectrum beta-lactamase-producing enterobacteria in hospitalised newborns. Int J Antimicrob Agents 2011;37(1):67–9.
117. Lee J, Kim HS, Jung YH, et al. Oropharyngeal colostrum administration in extremely premature infants: an RCT. Pediatrics 2015;135(2):e357–66.

118. Rodriguez NA, Vento M, Claud EC, et al. Oropharyngeal administration of mother's colostrum, health outcomes of premature infants: study protocol for a randomized controlled trial. Trials 2015;16:453.

119. Dettenkofer M, Wenzler S, Amthor S, et al. Does disinfection of environmental surfaces influence nosocomial infection rates? A systematic review. Am J Infect Control 2004;32(2):84–9.

120. Donskey CJ. Does improving surface cleaning and disinfection reduce health care-associated infections? Am J Infect Control 2013;41(5 Suppl):S12–9.

121. Swan JT, Ashton CM, Bui LN, et al. Effect of chlorhexidine bathing every other day on prevention of hospital-acquired infections in the surgical ICU: a single-center, randomized controlled trial. Crit Care Med 2016;44(10):1822–32.

122. Cleminson J, McGuire W. Topical emollient for preventing infection in preterm infants. Cochrane Database Syst Rev 2016;(1):CD001150.

123. Pabst RC, Starr KP, Qaiyumi S, et al. The effect of application of aquaphor on skin condition, fluid requirements, and bacterial colonization in very low birth weight infants. J Perinatol 1999;19(4):278–83.

124. Nopper AJ, Horii KA, Sookdeo-Drost S, et al. Topical ointment therapy benefits premature infants. J Pediatr 1996;128(5 Pt 1):660–9.

125. Mannelli I, Reigada R, Suarez I, et al. Functionalized surfaces with tailored wettability determine influenza a infectivity. ACS Appl Mater Interfaces 2016; 8(24):15058–66.

Personalized Decision Making

Practical Recommendations for Antenatal Counseling for Fragile Neonates

Marlyse F. Haward, MD[a], Nathalie Gaucher, MD, PhD[b,c],
Antoine Payot, MD, PhD[b,c,d,e], Kate Robson, MEd[f],
Annie Janvier, MD, PhD[b,c,d,e,g],*

KEYWORDS

- Antenatal consultation • Prematurity • Shared decision making palliative care
- NICU • Personalized decision making limit of viability • Ethics

KEY POINTS

- Personalized decision making during the antenatal consultation, as opposed to standardized and neutral transfer of information, empowers parents both during and after the decision-making encounter.
- Consultative approaches should establish trust, and include attention to emotional and intuitive aspects of decision making.
- Parents have varied preferences with regard to information, preferences for deliberation, and roles in decision making.
- Personalized decision making should replace shared decision making during antenatal consultations.

A. Janvier has no conflicts of interest.
Disclosure Statement: The authors have nothing to disclose.
[a] Department of Pediatrics, Albert Einstein College of Medicine, The Children's Hospital at Montefiore, New York, NY 10467, USA; [b] Department of Pediatrics, CHU Sainte-Justine Research Center, Sainte-Justine Hospital, University of Montreal, Montreal, Quebec H3T 1J4, Canada; [c] Clinical Ethics Unit, Sainte-Justine Hospital, University of Montreal, Montreal, Quebec H3T-1C5, Canada; [d] Palliative Care Unit, Sainte-Justine Hospital, Montreal, Quebec H3T-1C5, Canada; [e] Unité d'Éthique Clinique et de Partenariat Famille, Sainte-Justine Hospital, Montreal, Quebec H3T-1C5, Canada; [f] Canadian Premature Babies Foundation, Toronto, Ontario M4N 3M5, Canada; [g] Department of Pediatrics and Clinical Ethics, Sainte-Justine Hospital, University of Montreal, 3175 Chemin Côte-Sainte-Catherine, Montreal, Quebec H3T 1C5, Canada
* Corresponding author. Department of Pediatrics and Clinical Ethics, Sainte-Justine Hospital, University of Montreal, 3175 Chemin Côte-Sainte-Catherine, Montreal, Quebec H3T 1C5, Canada.
E-mail addresses: annie.janvier.hsj@ssss.gouv.qc.ca; anniejanvier@hotmail.com

Clin Perinatol 44 (2017) 429–445
http://dx.doi.org/10.1016/j.clp.2017.01.006
0095-5108/17/© 2017 Elsevier Inc. All rights reserved.
perinatology.theclinics.com

Fifty years ago, it was not rare for infants born with congenital anomalies or near-term to die. Neonatology is a recent specialty, emerging in the 1960s as a discipline dedicating itself to the care of sick neonates.[1] Rapid advancements, such as assessments of fetal lung maturity alongside consensus statements on antenatal steroids in the mid-1990s helped care for premature deliveries. Technological advances in ventilators, exogenous surfactants, and parenteral peripheral nutritional support improved management and survival for these young patients.[1,2] Neonatology was born and excelled in keeping young fragile infants alive.

DEVELOPMENTS IN NEONATOLOGY AND CLINICAL ETHICS

Coinciding with these medical advances, changes in the bioethical decision-making landscape, rising consumerism, and federal legislation regarding children with disabilities led to increased recognition of the role of parents as decision makers.[3,4] The climate in the medical arena, previously marked by maternal-infant separation both in terms of parental physical absence and exclusion from decision making,[5] evolved as seminal work championing maternal-infant bonding,[1,5] and patient-centered care emerged.[6] In North America, the President's Commission for the Study of Ethical Problems in Medicine and Biomedical and Behavioral Research[7] and the Royal College of Physicians and Surgeons of Canada[8] endorsed parents as surrogate decision makers for their infants when best interests were unclear, exploring moral boundaries of sanctity of life and quality of life. A landmark statement by the Institute of Medicine equated autonomous decision making and patient-centered care with "quality" of care so as to deliver "care that is respectful of and responsive to individual patient preferences, needs, and values."[3,6,9] In pediatrics, patient-centered care became synonymous with family-centered care, and the concept appeared in several policy statements, including Guidelines for Perinatal Care published jointly by the American Academy of Pediatrics (AAP) and American Congress of Obstetricians and Gynecologists.[3]

Concurrently, in bioethics, new models of decision making challenged physician authority and paternalism, as patients exercised their autonomy and demanded informed choices; physician obligations were defined and interactions between physicians and patients changed toward a more collaborative approach.[10,11] These partnerships between providers and parents became especially important in the neonatal intensive care unit (NICU) as younger infants were being resuscitated and evidence was mounting about risks of disabilities in survivors. Decision-making frontiers were propelled into areas of uncertainty, unpredictability, and value exploration. Evidence derived from neonatal outcome studies divided fragile neonates into "decision-making zones": (1) beneficial, where intervention was indicated because of good outcomes; (2) futile, where intervention was not recommended because of improbable survival; or (3) "gray zone," where outcomes could justify either life support or withholding of life support.[12,13]

INFORMING PARENTS AND DECISION MAKING

Shared decision making recommends that physicians and parents work together, requiring at a minimum physician-parent exchanges of medical information and explorations of values resulting in decisions attained through mutual consent.[11] Medical information considered essential to inform parents is based on presumptions of rational and informed decisional processes.[12,14–16] Reaffirmed as recently as 2015, this includes information about infant outcomes, with both local and national data, available options, and supplementing verbal communication with other modalities while being sensitive to parental values.[15] As stated by the AAP, the "primary goal of the antenatal consultation is to provide parents with information that will aid their decision making."[15]

However, prioritizing information exchange and suggesting a standardized set of facts is too simplistic. Decision making is multifaceted, and understanding risk information is dependent on relationships, trust, balances between cognitive and affective elements, life experiences, subjective interpretations of decisional outcomes, tolerance of risk/uncertainty, and other personal factors. Furthermore, a multitude of behavioral decisional processes, including biases, impact decision making.[17–19] In addition, information exchange/transfer represents only the first of 3 phases important in decision making, of which the other 2 include deliberation and defining roles involved in making a decision.[20,21] Patient preferences can vary in any of the 3 phases; in the amount and type of information desired,[22,23] preferred processes for deliberation,[24,25] and defining roles in assuming decisional responsibility.[20,25]

The goal of the antenatal consultation should not be to prioritize standardization of information nor to give it in a uniform/neutral fashion, but rather to adapt to parental needs and empower them through a personalized decision-making process, acknowledging individuality and diversity. In this article, we will describe why and how to personalize antenatal consultations and empower parents. The goal of this process is for parents to feel like parents and to feel like they are good parents, before birth, at birth and after, either in the NICU or until the death of their child.

Personalizing the Evaluation of the Situation: Avoiding Decisions Based on Gestational Age

Gestational age (GA), the framework on which these decisions are sometimes approached, is insufficient, inherently flawed, and simplistic as sole predictor of outcomes including neurodevelopmental disability and quality of life for extremely premature infants.[26–28] First-trimester ultrasound GA estimates incorporate an SD of ±4 to 7 days,[29–32] meaning for extremely premature infants GA can be miscalculated by a full week. This difference may result in foregoing resuscitation in more mature infants while resuscitating less mature infants. Furthermore, 4 other prognostic indicators, female sex, birthweight increment of 100 g, antenatal steroids, and singleton birth, have been shown equivalent to the arbitrary "1-week" prognostic milestone.[26] Although fetal estimations of weight before birth are flawed, the other 3 indicators can help refine antenatal counseling regarding the prognosis for the individual infant.

Categorizing care as beneficial, futile, or "gray" by GA alone carries important ethical considerations.[28,33] Arbitrary rules inevitably lead to self-fulfilling prophecies perpetuating outcomes and beliefs about futility.[34] Although some institutions report 32% survival at 22 weeks,[34] whole country cohorts, such as the French EPIPAGE study, describe 0% and 1% survival in France at 22 and 23 weeks, because of nonintervention.[35,36] There is tremendous variation in GA thresholds for resuscitation between professional societies.[37–46] It is comforting to observe that some professional associations, for example, the AAP, no longer have GA as the sole factor for judging whether life support is indicated for a preterm infant.[15] Although relying on GA boundaries in communicating prognostic uncertainty may seem to simplify information for the physician falsely implying a sense of certainty to the data,[28] there is no evidence that this simplification serves to empower parents, enhance decision making, and lead to better neonatal/parental outcomes. To the contrary, personalizing the situation by considering factors beyond GA is an essential first step in respecting each vulnerable patient as an individual and ensuring that reliable and accurate information serves as the basis for medical decisions.

Communicating with Prospective Parents: More than a Transfer of Information

In theory, communication of all options, outcomes, risks, and benefits empowers and informs patients by equalizing information asymmetry.[11] According to classic rational choice theories, this thorough transfer of information facilitates probability assessments and decision making.[17] However, the problem is that the facts considered important (outcome data) are chosen by physicians without parental input. For example, families are generally informed of the risk of severe neurodevelopmental impairment: cerebral palsy, visual impairment, hearing impairment, and low scores on a developmental screening test, most commonly more than 2 SDs below a standardized mean score on the Bayley Scales of Infant Development. Physicians should recognize that these classifications have been made using their own values; they have not asked parents of premature infants to categorize their children at 18 months, nor to describe their child's health. Some disabilities that are labeled "minor" in the medical literature, such as behavioral problems or conduct disorders, may be much harder for some families to cope with than "severe" disabilities, such as hearing loss or some forms of cerebral palsy. This leads to biases reflecting interpretation of risk.[12,14–16,34,47] In addition, those chosen facts are rarely based on an exploration of values or preferences of the individual parent at the time of consultation.[24,25,48–50] Yet unfortunately, in many investigations, assessments of information transfer, such as retention and comprehension of predetermined medical facts, often remain proxies for robust decision making, leading interventions to focus on improving complete transfer and recall of information, rather than personalizing the content of antenatal consultation and decision-making process.[15,51]

In neonatology, for prospective parents of unborn fragile neonates, transfer of information is often limited. Risk communication becomes increasingly challenging as prognostic uncertainty escalates and values diversify. It is known that risk communication can be influenced by framing effects when preferences are uncertain; for example, using percentages for mortality as opposed to percentages for survival.[52] It is also known that comprehension of statistical information and numeracy are difficult even for highly educated populations; for example, 4 out of 10 can mean something different from 40% for some individuals, depending on the risk it expresses.[53,54] When making decisions, there exists variability in the utility of risk information at baseline.[22,23,55] For some, risk information is dismissed in favor of more intuitive decision-making processes[19] if it does not conform to lived experiences, assumptions, or beliefs.[56] For example, a minimal-risk procedure may seem overwhelming to a family who lost a loved one in the operating room and may lead them to refuse treatment based on assessments other than probability. On the other hand, for others, it is an essential element in more analytical deliberations[17,57] and omission can be misinterpreted as an intentional nondisclosures or leave predetermined beliefs unchecked in the absence of a trusting physician-parent relationship.[58,59]

THE LIMITATIONS OF DECISION AIDS

Decision aids for antenatal counseling have attempted to overcome some of these challenges by using multiple modalities to improve comprehension of medical information and treatment options.[60–62] However, as with the professional guidelines, assumptions of rational decision processes prevail and only a few neonatal decision aids have been constructed with parental input.[60] None have been designed primarily, or only, by parents. In current neonatal decision aids, although survival and mortality statistics are generally balanced, depictions of long-term outcomes are not. In some, pictures of wheelchairs or of brain bleeds, as opposed to disabled children with their families, may reinforce fears of disability.[61] Furthermore, data representing parental perspectives, quality of life, and adjustment/resilience literature is missing[61]; these outcomes, rarely included in risk communication, frequently frame patients' decisions and perceptions of risk.[47,63]

Although decision aids assist comprehension of chosen medical risk information, the question remains whether standardized facts are sufficient and appropriate/optimal for all prospective parents. Given that neonatal decision aids have focused predominately on informational needs, and less on the processes of value exploration or how to be the parent of a sick infant, they may be most effective as a tool used after relationships have been built and specific informational needs determined. It also has been suggested that too much information, not considered central to the parent's deliberative needs, can be overwhelming or harmful.[22] Although some informational elements considered pertinent from parent perspectives[25,48] have been recently explored, it still remains unknown how information relative to medical risk is operationalized.

Decision Making: More than a Rational Process

Prenatal consultations with prospective parents, for prematurity and other serious antenatal problems, should move beyond exchanges of medical facts. Narratives have described these processes as complex deliberations between multiple interests, not reliant on medical information alone nor completely rational.[25] Emotions are increasingly recognized in neonatology, bioethics, and decision sciences to be critical for enabling robust decisions.[23,64,65] For example, patients often make decisions to avoid regret, rather than maximize benefits. Antenatal consultations that exclude discussion of complex emotional and social needs lead to decreased parental confidence in decisional outcomes.[24] For decisions of extreme emotional gravity, parents report reliance on intuitive processes[25] and frequently suggest attention to issues other than medical facts, such as the emotional climate and presence of both parents during the consultation.[25,60,66]

Decision-science theorists have argued that emotions are beneficial and help decision makers prioritize pertinent issues.[64] Neglecting feelings can inhibit questions, diminishing the ability to gather information and engage in successful patient-physician encounters.[67] Neuroscientific evidence has demonstrated poor decisions when emotions are hampered due to neurologic conditions.[68] Bioethical models of autonomy are calling for physicians to address emotions, thereby assisting patients in considering them when making choices.[65] Personalizing also means acknowledging these affective elements as integral in deliberations.

Certainly for highly complex, intense decisions related to life and death of an infant, disregarding emotions should be avoided. When preterm birth is imminent or inevitable, a multitude of feelings can predominate the parents' minds. Decisions are made as much with the heart as with the brain.[23] It has been suggested that incorporating these emotions, or at least acknowledging them for certain decision makers, leads to increased decisional competence by refining and clarifying moral values and personal priorities.[22,63] Personalizing information to correspond with a parent's primary concerns and fears, and addressing emotions alongside other nonmedical elements, strengthens relationships, facilitates clarity, and improves the comprehension and application of this information during deliberation.

PARENTAL EXPERIENCE AND CONCERNS

Women at risk of preterm birth report feeling powerless and experience a sense of loss of control.[69] As stated by one: *"Uncertainty, it's like vertigo or a precipice. And there is a lot of uncertainty. We don't know when I will deliver. We don't know how I will deliver. We don't know how it will go for the baby. We don't know what awaits the baby after. And we can get surprises, good or bad, for months after that.*"[69] Furthermore, individual families exist within their own social structure or microcosm influencing their ability to manage and cope with uncertainty and stress. Although their infant's well-being is generally their primary concern, they bring lived experiences and additional worries related to other children, maternal health, or finances.[69,70] In addition, each parent may have his or her own separate set of concerns and worries, influencing their personal experience with threatened preterm delivery.

Faced with the possibility of having a premature infant, prospective parents have the task of conceiving a new "parenthood vision."[24,69,70] Some may focus on the long-term well-being of their infant, some aspire to become primary decision makers and/or some want to be caregivers; bathing and singing to their infants. Despite these differences, most parents do not want to assume the role of a bystander.[71] They want to feel like they are a "real" parent, invested and present for their infant to the best of their ability.

PERSONALIZING THE AGENDA

In the antenatal consultation, neonatal providers have an opportunity to identify parental concerns and offer support. An evolution in consultation approaches has begun favoring a "controlled-improvised" agenda.[23] This contrasts strongly with the traditional physician-driven agenda, focused on conveying standardized medical risk information to all parents, supporting essentially rational decisional processes based on detailed information regarding outcomes. These new models of antenatal consultations favor a parent-driven agenda, and focus on building relationships permitting parental concerns to frame the conversation,[72] helping to diversify, strengthen, and personalize the consultation. Relationships begun in the antenatal consultation have been shown to be important determinants for future adaptation, by decreasing decisional regret and enhancing trust between physicians and parents.[73] Trust in turn improves risk comprehension.[74] Perceptions of risk are not constructed on rational assessments alone; therefore, building relationships and focusing on trust increases the credibility of the informant and the validity of the decision.[25,75,76]

RECOMMENDATIONS
Personalizing Conversations with Parents: a Controlled Improvisation Addressing what Matters to Parents

Personalizing conversations is not simple. It requires an assessment of the situation, an understanding of the parent and family, including previous experiences, emotions, and decision-making preferences, and an ability to support parental values and goals of the consultation. Approaching the consultation with an open and flexible mindset is essential; attempts to predict what parents want to discuss before meeting with them could compromise opportunities for a productive exchange. The consultation should not follow a prewritten script or an agenda, such as outcome boxes to tick or percentages to give; however, it can still be structured, for example, by using the SOBPIE[23] framework (Situation, Opinions, Basic politeness, Parents, Information, Emotions). By using the vignette in the next paragraph, the following section will be dedicated to practical recommendations to personalize antenatal consultations for fragile neonates in the gray zone. **Fig. 1** summarizes suggestions for guiding the consultation and teaching these skills, incorporating the SOBPIE framework and broadly defining the consultant's role as establishing trust and tailoring information.[23,24,69,70]

Prenatal Consultation Checklist   Mother's name: _____
___/___/___   ID:_____

Reason for consultation: _____   OB name: _____
☐ Communication with OB team: _____   Joint consultation with OB: ☐ yes ☐ no
Parent told about consultation: ☐ yes ☐ no   Significant person present: _____

Allow enough time / Limit interruptions (phone/pager) / Ensure privacy (# people) **/ Sit down**

Establish trust with parents
☐ Neonatologist introduction / role
☐ NICU team introduction
☐ Ask about the baby
  "Do you have a name?" _____
  "Tell me about your baby" _____
  "Does he/she have siblings?" _____
☐ Ask and Listen to parents' main concerns
  - "What is your greatest fear?"
  - "What is most important to you as a family?"
  - "Is anything worrying you at home or work?"
  - "What do you expect from this consultation?"
  - "What can I do for you?"

Address personalized parental concerns & questions
☐ Ask parents if they prefer statistical data,
  general terms, or both
☐ Discuss potential complications of prematurity
  relevant to them
☐ Explain their role as parents of a premature baby
  - Parental roles: touching, talking, family attachment
  - Baby appearance and behavior
  - Parent as caregiver: feeding/breastfeeding, clothing
  - Parental involvement in future decisions
☐ Explain how the NICU works
  - NICU visit offered ☐yes ☐no date: ___/___/___
  - Allied HCP visit offered ☐yes ☐no

Comments: _____

NICU team members (Name, role):_____

Follow-up
☐ NICU visit done (Date: ___/___/___)
☐ Allied HCPs consulted (Role & date):
  _____

☐ Follow-up visit (ideally) by same neonatologist
  - Date: ___/___/___ , GA: _____
☐ Written documents given
  Further comments: _____

Fig. 1. Antenatal consultation page 1. HCP, health care professional.

Josephine is in premature labor at 23 weeks. She had not planned this pregnancy, but when it happened, she felt it was fate. Her mother had just passed away a year ago, and as her caregiver, she had had a particularly difficult time adjusting. This pregnancy, however, had rejuvenated her spirits. When the contractions had begun she blamed a stomach flu and remained optimistic when her obstetrician suggested that with a little hydration they might stop. However, her optimism did not last, as her labor has progressed. Instead, she feels alone, anxious, angry, sad, and scared. The obstetrician tells her that she should prepare for the worst: delivering in the next few hours or days. She is alone in the hospital, as the father of the baby is out of the country for his work.

Inarguably, conversations related to life and death of children generally constitute the worst possible moments in a parent's life. No parents want to have this conversation, nor would they ever wish to be in this circumstance. Expectations suddenly and dramatically shift. Although many neonatal providers focus on the management of the unborn infant, prospective parents are also in a process of grieving their pregnancy and their parenthood project.[24] In this situation, they will generally focus on prolonging the pregnancy and stay in the pregnancy phase, as opposed to entering into the "baby phase."[24] Health care providers have to fulfill multiple roles at once; empathy toward the parent and compassion toward the infant within goals of a consultation that may either be known or unknown, and fluctuate between informative and supportive.

All providers, obstetricians, neonatologists, and nurses should take care to deliver the same message after assessing the Situation. We recommend that obstetricians and neonatologists meet to discuss these cases, if only briefly, before the antenatal consultations. This first assessment determines whether a decision needs to be or should be made; for example, if intervention is unlikely or likely to lead to survival.

Ideally, the antenatal consultation should include a member of the obstetrics team (staff, resident, or nurse). Conducting consultations in unison promotes trust through continuity and coherence of care. As depicted in **Fig. 1**, "establishing trust" is an important element of the antenatal consultation.

Next, Opinions and biases should be recognized by health care providers, taking care to examine the particularities of each consultation (for example, not making decisions based only on GA), with the aim to avoid interpretations of risk and values that would inappropriately frame the conversation or the decision.

Third, providers should practice Basic politeness. To optimize consultations, environmental factors should be considered; making sure to avoid distraction by cell phones and pagers, meeting in private locations with a limited number of individuals, staying sensitive to the nature and urgency of the consultation. In some hospitals, distractions are reduced to a minimum because a dedicated team, not responsible for intensive care patients and transport calls, is responsible for these consultations.

Nonmedical people usually do not know what a neonatologist is. Introducing oneself as a "baby doctor/nurse," taking care of babies being born too soon, for example, ensures that parents understand what neonatologists do.

Some sentences can help to set the stage of a personalized consultation. For example, asking parents:

-Have you been told the baby team would come and speak to you?

-What were you told?

The answer to these questions can help us understand what parents have heard from other providers. Josephine can give very different answers:

I was sent here from my village. They told me you can do miracles with the smallest babies;

The other doctor told me that all babies who are born at 23 weeks either die or are disabled; Are you here to convince me to resuscitate our baby? I don't want any experiments done on her;

You are supposed to give me information about small babies;

I don't want to hear bad things at the moment, I have heard enough. My baby will survive. She is kicking strong and she wants to live

Asking parents *"do you have a name?"* enables personalization of the conversation about their child, and understand the place of this child in their family. Here too, answers can be drastically different from

Samuel!;

She will die; I don't think I want to give her a name;

I don't even know if it is a boy or a girl…;

Me and my husband, we are not sure. We have a James in every family for generations, we do not know what to do in case he dies;

Her name is Amelia, we chose it years ago. We have waited for Amelia for the past 3 years;

In our religion, we name children after birth.

Questions such as *"Tell me about Samuel, what do you know about him?"* also help. If there are other children, asking who is taking care of them, shows interest in the family unit, providing insights into who the parents are and the context in which they live.

The neonatal provider can also ask Parents what their primary concerns are. Questions, such as *"What are your concerns?"* may help address misperceptions early on, and help team members understand parental expectations. Certain parents may have already decided on a course of action, so that the goals of the consultation shift from a decision-making deliberation toward one tailored around supporting coping mechanisms, or addressing fears and concerns. Questions, such as *"What can I do for you?"* or *"Tell me what you understand"* can help anchor conversations, as do investigations such as *"Do you have any experience with prematurity?"* Answers Josephine will give will help us to personalize information and the remainder of the consultation.

I don't know what you can do. Can you save my baby? Is my baby going to live? Why is this happening?

My mother died last year. She was very disabled. She had a trach and a G-tube. She was in and out of the hospital constantly. She could not live on her own. Can my baby be this disabled? I don't think I could handle that.

What do parents do in my situation?

I know this is in God's hands. I don't know why this is happening, but I know my mother up there is looking after me, she gave me this gift and I know she will help Lauren survive. She is a fighter and will beat the odds. She is a survivor, do what you have to do to help her.

I don't know. I'm scared. What should I know?

How long will she be in the hospital? Will I be able to see her, hold her, give her my milk, be there?

Each of these answers would prompt very different responses. Parents generally pay more attention to information addressing their pressing concerns. A question that is often helpful to frame the consultation is *"What are you most scared of?"* Parental answers can be very different.

I don't want her to die

I am afraid she will be in pain

What if she survives and is handicapped, and cannot have a normal life? Would this be fair?

Doctor, I wanted to speak to you just the 2 of us. I just arrived from the airport. I am afraid for Josephine, my wife. We have been going through 6 rounds of IVF. She is not very strong at the moment, physically and emotionally. And she is bleeding more. I am afraid she will die, can she? She wants a transfusion, but should the baby come out? She will choose the baby over her. But I am scared for her. I am not thinking about the baby right now, more about Josephine.

Sometimes, one parent is most afraid of death, while the other fears disability the most. Some parents will also have other concerns; some women may face deportation as illegal immigrants, others may be concerned about their potential loss of income, or for the other children at home. Addressing these "extreme" concerns is important. For example, telling partners that a woman's life is not in danger, or informing parents about how other parents cope with death or disability can help address their strongest fears. Dealing with their strongest fears often helps parents focus on other concerns they may have, or on information the medical team may give them.

Other questions that also can shape consultations include trying to ascertain the level of involvement desired in making decisions and what sorts of information are most useful: *"Some parents want a lot of numbers and information, and others want the big picture; what kind of parent are you?"* Some parents may prefer statistics and numbers, whereas others might not. Some would benefit from decision aids, whereas others may not. Based on qualitative research, most parents want to know about the complications of prematurity for their infant while simultaneously trying to understand how they can contribute as a "NICU parent,"[69,70] answering questions such as the following:

How can I help my baby?

What can I do for my baby?

Can I touch or hold him?

Can I breastfeed her?

What will she look like? Are the organs all formed?

How will he be fed, do I need to bring clothes?

As seen in **Fig. 1**, after establishing trust, the antenatal consultation can now focus on tailoring *Information* toward needs of the parents, individualized for the infant's condition, parental experiences, and goals of consultation. Parents strive for a "scientifically competent and humane medical team"[69,70]: trust is not only engendered by a knowledgeable and expert NICU team, but also by an open and compassionate approach to patient care.[24] Therefore, throughout the consultation, *Emotions* are important to support. Emotions can help to identify, explore, and construct values but also serve as a vehicle for building relationships. They provide opportunities for empathy, support, and trust between patients and physicians. The following sentence can help address/normalize parental emotions: *"I can see you are angry; many parents feel this way."* Asking parents if they want the team to leave and come back later is often helpful.

Sometimes, parents do not want to engage in conversations, others do not want to hear about "scary statistics," and others can also cry for a prolonged period. In these cases, it is important for neonatologists to be comfortable with silence and to tolerate it. There is some value in holding space with parents, being there in silence when parents cry, or giving parents time to process their situation or a difficult conversation. It is not rare that after a period of silence, parents communicate something that is important.

Additionally, it is helpful to inform parents that neonatologists are part of a larger allied health professional team and additional consultation with these professionals can optimize family-centered care. Follow-up visits by neonatologists and allied professionals are strongly encouraged, especially when pregnancies have progressed and the situation has evolved/improved, or when parents and providers are involved in complex decision-making processes.[24,70]

Last, attempts to minimize uncertainty and unexpected events before and after the consultation can help mitigate the stressors caused by threatened preterm birth, such as feelings of powerlessness and the "precipice of uncertainty."[69] Before consultation, parents should be made aware that a neonatology consultation will take place so they can prepare for it. They should know that a neonatal consultation does not mean an imminent delivery. They should also be told when the meeting will occur, so that both parents can be present.[70] Providing parents information about the NICU and how it functions, including written information and prenatal NICU visits are important steps in preparing parents[70] they decrease the double shock of meeting their premature baby for the first time, while discovering the NICU.[77] Neonatologists should be cognizant of the tone portrayed during the antenatal consultation. Allowing parents to maintain hope for a happy and healthy baby[24,78,79] and avoiding overly pessimistic outlooks on prematurity can temper unnecessary worries.[24,70,79]

In summary, a personalized approach to antenatal counseling seeks to meet the following objectives: (1) to respond to the stressful experiences of parents at risk for early preterm birth, (2) to address parents' authentic concerns, (3) to avoid creating additional stressors, and (4) to help them make a decision if there is one to be made.

INSTITUTIONAL PRACTICES

Simple institutional practices can encourage personalized antenatal consultations for threatened preterm birth. These include accommodations, such as dedicating one neonatologist to serve as the antenatal consultant without additional responsibilities of managing a busy NICU and systematically offering follow-up NICU visits and consultations with the neonatologist and allied health professionals including multidisciplinary meetings. Frequent discussions between obstetricians and neonatologists, as a team, also are recommended. Parent-centered tools can be created to teach and support personalized consultations (see **Fig. 1**), and consultation notes should reflect these practices, as proposed in **Fig. 2**.

PERSONALIZED DECISION MAKING

Deciphering preferences in decision making is important. For many, shared decision making implies that parents want to collaborate in decisions with physicians. In theory, clinicians should learn to discern between parents' informational needs for deliberation and their desires to be involved in making the decision, broadly defined as "problem solving" and "decision making."[80] Some parents may want information but not involvement in the decision, some parents may want both, or some may want neither, relinquishing the entirety of the process and decision by the medical team.[18,25] Assumptions about preferred role in decision making are often misjudged.[24,63,80–82] Evaluations that have surveyed parents involved in neonatal and pediatric end-of-life

```
Date: __/__/__                                    Mother's Name: _____
                                                  DOB: __/__/__
OB Name: _____                            Room nr.: _____
Reason for consultation:                          Hosp. ID:_____
  Prematurity  Other _____
BABY                                  MOTHER
GA:_____ ( U/S_____ LMP_____)  Age:_____ G___ P___ A___ Blood Gr: ___
  Singleton    Twin _____        Serol.: _____
EFW:_____ (__/__/__) Gender: _____  Habits: _____
ß-methasone __/__/__  __/__/__  __/__/__   _____
_____     Medications:_____
_____     PMH: _____
_____     _____
_____     OBST. H: _____
_____     _____
_____

CURRENT PREGNANCY
T1 _____
  T1 U/S(__/__/__)_____
T2 _____
  T2 U/S(__/__/__)_____
T3 _____
  T3 U/S(__/__/__)_____

DISCUSSION        Mother    Father       Other significant: _____
                  OB present: _____    NICU Team: _____
                  Baby's name: _____   _____
Parents' main concerns: _____
Family situation: _____
Information discussed relative to parents' needs:  Complications of prematurity    Parental roles
                                                   How NICU works
_____
_____
_____
_____
_____
☐ NICU visit offered              Written documentation provided : ☐ yes ☐ no

Follow-up
☐ NICU visit done (Date: __/__/___)        Neonatologist Name: _____
☐ Allied HCPs consulted (Role & date):
_____
☐ Follow-up visit by neonatologist: _____  Signature: _____ Date: __/__/__
   Date: __/__/__ , GA: _____
```

Fig. 2. Antenatal consultation page 2 (parent-centered).

decisions reveal heterogeneity; some prefer sharing the decision with physicians, some prefer making decisions independently, and some defer to the physician.[25,83] Decision-making preferences are influenced by age, gender, cultural norms, and specifics related to the decision.[84] Although those who participate in decision making for extremely premature infants find psychological short-term and long-term benefits,[73,85] excessive information or incorrect assumptions about decision-making roles may impede decisions for others.[84]

Problem-solving or deliberation processes not only differ between decision makers but preferences change with time and characteristics of the decision. True risk comprehension interprets objective information with subjective preferences to clarify choices leading to decisions consistent with values and beliefs. It is beyond the scope of this article to explore the multitude of cognitive biases and behavioral decisional processes that could potentially impact individual decision making, but it is important to personalize precisely because each person approaches decisions differently.[17–19,22,23]

A parent's approach to decision making has no relation to her or his ability as a parent. "Good" parents may choose to receive information so as to make decisions; "good" parents may choose to defer decision making to physicians, and "good" parents may choose to receive information alongside medical team recommendations sharing in the decision. And for other "good" parents, there is no decision to be made; rather, they feel "fate" or God is in control and to suggest a decision may in fact increase their distress. All of these "good" parents make reasonable decisions for their infants in a manner consistent with their preferences, frameworks, and beliefs.

SUMMARY

Decisions in the gray zone are complicated. They are reliant on personal viewpoints balancing sanctity of life and quality of life, reflect preferences for rational and intuitive processes, and roles in decision making. Instead of aspiring to achieve mutual consent in shared decision making, physicians should seek to practice personalized decision making. Personalized decision making would take into consideration a parent's preferences for decisional responsibility and deliberation and thereby informational and supportive needs. When relationships are built based on personalization, parents are empowered. For decisions of this magnitude and complexity, any decision made by a parent or physician, is one they never hoped to make. Parents and physicians try to make the best decision possible on behalf of fragile neonates under very difficult circumstances. Good clinical practice is contingent on both adequate clinical knowledge and support from compassionate, humane interactions between physicians and patients. A good outcome for the antenatal consultation is a successful interaction in which parents frame the consultation, and are empowered by support and resources to participate in problem solving or decision making to the extent with which they are comfortable.

REFERENCES

1. Philip AGS. The evolution of neonatology. Pediatr Res 2005;50(4):799–815.
2. Avery ME. A 50-year overview of perinatal medicine. Early Hum Dev 1992; 29(1–3):43–50.
3. Committee on Hospital Care. Family centered care and the pediatrician's role. Pediatrics 2003;112(3 Pt 1):691–6.
4. American Academy of Pediatrics. Patient and family centered care and the pediatrician's role. Policy statement. Pediatrics 2012;129(2):394–404.
5. Davis L, Mohay H, Edwards H. Mothers involvement in caring for their premature infants: an historical overview. J Adv Nurs 2003;42(6):578–86.
6. Barry MJ, Edgman-Levitan S. Shared decision-making: the pinnacle of patient centered care. N Engl J Med 2012;366(9):780–1.
7. President's Commission. Deciding to forego life-sustaining treatment: a report on the ethical, medical and legal issues in treatment decisions/President's

Commission for the Study of Ethical Problems in Medicine and Biomedical and Behavioral Research. Washington, DC: The Commission; 1983.

8. Gilmore A. Sanctity of life verses quality of life: the continuing debate. Can Med Assoc J 1984;130(2):180–1.

9. National Research Council. Crossing the Quality Chasm: a new health care system for the 21st century. Washington, DC: National Academies Press; 2001.

10. Emanuel E, Emanuel L. Four models of the physician-patient relationship. JAMA 1992;262(16):2221–6.

11. Charles C, Gafni A, Whelan T. Shared decision-making in the medical encounter: what does it mean? (or it takes at least two to tango). Soc Sci Med 1997;44(5): 681–92.

12. MacDonald H, American Academy of Pediatrics, Committee on Fetus and Newborn. Perinatal care at the threshold of viability. Pediatrics 2002;110(5): 1024–7.

13. Tyson JE, Stoll BJ. Evidence-based ethics and the care and outcome of extremely premature infants. Clin Perinatol 2003;30(2):363–87.

14. Batton DG, American Academy of Pediatrics, Committee on Fetus and Newborn. Clinical report—antenatal counseling regarding resuscitation at an extremely low gestational age. Pediatrics 2009;124(1):422–7.

15. Cummings J, American Academy of Pediatrics, Committee on Fetus and Newborn. Antenatal counseling regarding resuscitation and intensive care before 25 weeks of gestation. Pediatrics 2015;136(3):588–95.

16. Griswold KJ, Fnanaroff JM. An evidence-based overview of prenatal consultation with a focus on infants born at the limits of viability. Pediatrics 2010;125(4): e931–7.

17. Haward MF, Janvier A. An introduction to behavioural decision-making theories for paediatricians. Acta Paediatr 2015;104(4):340–5.

18. Bogardus S, Holmboe E, Jekel J. Perils, pitfalls and possibilities in talking about medical risk. JAMA 1999;281(11):1037–41.

19. Renjilian CB, Womer JW, Carroll KW, et al. Parental explicit heuristics in decision-making for children with life-threatening illnesses. Pediatrics 2013;131(2): e566–72.

20. Kon AA. The shared decision-making continuum. JAMA 2010;304(8):903–4.

21. de Vos MA, Bos AP, Plotz FB, et al. Talking with parents about end-of-life decisions for their children. Pediatrics 2015;135(2):e465–76.

22. Janvier A, Lorenz JM, Lantos JD. Antenatal counselling for parents facing an extremely preterm birth: limitations of the medical evidence. Acta Paediatr 2012;101(8):800–4.

23. Janvier A, Barrington K, Farlow B. Communication with parents concerning withholding or withdrawing of life sustaining interventions in neonatology. Semin Perinatol 2014;38(1):38–46.

24. Payot A, Gendron S, Lefebvre F, et al. Deciding to resuscitate extremely premature babies: how do parents and neonatologists engage in the decision? Soc Sci Med 2007;64(7):1487–500.

25. Caeymaex L, Speranza M, Vasilescu C, et al. Living with a crucial decision: a qualitative study of parental narratives three years after the loss of their newborn in the NICU. PLoS One 2001;6(12):e28633, 1–7.

26. Tyson JE, Parikh NA, Langer J, et al. National Institute of Child Health and Human Development Neonatal Research Network. Intensive care for extreme prematurity: moving beyond gestational age. N Engl J Med 2008;358(16):1672–81.

27. Lemyre B, Daboval T, Dunn S, et al. Shared decision-making for infants born at the threshold of viability: a prognosis based guideline. J Perinatol 2016;36(7): 503–9.
28. Dupont-Thibodeau A, Barrington KJ, Farlow B, et al. End of life decisions for extremely low-gestation-age infants: why simple rules for complicated decisions should be avoided. Semin Perinatol 2014;38(1):31–7.
29. Robinson HP. Sonar measurement of fetal crown-rump length as means of assessing maturity in first trimester of pregnancy. Br Med J 1973;4(5883):28–31.
30. Chervenak FA, Skupski DW, Romero R, et al. How accurate is fetal biometry in the assessment of fetal age? Am J Obstet Gynecol 1998;178(4):678–87.
31. Lynch CD, Zhang J. The research implications of the selection of a gestational age estimation method. Paediatr Perinat Epidemiol 2007;21(Suppl 2):86–96.
32. Salvedt S, Almstron H, Kublickas M, et al. Ultrasound dating at 12-14 or 15-20 weeks of gestation? A prospective cross-validation of established dating formulae in a population of in-vitro fertilized pregnancies randomized to early or late dating scan. Ultrasound Obstet Gynecol 2004;24(1):42–50.
33. Haward MF, Kirshenbaum NW, Campbell DE. Care at the edge of viability: medical and ethical issues. Clin Perinatol 2011;38(3):471–92.
34. Express Group. Incidence of and risk factors for neonatal morbidity after active perinatal care: extremely preterm infants study in Sweden (EXPRESS). Acta Paediatr 2010;99(7):978–92.
35. Perlbarg J, Ancel PY, Khoshnood B, et al, Epipage- 2 Ethics Group. Delivery room management of extremely preterm infants: the EPIPAGE-2 study. Arch Dis Child Fetal Neonatal Ed 2016;101(5):F384–90.
36. Janvier A, Lantos J. Delivery room practices for extremely preterm infants: the harms of the gestational age label. Arch Dis Child Fetal Neonatal Ed 2016;101: F375–6.
37. Pignotti MS, Berni R. Extremely preterm births: end-of-life decisions in European countries. Arch Dis Child Fetal Neonatal Ed 2010;95(4):F273–6.
38. de Leeuw R, Cuttini M, Nadai M, et al. Treatment choices for extremely preterm infants: an international perspective. J Pediatr 2000;137(5):608–15.
39. Taittonen L, Korhonen PH, Palomäki O, et al. Opinions on the counselling, care and outcome of extremely premature birth among healthcare professionals in Finland. Acta Paediatr 2014;103(3):262–7.
40. Khan RA, Burgoyne L, O'Connell MP, et al. Resuscitation at the limits of viability: an Irish perspective. Acta Paediatr 2009;98(9):1456–60.
41. Rysavy M, Li L, Bell E, et al. Between-hospital variation in treatment and outcomes in extremely preterm infants. N Engl J Med 2015;372(19):1801–11.
42. Lantos JD, Meadow W. Variation in the treatment of infants born at the borderline of viability. Pediatrics 2009;123(6):1588–90.
43. Seri I, Evans J. Limits of viability: definition of the gray zone. J Perinatol 2008; 28(Suppl 1):S4–8.
44. Itabashi K, Hiriuchi T, Kusuda S, et al. Mortality rates for extremely low birth weight infants born in Japan in 2005. Pediatrics 2009;123(2):445–50.
45. Verhagan AAE, Sauer PJJ. End of life decisions in newborns: an approach from The Netherlands. Pedaitrics 2005;116(3):736–9.
46. Meadow W, Lantos J. Moral reflections on neonatal intensive care. Pediatrics 2009;123(2):595–7.
47. Janvier A, Lantos J, POST group investigators. Stronger and more vulnerable: a balanced view of the impacts of the NICU experience on parents. Pediatrics 2016;138(3) [pii:e20160655].

48. Yee WH, Sauve R. What information do parents want from the antenatal consultation? Paediatr Child Health 2007;12(3):191–6.
49. Paul D, Epps S, Leef K, et al. Prenatal consultation with a neonatologist prior to preterm delivery. J Perinatol 2001;21(7):431–7.
50. Brazy JE, Anderson BM, Becker PT, et al. How parents of premature infants gather information and obtain support. Neonatal Netw 2001;20(2):41–8.
51. Kim UO, Basir MA. Informing and educating parents about the risks and outcomes of prematurity. Clin Perinatol 2014;41(4):979–91.
52. Haward MF, Murphy RO, Lorenz JM. Message framing and perinatal decisions. Pediatrics 2008;122(1):109–18.
53. Malenka DJ, Baron JA, Johanson S, et al. The framing effect of relative and absolute risk. J Gen Intern Med 1993;8(10):543–8.
54. Mazur DJ, Hickman DH. Patients' interpretations of probability terms. J Gen Intern Med 1991;6(3):237–40.
55. Bowling A, Ebrahim S. Measuring patients' preferences for treatment and perceptions of risk. Qual Health Care 2001;10(Supp 1):i2–8.
56. Holmber C, Waters EA, Whitehouse K, et al. My lived experiences are more important than your probabilities: the role of individualized risk estimates for decision-making about participation in the study of tamoxifen and raloxifene (STAR). Med Decis Making 2015;35(8):1010–22.
57. Plous S. The psychology of judgment and decision-making. New York: McGraw-Hill; 1993.
58. Aleszewski A, Horlink-Jones T. How can doctors communicate information about risk more effectively? BMJ 2003;327(7417):728–31.
59. Cox C, Fritz Z. Should non-disclosures be considered as morally equivalent to lies within the doctor-patient relationship? J Med Ethics 2016;42(10):632–5.
60. Guillen U, Suh S, Munson D, et al. Development and pretesting of a decision-aid to use when counseling parents facing imminent extreme premature delivery. J Pediatr 2012;160(3):382–7.
61. Kakkilaya V, Groome L, Platt D, et al. Use of a visual aid to improve counseling at the threshold of viability. Pediatrics 2011;128(6):e1511–9.
62. Muthusamy AD, Leuthner S, Gaebler-Uhung C, et al. Supplemental written information improves prenatal counseling: a randomized trial. Pediatrics 2012;129(5): e1269–74.
63. Godolphin W. The role of risk communication in shared decision-making. BMJ 2003;327(7417):692–3.
64. Slovic P, editor. The feeling of risk. London: Earthscan; 2001.
65. Walter J, Ross LF. Relational autonomy: moving beyond the limits of isolated individualism. Pediatrics 2014;133(Sup 1):S16–23.
66. Young E, Tsai E, O'Riordan A. A qualitative study of predelivery counselling for extreme prematurity. Peaediatr Child Health 2012;17(8):432–6.
67. Lerman C, Daly M, Walsh W, et al. Communication between patients with breast cancer and health care providers determinants and implications. Cancer 1993; 72(9):2612–20.
68. Bechara A, Tranel D, Damasio H. Characterization of the decision-making deficit of patients with ventromedial prefrontal cortex lesions. Brain 2000;12(pt11): 2189–202.
69. Gaucher N, Payot A. From powerlessness to empowerment: mothers expect more than information from the prenatal consultation for preterm labour. Paediatr Child Health 2011;16(10):638–42.

70. Gaucher N, Nadeau S, Barbier A, et al. Personalized antenatal consultations for preterm labor: responding to mothers' expectations. J Pediatr 2016;178: 130–4.e7.
71. McHaffie HE, Laing IA, Parker M, et al. Deciding for imperilled newborns: medical authority or parental autonomy? J Med Ethics 2001;27(2):104–9.
72. Haward MF, Janvier A, Lorenz JM, et al. Speaking to parents before premature birth: whose agenda? Poster session presented at Pediatrics Academic Society Meeting. Baltimore (MD), May 4, 2016.
73. Bohnhorst B, Ahl T, Peter C, et al. Parents' prenatal onward and postdischarge experiences in case of extreme prematurity: when to set the course for a trusting relationship between parents and medical staff. Am J Perinatol 2015;32(13): 1191–7.
74. Post DM, Cegala DJ, Miser WF. The other half of the whole: teaching patients to communicate with physicians. Fam Med 2002;34(5):344–52.
75. Paling J. Strategies to help patients understand risks. BMJ 2003;327(7417): 745–8.
76. Smith R. Communication risk: the main work of doctors. BMJ 2003;327(7417). 0 Editor's choice.
77. Arnold L, Sawyer A, Rabe H, et al. Parents' first moments with their very preterm babies: a qualitative study. BMJ open 2013;3(4) [pii:e002487].
78. Miquel-Verges F, Woods SL, Aucott SW, et al. Prenatal consultation with a neonatologist for congenital anomalies: parental perceptions. Pediatrics 2009;124(4): e573–9.
79. Boss RD, Hutton N, Sulpar LJ, et al. Values parents apply to decision-making for high-risk newborns. Pediatrics 2008;122(3):385–9.
80. Deber RB. Physicians in health care management: 8. The patient-physician partnership: decision-making, problem solving and the desire to participate. Can Med Assoc J 1994;151(4):423–7.
81. Perlman NB, Freedman JL, Abramovitch A, et al. Informational needs of parents of sick neonates. Pediatrics 1991;88(3):512–8.
82. Doron MW, Veness-Meehan KA, Margolis LH, et al. Delivery room resuscitation decisions for extremely premature infants. Pediatrics 1998;102(3):574–82.
83. Keenan HT, Doron MW, Seyda BA. Comparison of mothers' and counselors' perceptions of predelivery counseling for extremely premature infants. Pediatrics 2005;116(1):104–11.
84. Madrigal VN, Carroll KW, Hexem K, et al. Parental decision-making preferences in the pediatric intensive care. Crit Care Med 2012;40(10):2876–82.
85. Caeymaex L, Jousselme C, Vasilescu C, et al. Perceived role in end-of-life decision making in the NICU affects long-term parental grief response. Arch Dis Child Fetal Neonatal Ed 2013;98(1):F26–31.

Caring for Families at the Limits of Viability

The Education of Dr Green

Theophil A. Stokes, MD[a],*, Stephanie K. Kukora, MD[b],
Renee D. Boss, MD, MHS[c]

KEYWORDS

- Gestational age–based resuscitation • Antenatal counseling
- Shared decision-making • Neonatal Ethics • Individualized decision making
- Physician communication • End of life decision making

KEY POINTS

- Resuscitation decisions for infants born at the edges of viability are complicated moral dilemmas that cannot be simplified; the decision-making process must be individualized.
- Resuscitation guidelines based solely on estimates of gestational age are unscientific and unethical. Additional prognostic factors must be factored into the decision-making process.
- Advanced communication and counseling skills are necessary when assisting families in the process of making difficult medical decisions for their critically ill baby.

CASE STUDY

Dr Green is a first-year fellow in neonatology who is eager to learn and full of questions. It is a Friday night in the neonatal intensive care unit (NICU), and he is ready to begin his first overnight call. Early in his shift he receives a page from the obstetric resident, who has requested a "NICU consultation" for Mrs Evers, a 24-year-old G1 who has been admitted to the Labor and Delivery service in preterm labor at an estimated gestational age of 22 3/7 weeks. Dr Green has never before provided such a consultation, and he is understandably nervous about how to proceed.

Dr Green's attending neonatologist for the evening is Dr Gigante, a senior neonatologist who has practiced for more than 25 years. Dr Gigante is known for his rather blunt and matter-of-fact demeanor, and he seems annoyed by the obstetric resident's

[a] Walter Reed National Military Medical Center, 8901 Wisconsin Avenue, Bethesda, MD 20889, USA; [b] Division of Neonatal-Perinatal Medicine, Department of Pediatrics and Communicable Diseases, Floor 8, 1540 E Hospital Dr SPC 4254, Ann Arbor, MI 48109, USA; [c] Division of Neonatology, Johns Hopkins School of Medicine, Berman Institute of Bioethics, 600 North Wolfe Street, Baltimore, MD 21287, USA
* Corresponding author.
E-mail address: theophilstokes@gmail.com

Clin Perinatol 44 (2017) 447–459
http://dx.doi.org/10.1016/j.clp.2017.01.007
0095-5108/17/Published by Elsevier Inc.

perinatology.theclinics.com

request for a NICU consultation, as he states that neonates less than 23 weeks' gestation are "nonviable" and that the NICU's policy is to provide resuscitation only to infants of at least 23 weeks' estimated gestational age (EGA) at birth. He instructs Dr Green to remind his obstetric colleague that infants born less than 23 weeks EGA have a 100% mortality rate at their hospital, and believes that a NICU consultation is unwarranted at this time.

Dr Green is aware of the NICU's policy, but he is also uncomfortable with Dr Gigante's response. He finds himself questioning the merits of such a policy, and turns to the literature to investigate further.

GESTATIONAL AGE–BASED POLICY/PRACTICE GUIDELINES

The neonatology profession has frequently had local and/or national guidelines for resuscitation of infants born extremely prematurely. A number of these guidelines have focused exclusively, or significantly, on gestational age. In 2006, the Nuffield Council on Bioethics acknowledged that individual variability makes meaningful prognostication difficult, but went on to offer gestational age–based resuscitation guidelines as a tool to guide individual decision-making.[1] In the United States, the American Academy of Pediatrics and the American College of Obstetrics and Gynecology recommend using current morbidity and mortality data relevant to gestational age in helping the family make a decision in accordance with their values.[1–3]

Although professional guidelines offer support for clinicians and families faced with decisions regarding resuscitation, the intention of such guidelines to respect individualized decisions can be undermined in their translation into hospital protocols. This was exemplified in a 1990 case, ultimately upheld by the Texas Supreme Court, which did not find fault in the hospital for enacting a policy that led to resuscitation of an infant at 23 weeks' EGA over parental objections.[4] A 2008 survey of California neonatologists confirmed that practice site was a predictor of the gestational age at which individual clinicians were willing to initiate resuscitation, confirming that formal or informal local policies impact neonatologists' practices.[5]

THE LIMITATIONS OF GESTATIONAL AGE–BASED RESUSCITATION GUIDELINES

Estimates of gestational age clearly play an important role when prognosticating chances for survival among infants born preterm, as numerous studies have demonstrated a significant positive association between completed weeks of gestation and improved neonatal survival.[6–8] These data are useful and important, but alone insufficient to make determinations about whether or not intervention is warranted.

The first and most obvious flaw with treatment guidelines based solely on estimates of gestational age is that they do not account for inaccuracies inherent to dating of pregnancies. Compared with pregnancies with known dates based on in vitro fertilization (IVF), first trimester ultrasounds may vary by ± 7 days, and second trimester ultrasounds or last menstrual period estimates of gestational age may vary by ± 14 days.[9,10] This means that a pregnancy estimated to be 22 4/7 weeks' gestation may actually be closer to 24 weeks, an age in which some might argue that resuscitation attempts should be no longer optional, but mandatory. Clearly the uncertainty associated with dating pregnancies should be taken into account in the making of literal life and death decisions.

Even when pregnancies can be dated with absolute precision, we are still left to confront another major limitation of gestational age–based resuscitation protocols, namely their reliance on completed 7-day blocks of time. Embryologic development (like all human development) is a gradual process that varies between individuals, and viability does not simply get turned-on like a switch. Yet this line of thinking seems to be at the root of so many of our gestational age–based resuscitation guidelines. This can lead to inconsistent and seemingly ridiculous sounding scenarios in which a "nonviable" infant may be deemed worthy of resuscitation the next day, across town at a different hospital, or in a neighboring time zone. Hospitals that define viability at 23 weeks often withhold antenatal steroids until after midnight at 22 5/7 weeks' EGA, thus allowing completion of the 48-hour steroid course of therapy to coincide with "infant viability" at 23 weeks. In hospitals that set this threshold at 24 weeks, steroids may be withheld until 23 5/7 weeks. Or, as was recently demonstrated, infants born near the end of their 22nd or 23rd week of gestation were more likely to be resuscitated than their counterparts earlier in the week.[7]

Another flaw in the use of gestational age–based resuscitation protocols is the impact of the "self-fulfilling prophecy in intensive care."[11] Although survival rates of 5% or less are often quoted as a rationale for withholding antenatal steroids or resuscitation attempts for infants born less than 23 weeks' EGA,[3] such data are skewed by practices that withhold interventions before 23 weeks. Survival rates for infants born less than 23 weeks for whom resuscitation was attempted have been reported in the range of 20% to 25%.[7,8,12]

A final limitation of gestational age–based resuscitation guidelines is the discounting of additional prognostic factors that have clearly been demonstrated to affect neonatal outcomes. The use of antenatal steroids, female sex, singleton birth, and higher birth weight are each associated with reductions in the risk of death or death with neurodevelopmental impairment similar to those associated with a 1-week increase in gestational age.[6]

At this point, it is illustrative to return to the case of Mrs Evers described briefly at the outset of this article. Mrs Evers' pregnancy was deemed by Dr Gigante to be nonviable due to an EGA of 22 3/7 weeks. To evaluate this scenario more objectively, let us consider the following scenarios using the National Institute of Child Health and Human Development's (NICHD's) Neonatal Research Network Extremely Preterm Birth Outcome Data program (www.nichd.nih.gov/about/org/der/branches/ppb/programs/epbo/pages/epbo_case.aspx) to evaluate estimated outcomes (**Table 1**).

Table 1
Scenario A: Mrs Evers is carrying twin boys conceived via in vitro fertilization, thus her dates are certain

Outcomes	Outcomes for All Infants, %	Outcomes for Mechanically Ventilated Infants, %
Survival	2	6
Survival without profound neurodevelopmental impairment	1	3
Survival without moderate to severe neurodevelopmental impairment	0	1
Death	98	94
Death or profound neurodevelopmental impairment	99	97
Death or moderate to severe neurodevelopmental impairment	100	99

The estimated fetal weight each fetus is estimated to be 425 g. Antenatal steroids are being withheld per hospital policy.
From the National Institutes of Health. Available at: https://www.nichd.nih.gov/about/org/der/branches/ppb/programs/epbo/pages/epbo_case.aspx.

These numbers are indeed poor, and although mortality is not 100%, Dr Gigante's assessment that intervention is unwarranted might seem reasonable to many. Yet, if we alter the scenario slightly, we find a different set of outcomes (**Table 2**).

Survival estimates for this pregnancy at the same gestational age (22 3/7 weeks' EGA) are now as high as 30%. Furthermore, if we plausibly assume that Mrs Evers' dates may have been off by a few days, we arrive at these estimated outcomes (**Table 3**).

As demonstrated, the estimated survival outcomes in this scenario vary widely when variables beyond gestational age are included, with estimated survival rates ranging from as low as 2% in scenario A to as high as 44% in scenario C. This isn't to argue in favor or against an attempt at resuscitation, but rather to demonstrate the limitations in using EGA without other contextual factors, such as sex, plurality, or estimated fetal weight (which itself may be inaccurate) to make such decisions. These data rather definitively demonstrate that sweeping declarations of nonviability before 23 weeks' EGA are simply not true.

Dr Green talks to the obstetric resident, and learns that there is indeed some uncertainty about her dates. The 22 3/7 weeks' EGA is based on her first trimester ultrasound; however, she is 23 3/7 weeks' EGA based on her last menstrual period dating. The estimated fetal weight is 525 g, and she appears to be carrying a girl.

Dr Green updates Dr Gigante, with this new information, and he reluctantly agrees to proceed with antenatal counseling. Dr Gigante explains that the goal of the consultation will be to facilitate an informed decision from Mrs Evers about whether to proceed with delivery room resuscitation and NICU care for her infant. Dr Gigante familiarizes Dr Green with the NICU's decision-aid pamphlet that has been designed to inform families confronted with such decisions. The pamphlet includes a narrative and graphically detailed description of morbidity and mortality data, as well as discussion of intraventricular hemorrhage, periventricular leukomalacia, respiratory distress syndrome, bronchopulmonary dysplasia, and retinopathy of prematurity. Dr Gigante stresses the importance of clearly articulating the risks of long-term neurodevelopmental disability so that Mrs Evers can make a truly informed decision. He emphasizes the

Table 2
Scenario B: Mrs Evers is carrying a singleton female pregnancy

Outcomes	Outcomes for All Infants, %	Outcomes for Mechanically Ventilated Infants, %
Survival	11	30
Survival without profound neurodevelopmental impairment	6	18
Survival without moderate to severe neurodevelopmental impairment	3	11
Death	89	70
Death or profound neurodevelopmental impairment	94	82
Death or moderate to severe neurodevelopmental impairment	97	89

Her estimated gestational age is based on her recollection of her last menstrual period, although she admits that her periods are sometimes irregular. Her fetus is estimated to weigh 550 g, and her obstetrician (in a break from protocol) has started a course of antenatal steroids. Assuming her gestational age of 22 3/7 weeks' EGA, the following data are obtained.

From the National Institutes of Health. Available at: https://www.nichd.nih.gov/about/org/der/branches/ppb/programs/epbo/pages/epbo_case.aspx.

Table 3 Scenario C: same as B (Table 2), but here we assume that her dates are off by 4 days, and she is actually into her 23rd week of pregnancy		
Outcomes	**Outcomes for All Infants, %**	**Outcomes for Mechanically Ventilated Infants, %**
Survival	33	44
Survival without profound neurodevelopmental impairment	22	30
Survival without moderate to severe neurodevelopmental impairment	13	18
Death	67	56
Death or profound neurodevelopmental impairment	78	70
Death or moderate to severe neurodevelopmental impairment	87	82

From the National Institutes of Health. Available at: https://www.nichd.nih.gov/about/org/der/branches/ppb/programs/epbo/pages/epbo_case.aspx.

importance of respecting her autonomy as a parent, and stresses that this is a decision that she will need to make.

Antenatal Counseling and Periviable Decision-Making

Neonatologists possess medical knowledge and experience, and are duty-bound by a fiduciary relationship to their patients. Although they strive to serve their patients' best interest, their recommendations and practices may be influenced by their own personal experiences, values, and beliefs. Parents are socially bound to oversee the welfare and development of their children, are obligated to provide their care after discharge, and will live with the long-term emotional consequences of their infant's hospitalization, survival, or death.[13–17] They are presumed to share the values of their unborn child as well as the unique context of their family, and are tasked with advocating for their infant and giving him or her a voice.

The complexity of decision-making for infants with threatened delivery at the margins of viability stems from the existence of multiple ethically permissible options for resuscitative care, wide ranges of possible infant outcomes, and significant uncertainty in prognosis.[18] Although the roles of neonatologists and parents in this decision-making process are intertwined, attitudes vary regarding the degree to which parental preference should be factored into the decision-making process.[19–23] These differences in opinion underlie the spectrum of parental involvement in the decision-making process at the extremes of prematurity.

On the paternalistic end of the spectrum, parents are afforded little to no involvement in the perinatal decision-making process. This approach is rooted in a belief that physicians are uniquely qualified to make medical decisions that will be in the best interest of their patient. Advocates of a paternalistic approach argue that it can be excessively burdensome for parents to make such difficult decisions, and that paternalism is therefore a more compassionate approach.

An impartial, informed-consent approach to periviable decision-making falls on the opposite end of the spectrum. Rooted in the paradigm shifts that have occurred in physician-patient communication toward valuing patient autonomy, this approach assumes that parents are and should be the final arbiters in making life and death decisions for their infant. Antenatal counseling is therefore directed toward providing parents with nondirective medical information believed sufficient (by physicians) to inform a rational and autonomous decision while minimizing the physician's imposition of his or her own values.[24,25] This was found to be the most common approach to antenatal counseling in a 2002 survey of neonatologists practicing in the northeastern United States.[26] In the words of one neonatologist:

> I give them the most neutral information possible so that they could make the decision as to whether they want their child to be given care or not. I really want it to be neutral...it's really important to me that there be informed consent and I ask the parents: "Do you want us to take care of your child or not?" and that is the answer I am looking for.[27]

Shared decision-making (discussed later in this article) falls on the spectrum between a paternalistic, physician-centered model, and a nondirective, informative, parent-centered model.[28] Shared decision-making aims to incorporate the values and beliefs of the family with the knowledge and experience of the physician to promote the best possible patient outcome (beneficence), minimize burden (nonmaleficence), and incorporate patient preferences (autonomy).

It is important to note that none of the decision-making models described previously are inherently ethical. The appropriate model of decision-making will depend on the individual family's desired level of involvement in the process. This has been shown to vary among families, and physicians tend to be poor judges of how much or little involvement parents want.[20,23,29,30] Efforts to protect parental autonomy by assuming their desire to take full responsibility for such decisions are, ironically, paternalistic.

The Needs of Parents

A common recurring theme in the literature evaluating the decision-making experiences of NICU families is a desire to receive information that will enhance their meaningful participation in the decision-making process for their infant.[31–35] Yet the information that families believe important to inform such decisions can be highly variable based on the individual characteristics of the family being counseled. Although some families may seek truthful, direct, and uncomplicated medical information, others may rely on religion, hope, spirituality, and compassion to guide their decisions.[30,32–36] Some families may wish to avoid such decisions entirely, hoping instead for the neonatologist to advise them as to how to proceed.[29]

The uniform application of a neutral, informed-consent model of antenatal counseling and decision-making isn't appropriate for every family. Although rooted in a respect for parental autonomy and presumably well intended, it may instead leave families feeling unsupported or even abandoned by the process. In the words of prospective parents:

> The doctor comes, gives information, and leaves, it's like there is no relationship, someone you could rely on. If you are ill, you need to rely on someone and say "help me"...he/she just comes, gives information, and leaves.

> We don't expect the physician to make the decision for us. But we need to feel that, well, that the physician...treats us more humanely...not like a client.[27]

Neonatologists have an obligation to provide care that is in the best interest of their patients. When providing antenatal counseling, the neonatologist's patient is not only the yet-to-be born infant, but the family being counseled as well. Although it is important to be respectful of parental autonomy, it is also important to provide counseling that is beneficent and nonmaleficent. The risk of doing harm isn't simply theoretic, as poor communication with intensive care unit (ICU) physicians and participation in end-of-life decision-making have been found to correlate with symptoms of posttraumatic stress disorder in family members of ICU patients.[37,38] An ethical approach to antenatal counseling requires a willingness and ability to tailor the approach so that it can be provided in a manner best suited to the individual family. Frequently, neonatologists will need to be prepared to share in the decision-making process.

Shared Decision-Making

Shared decision-making has been described as "The Pinnacle of Patient-Centered Care," and has become the norm for many medical scenarios in the United States and elsewhere.[39] Shared decision-making is appropriate for clinical situations involving values-based decisions, meaning that, in an identical clinical scenario, different individuals might weigh the outcomes differently based on their own deeply held personal beliefs.

Effective shared decision-making begins with clarity regarding the choices to be discussed with a family. Some clinician groups have a process to reach and enforce management consensus based on neonatal outcomes, such that every clinician offers similar treatment choices at particular gestational ages.[40] Some hospital regulations or religious affiliations dictate physician management for periviable infants, limiting the available treatment options. Tools like the NICHD calculator are used by some to determine treatment choices for individual families.[6] But in general, we know little about how individual clinicians in different settings decide which options will be shared with families.

Once it is clear which choices will be shared with the family, the next step is to determine who will participate in the decision. When these conversations occur in teaching institutions, it is clear delineation of which portions are appropriate for trainees to lead and which are the responsibility of more experienced clinicians is vital. Parents should be asked who they would like to have a voice in the discussion, whether that be other family members, friends, or other clinicians. Individual family members may hold different values related to the decisions at hand, and which family member(s) will have the ultimate say must be determined. Individual health care team members may also hold different values. Such variability is expected and common, but it can lead to conflict and moral distress if timely opportunities for discussion and conflict mediation are not offered.[18]

The process of shared decision-making is easily shaped by the power imbalance inherent to the parent-clinician relationship. Clinicians must learn to avoid abdication of all decisional authority (eg, objectively describing treatment options and asking the parents to make the decision), and the other extreme of paternalism (eg, not telling parents that treatment options exist). Sharing decisions means being curious about who the parents are as people, assessing their experiences and beliefs relevant to the current decision. It means offering insights into how different families weigh similar decisions, and possibly recommending the treatment option most aligning with the goals and values described by the parents. Data suggest that although most families wish to participate to some degree in these decisions, most want to hear physician recommendations and to then have the option to follow or decline those recommendations.[41] Clinicians, however, are often uncomfortable making recommendations, which suggests an area for further training.[42,43]

Neonatologists are not commonly trained to help families articulate personal values and preferences, and are rarely trained in skills to navigate values conflicts.[44] This lack of training is in contrast to the skills demanded by antenatal counseling. Often, antenatal counseling for extreme prematurity entails consideration of the infant's potential quality of life and how it is intertwined with, yet separate from, the family's quality of life. How, for example, should we counsel a couple whose 4-year-autistic son engages in self-harming without his mother's presence, as they consider the possibility that resuscitation of their 23-week infant could lead to months in the NICU? Incorporating interdisciplinary team members from social work, chaplaincy, and palliative care may sometimes be needed to help families navigate these conflicts.

Dr Green accompanies Dr Gigante to Mrs Evers hospital room. Mrs Evers appears uncomfortable from her contractions, which are occurring every 4 to 5 minutes. After a brief introduction, Dr Gigante provides Mrs Evers with a copy of the NICU's decision-aid pamphlet, and then proceeds with a detailed account of possible morbidities and mortality data.

Dr Gigante then asks Mrs Evers whether she desires for her infant to be resuscitated should delivery occur at this premature gestation, and explains that comfort care would also be an option. Mrs Evers asks Dr Gigante what he thinks would be best, to which he replies, "This is a decision that you will have to make."

Exasperated and seemingly angry, Mrs Evers replies, "Just save my baby!"

Dr Green was a silent observer of the conversation. He noted that Mrs Evers appeared distracted by her painful contractions, and that she didn't ask many questions of Dr Gigante even though he repeatedly paused and asked her if she had any. He wonders how much information she actually heard or was able to process, as she seems to have had a blank look on her face after being told that her infant might die.

Neonatologists Need a Better Understanding of what It Means to Counsel

The Mirriam-Webster Dictionary defines counseling as "*advice and support that is given to people to help them deal with problems, make important decision, etc.*" Neonatologists tasked with providing antenatal counseling to families must recognize that the challenges inherent in counseling are far greater than relaying complicated medical information at a comprehensible level. True counseling requires that families be engaged in a conversation that will illuminate the *advice and support* needed by the individual family at hand. Navigating the raw and sometimes unpredictable emotionality of the situation, acknowledging and embracing the clinical uncertainty, and identifying and offsetting the physician/patient power differential are all components that impel the success or failure of a counseling session.[45]

Among the most difficult aspects of these conversations is that they typically occur between neonatologists and family members who have never met. This lack of familiarity presents an immediate obstacle to communication, particularly in the emotionally charged setting of a threatened preterm delivery. As social psychologists have demonstrated, human beings tend to make 2 basic judgments on meeting someone for the first time. People will typically first make an assessment of the other person's warmth or trustworthiness, followed by a judgment of the other person's competence or intelligence.[46] An understanding of these evolutionarily rooted behavioral patterns is of critical importance to the antenatal counseling practice. Neonatologists who are judged by parents to be warm and trustworthy create an environment conducive to the sharing of information, whereas neonatologists who are judged to be cold and uncaring may trigger a primal threat response that can inhibit trust and create a climate ill-suited to productive communication. This helps explain the negative reactions some parents express toward the neutral, standardized informed-consent model of antenatal consultations.

Conveying warmth in the setting of antenatal counseling is in large part related to the neonatologist's ability to demonstrate care and compassion for the difficulties they are confronting as a family. Simple strategies that can help demonstrate your awareness of the hardships being experienced by the family include the following:

- Reviewing the medical record and learning what you can from the doctors or nurses who know the family better

- Taking a moment to reflect on the gravity of the situation before walking into the room and trying to imagine how you might feel if the person behind the door was someone you knew and cared about

- Limiting the number of health care providers in the room for such conversations

- Doing what you can to prevent or minimize interruptions (ask a colleague to cover phone/ pager; silence your own phone)

- Asking the parent's nurse to limit distractions in the room while you are talking

- Making sure that everyone has the ability to sit

- Asking the family if there are others who should be present for the conversation, and waiting for them if time permits

- Introducing yourself to everyone in the room, and learning the names and the roles of everyone in the room who you are talking to

---

Learning about the values, beliefs, experience, and situation of each specific family is a crucial objective of this initial meeting. Ideally, most of the talking at the outset of these conversations will be done by the family, which can allow the neonatologist to learn about who they are and what they do and what they understand. Taking the time to listen to a family's story demonstrates care and concern, and allows the neonatologist to assess how best to individualize communication. The neonatologist who is judged to be warm and trustworthy can then demonstrate his or her competence and understanding of neonatology in a manner best suited to the individual family.

Individualizing antenatal counseling requires that neonatologists be able to elicit the specific needs of the family. It requires an understanding of the family's desired level of involvement in the decision-making process, with appropriate tailoring of the decision-making model according to these preferences. For families wishing to have a role in the decision-making process, it requires the ability to elicit this and provide appropriate information to support the individual family's decision. Some families will make decisions based on their own spiritual beliefs,[36] whereas for others, morbidity and mortality information may be of great importance. Each family is different, and neonatologists must have flexibility in conducting such conversations. It is not a process conducive to protocolization or a standardized approach.

STRATEGIES FOR TEACHING COUNSELING SKILLS

Little formal training is dedicated to teaching obstetricians and neonatologists how to guide this collaboration with parents who are often highly emotional and overwhelmed.[44] How can we learn to talk with families, and with each other, about the values inherent in decisions about treatment interventions at the extremes of prematurity?

Neonatology fellows often learn prenatal counseling skills by observing more senior clinicians counsel families, and by participating in counseling sessions themselves. This experiential learning has value in that it can illuminate some of the breadth of parents' questions and responses that one may encounter during antenatal counseling. But data suggest that this unstructured training does not regularly incorporate the supervision and feedback that are essential to improving trainees' skills.[36] Supplementation of these clinical experiences with targeted communication training is therefore necessary.

Additional approaches to teaching prenatal counseling skills include readings or didactic lectures on the topic. Written materials are often helpful to trainees who can refer to them over time, such as immediately before performing a prenatal consult. Online modules are another tool that the trainee can use whenever needed; online modules that incorporate learner participation and skills evaluations may be even more effective.[47]

None of these tools, however, substitutes for the value of role-play and simulation for learning the advanced communication skills relevant to antenatal counseling. A growing body of research confirms that these forms of active learning improve trainee confidence and preparation to engage in complex conversations with patients and families. Role-play and simulation trainings result in behavior changes immediately and over time.[48–50] Successful communication skills simulation trainings and role-plays allow trainees to practice a range of communication skills (such as Ask-Tell-Ask) with real-time feedback from the "parents" (who may be standardized patients, actors, or trained volunteers) and from faculty. There are existing trainings that simulate counseling by individual clinicians and by interdisciplinary neonatal teams.[49,50] Trainings can occur as intensive courses, for example, over 2 to 3 days, and/or episodically over months. The optimal approach to teaching such skills will likely vary, and continued research into the efficacy of different models is necessary.

A few hours after the initial meeting, Mrs Evers is still in labor. Dr Green is uncertain how to proceed, and decides to go back to Mrs Evers room. Her husband is now with her at the bedside.

Dr Green sits down and introduces himself. He then asks Mr and Mrs Evers how they are feeling about what is happening. For the next 20 minutes, Mr and Mrs Evers share the story of their pregnancy. They share their hopes and their fears for their daughter, and their uncertainty about how best to proceed. They share their intention to name their daughter Elizabeth, after Mrs Evers' grandmother.

Dr Green listens and empathizes as Mr and Mrs Evers share their story. He acknowledges the uncertainty of the situation, and provides statements of support. He answers their questions about what the resuscitation process will entail, and acknowledges their sadness over how different an experience this will be from what they had been hoping for. He does his best to answer their questions about possible NICU morbidities and long-term outcomes.

Mr and Mrs Evers share with Dr Green their spiritual beliefs about life's sacredness. They express that they want to give their infant a chance, but that they do not want her to suffer unnecessarily. Ultimately Dr Green proposes a plan for the NICU team to attend the delivery and to attempt resuscitation, with a reassessment to be made after evaluating Elizabeth's response to airway management. Mr and Mrs Evers both agree that this is how they would like to proceed. They express their appreciation for Dr Green's help, and thank him for caring for their infant.

Dr Green's emotions are mixed as he walks back to the NICU. He is anxious about whether he may have overstepped his bounds, and fearful of Dr Gigante's response. He is also worried about whether the Evers family truly understood the ramifications of their decision to proceed with resuscitation. Yet these feelings are contrasted with a positive sense of having helped a family at a time when they needed it most. The gratitude they expressed toward him was genuine, and Dr Green is determined to do all that he can to help the family navigate the complexities of their impending pre-mature childbirth.

Dr Green feels like he did the best that he could under the circumstances.

SUMMARY

Resuscitation decisions for infants born at the edges of viability are complicated moral dilemmas, and the process of making these decisions can be emotionally exhausting and morally distressful for families and physicians alike. Efforts to simplify the process with gestational age–based resuscitation guidelines or standardized approaches to antenatal counseling and decision-making belie that there are no simple answers. An ethical approach to making these types of decisions requires input from both physicians and parents, and individuals tasked with facilitating such decisions must possess the communication and counseling skills needed to assist families with these painful and life-altering decisions.

Although challenging, these ethical dilemmas present physicians with an opportunity to develop a therapeutic relationship with families during a time of intense need; an opportunity to use "their personal qualities, together with the scientific and technologic tools of medicine, to provide individualized help…"[51] Moving forward, it is incumbent on all of us to continue our investigation into how we can better assist families in this process while maintaining our goal of providing care that is in the best interest of our families.

REFERENCES

1. Brazier M, et al. Critical care decisions in fetal and neonatal medicine: ethical issues. Nuffield Counc Bioeth 2006;1–276.
2. American Academy of Pediatrics Committee on Fetus and Newborn, Bell EF. Noninitiation or withdrawal of intensive care for high-risk newborns. Pediatrics 2007;119:401–3.
3. American College of Obstetricians and GynecologistsSociety for Maternal-Fetal Medicine. ACOG obstetric care consensus No. 3: periviable birth. Obstet Gynecol 2015;126:e82–94.
4. Texas Supreme Court. Miller v. HCA, Inc. Wests South West Report 2003;118: 758–72.
5. Partridge JC, Sendowski MD, Drey EA, et al. Resuscitation of likely nonviable newborns: would neonatology practices in California change if the Born-Alive Infants Protection Act were enforced? Pediatrics 2009;123:1088–94.
6. Tyson JE, Parikh NA, Langer J, et al. Intensive care for extreme prematurity–moving beyond gestational age. N Engl J Med 2008;358:1672–81.
7. Rysavy MA, Li L, Bell EF, et al. Between-hospital variation in treatment and outcomes in extremely preterm infants. N Engl J Med 2015;372:1801–11.
8. Stoll BJ, Hansen NI, Bell EF, et al. Neonatal outcomes of extremely preterm infants from the NICHD Neonatal Research Network. Pediatrics 2010;126:443–56.
9. Sladkevicius P, Saltvedt S, Almström H, et al. Ultrasound dating at 12-14 weeks of gestation. A prospective cross-validation of established dating formulae in in-vitro fertilized pregnancies. Ultrasound Obstet Gynecol 2005;26:504–11.
10. Wennerholm UB, Bergh C, Hagberg H, et al. Gestational age in pregnancies after in vitro fertilization: comparison between ultrasound measurement and actual age. Ultrasound Obstet Gynecol 1998;12:170–4.
11. Wilkinson D. The self-fulfilling prophecy in intensive care. Theor Med Bioeth 2009; 30:401–10.

12. Carlo WA, McDonald SA, Fanaroff AA, et al. Association of antenatal corticosteroids with mortality and neurodevelopmental outcomes among infants born at 22 to 25 weeks' gestation. JAMA 2011;306:2348–58.

13. Singer LT, Salvator A, Guo S, et al. Maternal psychological distress and parenting stress after the birth of a very low-birth-weight infant. JAMA 1999;281:799–805.

14. Singer LT, Fulton S, Kirchner HL, et al. Parenting very low birth weight children at school age: maternal stress and coping. J Pediatr 2007;151:463–9.

15. Golish TD, Powell KA. 'Ambiguous loss': managing the dialectics of grief associated with premature birth. J Soc Pers Relat 2003;20:309–34.

16. McGettigan MC, Greenspan JS, Antunes MJ, et al. Psychological aspects of parenting critically ill neonates. Clin Pediatr (Phila) 1994;33:77–82.

17. Glaser A, Bucher HU, Moergeli H, et al. Loss of a preterm infant: psychological aspects in parents. Swiss Med Wkly 2007;137:392–401.

18. Carter BS. End of life decisions for newborns: an ethical and compassionate process? Arch Dis Child Fetal Neonatal Ed 2016;101:F92–3.

19. Doron MW, Veness-Meehan KA, Margolis LH, et al. Delivery room resuscitation decisions for extremely premature infants. Pediatrics 1998;102:574–82.

20. McHaffie HE, Laing IA, Parker M, et al. Deciding for imperilled newborns: medical authority or parental autonomy? J Med Ethics 2001;27:104–9.

21. Singh J, Fanaroff J, Andrews B, et al. Resuscitation in the 'gray zone' of viability: determining physician preferences and predicting infant outcomes. Pediatrics 2007;120:519–26.

22. Brinchmann BS, Førde R, Nortvedt P. What matters to the parents? A qualitative study of parents' experiences with life-and-death decisions concerning their premature infants. Nurs Ethics 2002;9:388–404.

23. Kavanaugh K, Savage T, Kilpatrick S, et al. Life support decisions for extremely premature infants: report of a pilot study. J Pediatr Nurs 2005;20:347–59.

24. Emanuel EJ, Emanuel LL. Four models of the physician-patient relationship. JAMA 1992;267:2221–6.

25. Charles C, Gafni A, Whelan T. Shared decision-making in the medical encounter: what does it mean? (or it takes at least two to tango). Soc Sci Med 1997;44: 681–92.

26. Bastek TK, Richardson DK, Zupancic JAF, et al. Prenatal consultation practices at the border of viability: a regional survey. Pediatrics 2005;116:407–13.

27. Payot A, Gendron S, Lefebvre F, et al. Deciding to resuscitate extremely premature babies: how do parents and neonatologists engage in the decision? Soc Sci Med 2007;64:1487–500.

28. Schumacher RE. Myth: neonatology is evidence-based. Semin Fetal Neonatal Med Ed 2011;16:288–92.

29. Zupancic JAF, Kirpalani H, Barrett J, et al. Characterising doctor-parent communication in counselling for impending preterm delivery. Arch Dis Child Fetal Neonatal Ed 2002;87:F113–7.

30. Wocial LD. Life support decisions involving imperiled infants. J Perinat Neonatal Nurs 2000;14:73.

31. Pinch WJ, Spielman ML. Ethical decision making for high-risk infants. The parents' perspective. Nurs Clin North Am 1989;24:1017–23.

32. Pinch WJ, Spielman ML. The parents' perspective: ethical decision-making in neonatal intensive care. J Adv Nurs 1990;15:712–9.

33. Pinch WJ, Spielman ML. Ethics in the neonatal intensive care unit: parental perceptions at four years postdischarge. ANS Adv Nurs Sci 1996;19:72–85.

34. Pepper D, Rempel G, Austin W, et al. More than information: a qualitative study of parents' perspectives on neonatal intensive care at the extremes of prematurity. Adv Neonatal Care 2012;12:303–9.
35. Xafis V, Wilkinson D, Sullivan J. What information do parents need when facing end-of-life decisions for their child? A meta-synthesis of parental feedback. BMC Palliat Care 2015;14:19.
36. Boss RD, Hutton N, Sulpar LJ, et al. Values parents apply to decision-making regarding delivery room resuscitation for high-risk newborns. Pediatrics 2008; 122:583–9.
37. Azoulay E, Chevret S, Leleu G, et al. Half the families of intensive care unit patients experience inadequate communication with physicians. Crit Care Med 2000;28:3044–9.
38. Azoulay E, Pochard F, Kentish-Barnes N, et al. Risk of post-traumatic stress symptoms in family members of intensive care unit patients. Am J Respir Crit Care Med 2005;171:987–94.
39. Barry MJ, Edgman-Levitan S. Shared decision making–pinnacle of patient-centered care. N Engl J Med 2012;366:780–1.
40. Kaempf JW, Tomlinson M, Arduza C, et al. Medical staff guidelines for periviability pregnancy counseling and medical treatment of extremely premature infants. Pediatrics 2006;117:22–9.
41. Caeymaex L, Speranza M, Vasilescu C, et al. Living with a crucial decision: a qualitative study of parental narratives three years after the loss of their newborn in the NICU. PLoS One 2011;6:e28633.
42. Edmonds BT, et al. Patient education and counseling. Patient Educ Couns 2015; 98:49–54.
43. Einstein DJ, Einstein KL, Mathew P. Dying for advice: code status discussions between resident physicians and patients with advanced cancer–a national survey. J Palliat Med 2015;18:535–41.
44. Boss RD, Hutton N, Donohue PK, et al. Neonatologist training to guide family decision making for critically ill infants. Arch Pediatr Adolesc Med 2009;163:783–8.
45. Haward MF, Janvier A. An introduction to behavioural decision-making theories for paediatricians. Acta Paediatr 2015;104:340–5.
46. Fiske ST, Cuddy AJC, Glick P. Universal dimensions of social cognition: warmth and competence. Trends Cogn Sci 2007;11:77–83.
47. Lee AL, Mader EM, Morley CP. Teaching cross-cultural communication skills online: a multi-method evaluation. Fam Med 2015;47:302–8.
48. Back AL, Arnold RM, Baile WF, et al. Efficacy of communication skills training for giving bad news and discussing transitions to palliative care. Arch Intern Med 2007;167:453–60.
49. Boss RD, Urban A, Barnett MD, et al. Neonatal Critical Care Communication (NC3): training NICU physicians and nurse practitioners. J Perinatol 2013;33:1–5.
50. Meyer EC, Brodsky D, Hansen AR, et al. An interdisciplinary, family-focused approach to relational learning in neonatal intensive care. J Perinatol 2011;31:212–9.
51. Schei E. Doctoring as leadership: the power to heal. Perspect Biol Med 2006;49:393–406.

Index

Note: Page numbers of article titles are in **boldface** type.

Clin Perinatol 44 (2017) 461–468
http://dx.doi.org/10.1016/S0095-5108(17)30029-5
0095-5108/17

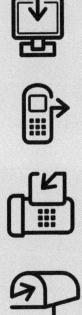
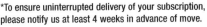

Printed and bound by CPI Group (UK) Ltd, Croydon, CR0 4YY

07/10/2024

01040504-0002